Simkin's Labor Progress Handbook

Early Interventions to Prevent and Treat Dystocia

Fifth Edition

Edited By

Lisa Hanson
Klein Professor and Associate Director, Midwifery Program
Marquette University
College of Nursing
Milwaukee, WI, USA

Emily Malloy
Certified Nurse Midwife
Director of Midwifery Research
Midwifery and Wellness Center
Participating Faculty
Marquette University
College of Nursing
Milwaukee, WI, USA

Penny Simkin
Certified Birth Doula and Certified Childbirth Educator
USA

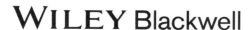

Registered Offices
John Wiley & Sons, Inc., 111 River Street, Hoboken, NJ 07030, USA
John Wiley & Sons Ltd, The Atrium, Southern Gate, Chichester, West Sussex, PO19 8SQ, UK

For details of our global editorial offices, customer services, and more information about Wiley products visit us at www.wiley.com.

Wiley also publishes its books in a variety of electronic formats and by print-on-demand. Some content that appears in standard print versions of this book may not be available in other formats.

Trademarks: Wiley and the Wiley logo are trademarks or registered trademarks of John Wiley & Sons, Inc. and/or its affiliates in the United States and other countries and may not be used without written permission. All other trademarks are the property of their respective owners. John Wiley & Sons, Inc. is not associated with any product or vendor mentioned in this book.

Library of Congress Cataloging-in-Publication Data
Names: Hanson, Lisa, 1958- editor. | Malloy, Emily, 1983- editor. | Simkin, Penny, 1938- editor.
Title: Simkin's labor progress handbook : early interventions to prevent and treat dystocia / edited by Lisa Hanson, Professor and Director, Midwifery Program, Marquette University, USA, Emily Malloy, Penny Simkin.
Other titles: Labor progress handbook | Labor progress handbook
Description: Fifth edition. | Hoboken, NJ : John Wiley & Sons, 2024. | Revised edition of: Labor progress handbook / Penny Simkin, Lisa Hanson, Ruth Ancheta. Fourth edition. [2017]. | Includes bibliographical references and index.
Identifiers: LCCN 2023026403 (print) | LCCN 2023026404 (ebook) | ISBN 9781119754466 (paperback) | ISBN 9781119754428 (pdf) | ISBN 9781119754497 (epub)
Subjects: LCSH: Labor (Obstetrics)--Complications--Prevention--Handbooks, manuals, etc. | Birth injuries--Prevention--Handbooks, manuals, etc. | Shoulder dystocia--Prevention--Handbooks, manuals, etc.
Classification: LCC RG701 .S57 2024 (print) | LCC RG701 (ebook) | DDC 618.4--dc23/eng/20230623
LC record available at https://lccn.loc.gov/2023026403
LC ebook record available at https://lccn.loc.gov/2023026404

Cover Image: © RuslanDashinsky/Getty Images
Cover design by Wiley

Set in 9/11pt PlantinStd by Integra Software Services Pvt. Ltd, Pondicherry, India

SKY10075769_052224

Dedication

We dedicate this book to childbearing people, their families, and caregivers in the hope that some of the suggestions offered reduce the need for interventions and promote normal physiologic labor and birth. This book is named in honor of Penny Simkin, the original author, a leader innovator, activist, author, childbirth educator and doula.

Contents

Chapter 4:   Assessing Progress in Labor   41
Wendy Gordon, DM, MPH, CPM, LM, with contributions by Gail Tully, BS, CPM, and
Lisa Hanson, PhD, CNM, FACNM, FAAN

List of Contributors

Editors:

Lisa Hanson PhD, CNM, FACNM, FAAN
Klein Professor
Associate Director, Midwifery Program
Marquette University, USA
College of Nursing
Milwaukee, WI

Emily Malloy PhD, CNM
Certified Nurse Midwife
Director of Midwifery Research
Midwifery and Wellness Center
Aurora Sinai Medical Center
Participating Faculty
Marquette University, USA
College of Nursing
Milwaukee, WI

Penny Simkin BA, PT, CCE, CD(DONA)
Certified Birth Doula and Certified Childbirth Educator,
USA

Contributing Authors:

Nicole Carlson PhD, CNM, FACNM, FAAN
Associate Professor
Nell Hodgson Woodruff School of Nursing
Emory University Atlanta, Georgia, USA

Joyce K. Edmonds, PhD, MPH, RN
Senior Research Scientist
Ariadne Labs
Harvard T.H. Chan School of Public Health
Boston, MA, USA

Elise Erickson PhD, CNM, FACNM
Assistant Professor
The University of Arizona AZ, USA
College of Nursing: Advanced Nursing Practice & Science
College of Pharmacy: Pharmacy Practice & Science
College of Medicine: Department of Obstetrics &
Gynecology

Wendy Gordon, DM, MPH, CPM, LM
Chair & Associate Professor
Department of Midwifery
Bastyr University
WA, USA

Amy Marowitz, DNP, CNM
Associate Professor
Department of Midwifery and Women's Health
Frontier Nursing University
Kentucky, USA

Sharon Muza, BS, CD/BDT(DONA), LCCE,
FACCE, CLE
Seattle Area Certified Birth Doula and Lamaze
Certified Childbirth Educator

Kathryn Osborne PhD, CNM, FACNM
Associate Professor
Department of Women, Children and Family Nursing
College of Nursing
Rush University
Chicago, USA

Amber Price DNP, CNM, RN
President
Sentara Williamsburg Regional Medical Center
Williamsburg, VA, USA

Jesse Remer, BS, CD(DONA), BDT(DONA),
LCCE, FACCE
Founder, Mother Tree International

Karen Robinson, PhD, CNM, FACNM
Interim Assistant Dean of Graduate Programs
Associate Professor
Marquette University College of Nursing

Venus Standard MSN, CNM, LCCE, FACNM
Director, DEI Education and Community Engagement
Director and Co-Principal Investigator of LEADoula
program
University of North Carolina School of Medicine
Columbia, USA
Department of Family Medicine
Women's Health - Maternal and Child Health

Ellen L. Tilden, PhD, RN, CNM, FACNM, FAAN
Associate Professor
Oregon Health and Science University Portland,
Oregon, USA

School of Nursing, Nurse-Midwifery Department
School of Medicine, OBGYN Department
Center M Co-Founder and CSO

Gail Tully, BS, CPM
Spinning Babies®

Robin Elise Weiss, Ph.D., MPH, CLC, LCCE,
FACCE, AdvCD/BDT(DONA)
DONA International

Foreword

Writing a Forward to the 5th edition of Simkin Penny's *Labor Progress Handbook* brings to mind many of Penny's workshops that I attended either as an attendee or rarely a co-teacher. Penny's genius is her ability to present in a way that is accessible and pertinent to childbirth educators, doulas, family doctors, midwives, maternity nurses, and obstetricians. The Simkin's Labor Progress Hanbook evokes memories of Penny's workshops, where a mélange of maternity professionals of all kinds working, together on the floor and on birthing balls, or squeezing each other's pelvises or squatting in the correct position, with heels down or incorrect, heels up—demonstrating how the former opens the pelvic floor while the latter does not. What a collaborative scene!

How did Penny do it, when the normally separate but obviously related disciplines rarely learn together? Penny's understated and matter-of-fact, just-get-on-with-it approach engaged participants in an uplifting experience—an exercise based on her long-acquired knowledge as a physiotherapist applying her understanding of anatomy to birthing. No wonder Penny's workshops were always full. The Simkin's Labor Progress Handbook is deeply reflective of this experience, and the collaboration of the many birth disciplines is reflected in the authorship.

Penny was one of the founders of the doula movement, who, along with Marshall Klaus, Phyllis Klaus, John Kennel, and Annie Kennedy, embraced this new collaborator, and worked to bring doulas into the mainstream—fully appreciating how difficult that was going to be.[1] That doulas were part of the workshops made a statement that doulas could add their knowledge, as demonstrated in the Simkin's Labor Progress Handbook, to that of the other birth providers, even while the doula's allegiance and responsibility was to the laboring person only–and not the hospital or other institution.[2]

Reading Simkin's Labor Progress Handbook, one comes to the realization that it fits into the knowledge gap between a dry obstetrical textbook, cold evidence from a randomized controlled trial (with all its issues of generalizability)[3] and the bedside or floor side of real laboring persons and their supporters. Reading Simkin's Labor Progress Handbook is like being in one of Penny's workshops, navigating between evidence coming from multiple conventional sources and the lived experience of the multidisciplinary participants–respectfully appreciating the practice lives of all. I am especially excited to see so many midwifery scientists and doula clinical experts carry on the legacy of Penny's book and renaming it in her honor.

As in the introductory chapter, I too grappled with the narrow perspective of the three Ps, and in appreciation of Penny's many contributions, I offer my version of the three Ps:

The 3 Ps Expanded★★

1. **Power** – strength, length, duration of contractions
2. **Passage** – the pelvis; shape, size, angles
3. **Passenger** – the baby; size, position, and attitude.

These are the commonly recognized "P's," to which we add nine more to consider:

4. **Person** – the laboring person's beliefs, preparation, knowledge, and "capacity" for doing the work of labor and birth

5. **Partner** – how the laboring person is supported and their knowledge, beliefs and preparation for the labor is integrated
6. **People** – the "entourage" – others who may be involved in the birth process and their beliefs, preparation, and knowledge of the process
7. **Pain** – the *laboring person's* past experiences of pain and the experience of pain in psychological and cultural terms: beliefs, environment, on the laboring person's capacity for coping with labor and birth.
8. **Pain** – *OURS*: how we professionals think of pain and manage it—seeking to abolish it or use it; how we professionals time the pain management tools at our disposal to minimize further interventions
9. **Professionals** –the manner in which all members of the healthcare team support, inform, and collaborate in care and information-sharing with the woman and her partner.
10. **Passion** – the *Laboring Person's*. The experienced journey of pregnancy, labor, and birth is one that is special and unique to each participant. It is crucial for all parties involved in the care to be recognized and honored, and that this principle guide us in our practice.
11. **Passsion** – *OURS*. The passion toward maternity care that drives us
    a) But for the woman and her supports, we need to recognize the importance of intimacy in this life-changing experience.
    b) We need to control our anxiety and need for perfection so that the laboring person can fully experience the passion – even when the birth is complex and requires considerable help from us.
12. **Politics** – enough said –You know it's true!

**MCK: Borrowed, stolen and modified from too many people to mention

Michael C Klein CM, MD, FCFP CCFP FAAP (neonatal-perinatal)
Emeritus Professor
Family Practice & Pediatrics
University of British Columbia
Senior Scientist Emeritus
BC Children's Hospital Research Institute, Vancouver
Recipient The Order of Canada
mklein@mail.ubc.ca
www.michaelcklein.ca
Author Dissident Doctor—catching babies and challenging the medical status quo.
2018. Douglas and McIntyre. ISBN 978–1–77162–192–2

REFERENCES

1. Eftekhary S, Klein, MC, Xu, S. (2010) The life of a Canadian doula: Successes, confusion, and conflict. *Journal of Obstetrics and Gynaecology Canada* 32(7), 642–649.
2. Amram N, Klein, MC, Mok, H, Simkin, P, Lindstrom, K, Grant, J. (2014) How birth doulas help clients adapt to changes in circumstances, clinical care, and client preferences during labor. *The Journal of Perinatal Education* 23(2), 96–103.
3. Klein MC. (2023) Homage to Dr. Murray Enkin and the complexity of evidence-based medicine. *Birth* 50(2), 255–257. doi: 10.1111/birt.12723.

Chapter 1

Introduction

Lisa Hanson, PhD, CNM, FACNM, FAAN and Emily Malloy, PhD, CNM

CAUSES AND PREVENTION OF LABOR DYSTOCIA: A SYSTEMATIC APPROACH

Labor dystocia, dysfunctional labor, failure to progress, arrest of labor, arrested descent—all these terms refer to slow or no progress in labor, which is one of the most vexing, complex, and unpredictable complications of labor. Labor dystocia is the most common medical indication for primary cesarean sections.[1] Some have suggested that the use of the term "dystocia" be abandoned in favor of more precise definitions since one clear explanation is lacking.[1] The modern course of labor is very different than in the past, and optimal strategies to reduce unnecessary interventions while providing interventions when needed and appropriate are still under investigation.[2] Dystocia also contributes indirectly to the number of repeat cesareans, especially in countries where rates of vaginal births after previous cesareans (VBAC) are low. Thus, preventing primary cesareans for dystocia decreases the total number of cesareans. The prevention of dystocia also reduces the need for many other costly, time-intensive, and possibly risky interventions, and spares the laboring person from discouragement and disappointment that often accompany a prolonged or complicated birth.[3]

The possible causes of labor dystocia are numerous. Some are *intrinsic*:

- The powers (uterine contractions).
- The passage (size, shape, and joint mobility of the pelvis and the stretch and resilience of the vaginal canal).
- The passenger (size, shape, and flexion of fetal head, fetal presentation, and position).
- The pain (and the laboring person's ability to cope with it).
- The psyche (emotional state of the laboring person).

Others are *extrinsic*:

- Environment (the feelings of physical and emotional safety generated by the setting and the people surrounding the laboring person).
- Ethno-cultural factors (the degree of sensitivity and respect for the person's culture-based needs and preferences).
- Hospital or caregiver policies (how flexible, family- or person-centered, how evidence-based).
- Psycho-emotional care (the priority given to non-medical aspects of the childbirth experience).

The focus of Simkin's Labor Progress Handbook is on prevention, differential diagnosis, and early interventions to use to prevent labor dystocia. We emphasize relatively simple care measures and low technology approaches designed to help maintain normal labor progress, and to manage and correct minor deviations before they become serious enough to require technologic interventions. We believe this approach is consistent with worldwide efforts, including those of the World Health Organization, to reserve the use of medical interventions for situations in which they are needed: "The aim of the care [in normal birth] is to achieve a healthy mother [birth parent] and baby with the least possible level of intervention that is compatible with safety."[4]

The suggestions in this book are based on the following premises:

- The timing of dystocia is an important consideration when establishing cause and selecting interventions.
- Sometimes several causal factors can occur simultaneously.
- Clinicians and caregivers are often able to enhance or maintain labor progress with simple non-surgical, non-pharmacological physical, and psychological interventions. Such interventions have the following advantages:
  ◦ Compared to most obstetric interventions for dystocia, they carry less risk of harm or undesirable side effects to laboring person or fetus;
  ◦ The laboring persons is autonomous with the right to accept or refuse interventions. These suggestions treat the laboring person as the key to the solution, not part of the problem;
  ◦ They build or strengthen the cooperation between the laboring person, their support people (loved ones, doula), and their clinicians;
  ◦ they reduce the need for riskier, costlier, more complex interventions;
  ◦ They may increase the person's emotional satisfaction with their experience of birth.
- The choice of solutions depends on the causal factors, if known, but trial and error is sometimes necessary when the cause is unclear. The greatest drawbacks are that the laboring person may not want to try some interventions; they may take time; and/or they may not correct the problem.
- Time is usually an ally, not an enemy. With time, many problems in labor progress are resolved. In the absence of medical or psychological contraindications, patience, reassurance, and low- or no-risk interventions may constitute the most appropriate course of management.
- The clinician may use the following to determine the cause of the problem(s):
  ◦ Objective data: vital signs; fetal heart rate patterns; fetal presentation, position, and size; cervical assessments; assessments of contraction strength, frequency, and duration; membrane status; and time;
  ◦ Subjective data: person's affect, description of pain, level of fatigue, ability to cope using self-calming techniques:
  ◦ Essential components:
    – Attentive listening
    – Informed consent and refusal
    – Shared decision-making with the laboring person

Chart 1.1 illustrates the step-by-step approach followed in this book—from detection of little or no labor progress through graduating levels of interventions (from simple to complex) to correct the problem.

If the primary physiologic interventions are contraindicated or if they are unsuccessful, then secondary—relatively low-technology—interventions are used, and only if those are unsuccessful are tertiary, high-technology obstetrical interventions instituted under the guidance of the physician or midwife. Other similar flow charts appear throughout this book showing how to apply this approach to a variety of specific causes of dysfunctional labor.

Many of the interventions described here are derived from the medical, midwifery, nursing, and childbirth education literature. Some of the strategies described in this book lend themselves to randomized controlled trials, others do not. Others come from the psychology, sociology, and anthropology literature. Suggestions also come from the extensive wisdom and experience of nurses, midwives, physicians, and doulas and other labor support providers. Many are applications of physical therapy principles and practices. The fields of therapeutic massage and chiropractic provide methods to assess and correct soft tissue tension and imbalance that can impair labor progress. We have provided references for these, when available. Some items fall into the category of "shared wisdom," where the original sources are unknown.

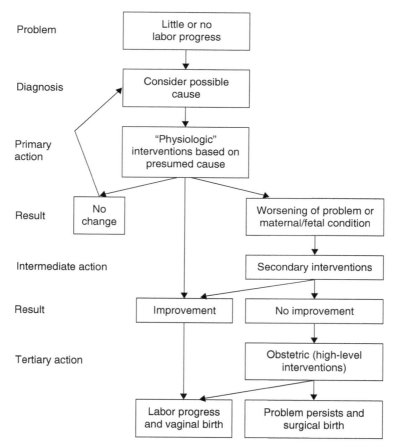

Chart 1.1. Care plan for the problem of "little or no labor progress."

During the past half-century, extensive scientific evaluation of numerous entrenched medical customs, policies, and practices, intended to improve birth outcomes, has determined that many are ineffective or even harmful. Routine practices, such as enemas, pubic shaving, routine continuous electronic fetal monitoring, maternal supine and lithotomy positions in the second stage of labor, routine episiotomy, immediate clamping of the umbilical cord, routine suctioning of the newborn's airway after birth, and separation of the newborn from parent/s are examples of care practices that became widespread before they were scientifically evaluated. Scientific study now shows that these common practices were not only ineffective, they increased the risks for the birthing person and neonate.[5]

Other valid considerations, such as the laboring person's needs, preferences, and values, also play a large role in the selection of approaches to their care. Our paradigm is one of respectful maternity care, although we recognize that throughout history and around the world, laboring people have been subject to racism, sexism, gender discrimination, disrespect, and other abusive and harmful behaviors. It is our expectation that laboring people are treated using a respectful maternity care and human rights model.

Racism and white supremacy are pervasive in obstetric care. Scholars have identified that many of the people identified as early founders of obstetrics and gynecology learned their skills through experimentation, coercion, and abuse of black, brown, and poor birthing people.[6] Therefore, in this book, we will avoid using the names of those early experimenters in favor of descriptive terminology, for example, left side lying, or runner's lunge for the position formerly called by a gynecologist's name. Additionally, for one hundred years, nurses, midwives, and physicians were taught a system of pelvic classification with the aim of predicting difficult births that was overtly racist, and based only on pseudoscience.[7] Therefore, in this book, we recognize that humans and pelvises are dynamic, and there is not one perfect pelvis. Rather, our goal is to help birthing people and birth workers take advantage of the mobility of the pelvis. The interventions and positions shown throughout this book are offered to provide many options in one place, rather than a "one size fits all" approach.

Maternity care practices, providers, and outcomes differ around the world. Many counties have recognized the importance of improving maternal and neonatal care, although progress has been slow.[8,9] During the past decade, increasing evidence has pointed to the importance of midwives to improve outcomes. In 2014 the *Lancet* published a series on midwifery in four papers.[10–13] The goal of the series was to correct misunderstandings about the midwifery profession. An important conclusion of the series was that better utilization of midwives could prevent a significant portion of perinatal morbidity, including stillbirth. Many countries are working toward a goal of strengthening their midwifery workforce and increasing access to midwifery care to decrease maternal morbidity and mortality.[14] Midwifery care is associated with more spontaneous vaginal birth, less preterm birth, less epidural use, less episiotomy use, fewer instrumental births.[15] Currently, we must find the balance between intervention and non-intervention. There is a time and place for both, but around the world more labor interventions are occurring without an improvement in outcomes for pregnant and birthing people and their newborns.

Depending on healthcare setting, midwifery training and availability, the World Health Organization makes a recommendation for Midwifery Led Continuity of Care models (MLCC).[16] MLCC involves care by a midwife or team of midwives during the antenatal, intrapartum, and postpartum period.[16] MLCC does not exclude other caregivers from providing care, but rather starts most pregnant people with the midwifery model, and those who need care by other professionals are referred based on their specific needs or conditions. While high-risk pregnant people benefit from the care of an obstetrician, low-risk pregnant people generally benefit from less invasive approaches to care provided by a midwife or family/general physician. Midwifery care is rooted in evidence-based care—a combination of research evidence, clinical experience, and the needs and wishes of the pregnant, laboring, or birthing person.[17]

May 5 is the International Day of the Midwife; in 2021 the theme of the day was "follow the data and invest in midwives."[14] Midwifery care varies widely by country. In the UK midwives and general practice providers deliver 80% of maternity care while in the United States midwives deliver approximately 10% of maternity care.[18,19] In some countries, such as Germany and Japan, there are many more midwives than obstetricians.[20] Many countries are working to increase their midwifery workforce, such as India, which has developed the Nurse Practitioner in Midwifery credential and Mexico which started an Initiative to Promote Professional Midwifery in 2015.[21,22]

The intention of this book is to be widely applicable in many different settings and to many different clinicians and support people, including nurses, midwives, physicians, doulas, and others. The differences in clinicians and their differing approaches to childbirth are reflected in the varying rates of interventions and cesarean births when labor is considered low risk. We hope that this book will offer tools for use in many different settings and situations.

NOTES ON THIS BOOK

This book is directed toward caregivers—midwives, nurses, doulas, and physicians—who want to support and protect the physiological process of labor, with the objective of avoiding complex, costly, and more risky interventions. It will also be helpful for students in midwifery, maternity nursing, and obstetrics; for childbirth educators (who can teach many of these techniques to expectant parents); and for doulas (trained labor support providers whose scope of practice includes use of many of the non-clinical techniques). The chapters are arranged chronologically according to the phases and stages of labor.

NOTE FROM THE AUTHORS ON THE USE OF GENDER-INCLUSIVE LANGUAGE

We acknowledge that pregnant and birthing people may or may not identify with the gendered terms woman/women/she/her/hers. Therefore, in this edition we include the use of gender-inclusive language and use the terms pregnant, laboring, or birthing person. This is to avoid making assumptions about those who give birth. There remain references to women and/or mothers when citing scientific literature where participants described themselves as female or the researchers identified the person as a woman or mother.

CONCLUSION

The fifth edition of this book is named to honor Penny Simkin, the original author of this book. She is a world-famous doula, childbirth educator, and author of numerous articles and books. Simkin's Labor Progress Handbook welcomes many new chapter authors and contributors who are expert midwifery clinicians, doulas, childbirth educators and/or scientists. This book focuses on prevention of labor dystocia, and a stepwise progression of interventions aimed at using the least invasive approaches that will result in safe delivery. To our knowledge, this is the first book that compiles labor progress strategies that can be used by a variety of clinicians and support people in a variety of locations. Most of the strategies described can be used for births occurring in hospitals, at home, and in free-standing birth centers.

Knowledge of appropriate early interventions may spare pregnant people from long, discouraging, or exhausting labors, reduce the need for major interventions, and contribute to safer and more satisfying outcomes. The laboring person may not even recognize the intervention done for them, but they will appreciate and always remember your attentiveness, expertise, respect, and support as they brought their child into the world. This will contribute so much to their satisfaction and positive long-term memories of their childbirths.[23] We wish you much success and fulfilment in your important work.

REFERENCES

1. Neal JL, Ryan SL, Lowe NK, Schorn MN, Buxton M, Holley SL, Wilson-Liverman AM. (2015) Labor dystocia: Uses of related nomenclature. *Journal of Midwifery & Women's Health* 60(5), 485–498.
2. Myers ER, Sanders GD, Coeytaux RR, McElligott KA, Moorman PG, Hicklin K, Grotegut C, Villers M, Goode A, Campbell H, Befus D, McBroom AJ, Davis JK, Lallinger K, Fortman R, Kosinski A. (2020) *Labor Dystocia*. Agency for Healthcare Research and Quality (US).
3. (2019 Feb) ACOG Committee Opinion No. 766: Approaches to Limit Intervention During Labor and Birth. *Obstetrics and Gynecology* 133(2), e164–e173. doi: 10.1097/AOG.0000000000003074. PMID: 30575638.N.
4. World Health Organization. (1996) *Care in Normal Birth: A Practical Guide*. Geneva: WHO. Chapter 1. Available from: http://apps.who.int/iris/bitstream/10665/63167/1/WHO_FRH_MSM_96.24.pdf
5. Block J. (2007) *Pushed: The Painful Truth about Childbirth and Modern Maternity Care*. Cambridge, MA: Da Capo Lifelong.
6. Cooper Owens D. (2017) *Medical Bondage. Race, Gender, and the Origins of American Gynecology*. Athens, GA: University of Georgia Press. ISBN-10: 9780820351353.
7. VanSickle C, Liese KL, Rutherford JN. (2022) Textbook typologies: Challenging the myth of the perfect obstetric pelvis. *Anatomical Record (Hoboken, N.J.: 2007)* 305(4), 952–967. doi: 10.1002/ar.24880
8. Kennedy HP, Cheyney, M, Dahlen, HG, Downe, S, Foureur, MJ, Homer, C, Jefford, E, McFadden, A, Michel-Schuldt, M, Sandall, J, Soltani, H, Speciale, AM, Stevens, J, Vedam, S, Renfrew, MJ. (2018) Asking different questions: A call to action for research to improve the quality of care for every woman, every child. *Birth (Berkeley, Calif.)* 45(3), 222–231. doi: 10.1111/birt.12361
9. Kennedy HP, Balaam MC, Dahlen H, Declercq E, de Jonge A, Downe S, Ellwood D, Homer C, Sandall J, Vedam S, Wolfe I. (2020) The role of midwifery and other international insights for maternity care in the United States: An analysis of four countries. *Birth (Berkeley, Calif.)* 47(4), 332–345. doi: 10.1111/birt.12504
10. Homer CS, Friberg, IK, Dias, MA, ten Hoope-Bender, P, Sandall, J, Speciale, AM, Bartlett, LA (2014) The projected effect of scaling up midwifery. *Lancet (London, England)* 384(9948), 1146–1157. doi: 10.1016/S0140-6736(14)60790-X

11. Renfrew MJ, McFadden, A, Bastos, MH, Campbell, J, Channon, AA, Cheung, NF, Silva, DR, Downe, S, Kennedy, HP, Malata, A, McCormick, F, Wick, L, Declercq, E. (2014) Midwifery and quality care: Findings from a new evidence-informed framework for maternal and newborn care. *Lancet (London, England)* 384(9948), 1129–1145. doi: 10.1016/S0140-6736(14)60789-3

12. ten Hoope-Bender P, de Bernis, L, Campbell, J, Downe, S, Fauveau, V, Fogstad, H, Homer, CS, Kennedy, HP, Matthews, Z, McFadden, A, Renfrew, MJ, Van Lerberghe, W. (2014) Improvement of maternal and newborn health through midwifery. *Lancet (London, England)* 384(9949), 1226–1235. doi: 10.1016/S0140-6736(14)60930-2

13. Van Lerberghe W, Matthews Z, Achadi E, Ancona C, Campbell J, Channon A, de Bernis L, De Brouwere V, Fauveau V, Fogstad H, Koblinsky M, Liljestrand J, Mechbal A, Murray SF, Rathavay T, Rehr H, Richard F, ten Hoope-Bender P, Turkmani S. (2014) Country experience with strengthening of health systems and deployment of midwives in countries with high maternal mortality. *Lancet (London, England)* 384(9949), 1215–1225. doi: 10.1016/S0140-6736(14)60919-3

14. International Confederation of Midwives (ICM). (2021) Follow the data: Invest in midwives. Retrieved from https://www.internationalmidwives.org/icm-events/international-day-of-the-midwife-2021.html

15. Sandall J, Soltani H, Gates S, Shennan A, Devane D. (2015) Midwife-led continuity models versus other models of care for childbearing women. *The Cochrane Database of Systematic Reviews* (9), CD004667. doi: 10.1002/14651858.CD004667.pub4

16. WHO. (2018) *WHO Recommendations: Intrapartum Care for a Positive Childbirth Experience.* Geneva: World Health Organization. License: CC BY-NC-SA 3.0 IGO.

17. Pape TM. (2003) Evidence-based nursing practice: To infinity and beyond. *The Journal of Continuing Education in Nursing* 34, 154–161.

18. American College of Nurse Midwives. (2021). Evidence base practice definition. Retrieved from: https://www.midwife.org/Evidence-based-Practice-Definition. (accessed October 9, 2021).

19. American College of Nurse Midwives. (2019). Fact Sheet: Essential facts about midwives. (accessed October 9, 2021).

20. Dekker R. (2021) EBB 175: The evidence on midwifery care. *Evidence Based Birth Evidence that Empowers.* Retrieved from: https://evidencebasedbirth.com/evidence-on-midwives

21. Akins L, Keith-Brown K, Rees M, Sesia P, Blanco G, Coronel D, Cuellar G, Hernandez R, Yang C. (2019). Strengthening midwifery in Mexico: Evaluation of progress 2015–2018. Retrieved from: https://www.macfound.org/media/files/strengthening_midwifery_in_mexico_three-year_progress_report_revised_7_junio2019.pdf

22. Lalchandi K. (2021). India's investment in midwives: A step in the right direction to achieving universal health coverage. Retrieved from: https://www.jhpiego.org/story/indias-investment-in-midwives-a-step-in-the-right-direction-to-achieving-universal-health-coverage-for-all-by-2030

23. Simkin P. (1992) Just another day in a woman's life? Part 11: Nature and consistency of women's long-term memories of their first birth experiences. *Birth* 19(2), 64–81. doi: 10.1111/j.1523-536X.1992.tb00382.x

Chapter 2
Respectful Care
Amber Price, DNP, CNM, RN

Almost everywhere on the planet, people seek out others for assistance during the birth process. Rarely does birth happen in complete isolation, unless it is by choice or necessity. In years past, birth took place inside the home, visible and audible to all. When people lived in small communities, they relied on others in their communities to assist them. Few people had babies who had not been present at the births of siblings, grandmothers, neighbors, or friends. Demystifying birth having seen it left people prepared, with memories of the sounds and work of labor and birth, and of others successfully completing the journey.[1] Attending birth fosters belief in the ability of the body to give birth, grows confidence, and normalizes the event. We are now in a time in history where people about to give birth have rarely witnessed it. Those who witnessed a birth on television likely saw a medicalized birth, in a hospital, with technology as a central feature.[1] How a person witnesses birth shapes their belief of it. Every culture has its beliefs and rituals around birth, and while it is shrouded in mystery in some cases, it is a universal equalizer.

In most cultures, the societal norm is to present to a health care provider for confirmation of pregnancy as soon as possible.[1] In some cultures, there are a lot of different birth attendants from which to choose. Rarely do pregnant people choose a provider based on attributes like approximation of their communication style, shared cultural or personal beliefs, or the ability to foster confidence and autonomy. Pregnant people may assume that the person who managed their contraception is going to be great at managing their pregnancy. It is very difficult for people to change providers during pregnancy, or they may not have an option to change, and therefore may end up giving birth with someone who does not understand their culture, read their body language well, communicate in a way that makes sense or feels comforting and respectful, or honor their wishes. It is sometimes easier for people to tell themselves that it will be okay, that a safe outcome is all that matters. A "healthy mom and baby" is often repeated by caregivers as the goal of pregnancy, but that is a very low bar to set. The experience of birth can contribute to a person's physical and emotional wellbeing for life.

Simkin's Labor Progress Handbook: Early Interventions to Prevent and Treat Dystocia, Fifth Edition. Edited by Lisa Hanson, Emily Malloy, and Penny Simkin.
© 2024 John Wiley & Sons Ltd. Published 2024 by John Wiley & Sons Ltd.

Childbearing is a rite of passage in every nation, but it is also universally a time of intense vulnerability. Many people report fear in early pregnancy and seek out immediate medical care for reassurance and guidance. It is this same fear, however, that makes pregnant people uniquely vulnerable to coercion. The cultural and social norms surrounding birth are vastly different around the globe, and stories of beautiful, empowered, and safe birth intermingle with stories of abuse and despair. Examples of giving birth on the floor and having to clean your own space afterward, and of being beaten and scolded by birth attendants, come from nations where unequal treatment in daily life mimics this reality.[2] In other nations, abuse is more subtle, but just as harmful, and can result in trauma even without visible bruises. The culture and belief of the individual giving birth tends to determine the experience. In cultures where gender imbalances are the norm, this imbalance will be amplified in the birth space. All ills in society, from racism to gender inequality and abuse, are amplified in birth settings.

Human rights are fundamental entitlements due to all people. Every culture on earth reports violations of these rights during pregnancy and birth.[2] The term *Respectful Maternity Care* (RMC) is an umbrella term that engulfs a wide range of issues commonly encountered in the birth space. The categories of disrespectful and abusive care during childbirth include[2,3]:

- Physical abuse
- Non-consented clinical care
- Non-confidential care
- Non-dignified care
- Abandonment and detention in healthcare facilities
- Sexual abuse
- Verbal abuse
- Stigma and discrimination
- Failure to meet professional standards of care
- Poor rapport between women and providers

HEALTH SYSTEM CONDITIONS AND CONSTRAINTS

"There is no circumstance where abuse, coercion, or a violation of your rights is acceptable. Every person has the right to self determination, in a safe, respectful, and supportive birth environment, free from harm. We strongly condemn any and all physical and verbal abuse of birthing persons and demand an immediate cessation of the antiquated harmful obstetric practices of years past. This includes intervention by force, coercion, or legal threat."[4]

Examples of violations of the principles of Respectful Maternity Care can be found in our daily lives. Most births are completely normal and uncomplicated. However, there are numerous examples of birth being portrayed as humorous, normalizing screaming and bodily harm. In movies, birthing people are almost always screaming, and birth is usually an emergency, because that keeps viewers on the edge of their seats. Many people therefore go into their birth experience expecting it to be traumatic, and have a great fear of birth, which is referred to as *tokophobia*.[5] Making light of suffering, exhaustion, and injury is not something we see portrayed in any other aspect of healthcare. If these are your only exposures to birth, it primes you to be afraid, and fear is the worst possible deterrent to self-advocacy.

While healthcare systems should strive to be safe spaces for birthing families, and minimize instances where crucial conversations are necessary, it is common for pregnant people to be challenged on birthing wishes that go counter to the culture of the clinician, birth setting, or the local region.[6] Memories of birth last a lifetime and are widely shared. A birth story may inspire fear or confidence in a birthing community, firmly rooting cultural norms and birth practices in a region.

Among the populations most vulnerable to disrespectful care are prisoners, people of color, LGBTQ people, obese people, and people with addiction issues or mental health conditions. While disrespect and abuse may happen to anyone, those who are more vulnerable to it have likely had prior negative experiences with healthcare providers, are less likely to seek care, and are uncomfortable in a medical setting.

LGBTQ BIRTH CARE

The sex a person is assigned at birth may not correspond to the individual's personal identity. "Sexual orientation"—loosely defined as who someone is attracted to sexually—and gender identity may define people's life and birth experiences. Choosing to love someone who is not of an opposite sex is still taboo in some cultures and can be intensely triggering to some people. "Gender identity" reflects a deeply felt and experienced sense of one's own gender. A person's gender identity is typically consistent with the sex assigned to them at birth. "Gender expression" refers to the way in which an individual outwardly chooses to presents their gender. Expressions of gender may be expressed through dress, body language, and other enhancers/modifications that may include make-up and hair choices that do not conform to the sex assigned at birth. According to the World Health Organization, "heteronormativity" is defined as the assumption that everyone is heterosexual, and that heterosexuality is superior to all other sexualities. Among both individuals and institutions, this can lead to invisibility and stigmatization of other sexualities and gender identities. Often included in this concept is a level of gender normativity and gender roles, the assumption that individuals *should* identify as men and women, and be masculine men and feminine women. In some cultures, the stigma of being non-normative to the culture is so strong that people experience significant discrimination and abuse at the hands of society and healthcare providers. Gender identity is not static and limited to male/female identities, but rather exists on a spectrum.[7]

Birthing people who do not identify as women struggle with a world where birth has traditionally been the "realm of the woman." Most images of pregnancy in media and literature feature traditional female-identifying persons and language. The pregnant person is almost exclusively referred to as "she," and is usually featured with breasts. Birth terminology is sex-specific, and often excludes people who do not identify as female. Even the terminology of Maternity care, identifying a pregnant person as "mother," may not feel accurate to the person. This trigger-language is everywhere for people who do not identify as female, and can cause significant distress and a feeling of being "other" during an intensely vulnerable time that should be exciting and enjoyable.

When a person or couple does not conform to the cultural norm attributed to childbearing people, there may be situations where Respectful Care is compromised. Sometimes this is done without malice or intent, such as when someone refers to the baby's parents as "mother and father," though sometimes the intent is to chastise and harm due to an intense personal reaction from the provider rooted in their own beliefs about sex and gender identity. For people who encounter a system where they are likely to be marginalized or encounter abuse, it is important to find a provider who respects personal wishes, and to communicate expectations about sex/gender specific language for themselves, their partner, and their baby. The birth experience itself may trigger intense feelings, and predispose the gender non-normative birthing person to trauma. It is important to process the birth experience with a trusted person who is privy to the specific circumstances and identity within a few weeks of the birth. When caring for someone who identifies as LGBTQ+, it is important to ask how they want to be addressed, what the important things are for you to remember and share with the rest of the team, and how they envisioned their birth. Making assumptions about who receives the baby at birth, culture-specific parenting and sex terminology (i.e., "it's a girl," "she," "mother") may not only be offensive and upsetting to the birthing person, but may lead to a trauma response. Not using the word "woman" has been a hotly debated issue in women's healthcare, where the perception is that women are erased from birth by eliminating this gendered term. However, the word "woman" is perfectly fine and appropriate to use with anyone who identifies as such. The care we must take is to follow *The Platinum Rule*—to do unto others as they would have done unto themselves, rather than *The Golden Rule*, which assumes we should care for others the way we wish to be cared for ourselves[8]. This principle extends to the language people prefer us to use.

RMC AND PREGNANT PEOPLE IN LARGER BODIES

The World Health Organization estimates that 52% of the world's people have a BMI over 25. During pregnancy, 73% of pregnant people gain more weight than recommended.[9] People in a large body face significant bias in society, but particularly in the healthcare setting, where weight is quickly blamed for all health problems and risks. Equipment is designed for people of average weight. Monitors used to listen to baby hearts rely on ultrasound technology, which does not penetrate adipose tissue well. Beds have weight limits, as do MRI machines, OR tables, and CT scans. Gowns are rarely big enough to comfortably fit a person in a larger body. Blood pressure cuffs, fetal monitor bands, toilets, and chairs are also not designed for larger bodies. It is very difficult for people to feel comfortable in an environment where nothing fits, and where most things are not usable.

Healthcare providers have a bias against patients with a high BMI. There is a societal bias, but in healthcare this is amplified due to the lack of appropriate tools to safeguard patients of size. It is difficult to move a large patient. It is challenging to complete all of the tasks asked of nurses when the person has significant support needs due to their size. In some cultures, and certain communities, size is acceptable and is seen as a variation of normal. In the healthcare setting, it is seen as a high-risk medical condition. Bradford and colleagues[10] state that weight stigma is a culturally acceptable form of discrimination. Because of the impact and importance of language, they suggest using the following terms: Larger body/person in larger body, smaller body/person in a smaller body, higher body weight, person with thin privilege, higher BMI, Lower BMI, and Obesity.[10]

For people who have felt very comfortable in their communities as a person of size, it is hard to adjust to being labeled high-risk, and they may feel acutely out of place. There are health practitioners who refuse to care for pregnant people with a high BMI because of liability issues. The larger the patient, the more difficult it becomes to find a care provider, particularly one who is comfortable and skilled in taking care of people of size. There are very real safety issues to consider. If the laboring person's BMI is over 50, the hospital may not be able to provide life-saving care in an emergency due to lack of equipment. There are many hospitals which have adjusted their inventory to accommodate people of size. There are monitors that work on people with a high BMI (Fig. 2.1a), and allow them to stay mobile (Fig. 2.1b). Birth providers who care for large pregnant people need to have crucial conversations around how things may need to change just because of size.

SHARED DECISION-MAKING

A key component of patient-centered care during childbirth is *Shared Decision-Making*. It is a process whereby birthing people and clinicians make decisions that are in the best interest of the patient, and are individualized to the person. Shared decision-making incorporates clinical evidence that balances risks and expected outcomes with people's preferences and values.[11] It requires people to actively participate in discussions and decisions with healthcare providers. Being an active participant in birth does not require expertise in birthing. It only requires two people who are willing to communicate effectively, with a shared goal.[11] Clinicians have a duty of care for the adequacy of the pregnant person's knowledge, which can only happen when relevant knowledge is offered freely, and when personal beliefs and biases—which are potential defeaters—that may impinge on decision-making are disclosed.

Informed Consent is not the same thing as shared decision-making.[11] The way someone pictures their birth is important. If a person does not get the moment they envisioned because their birth was not ideal, they will feel somewhat disappointed, and will grieve the loss of that image. If people have decision-making power along the way, are given options, choices, counseling, and time to think and decide, they will likely feel positive about their birth experience even if it did not go as planned.

Shared decision-making is becoming more common in medicine, but it needs to be practiced at every opportunity. The idea that a pregnant person—a non-medical provider—can make decisions for themselves is a newer concept for some in healthcare, and a hard adjustment for some clinicians and providers. Sometimes when a provider is told "I do not want that done" their response is to be upset at being challenged on years of expertise, and the response can be very defensive and directive. Clinicians can develop the tools to have difficult conversations, and learn to use the words and behaviors that make these discussions non-confrontational, fostering an environment where both parties feel heard. In crucial conversations, emotions usually run high, there are differing opinions, and there is a lot at stake. When conversations go awry, people tend to do the exact wrong thing, and derail any progress.[12] Our bodies react with hormonal responses that make it hard to listen, and evoke anger, making us want to run away from the situation. Remember that individuals cannot control how the others will communicate, but individuals can have full control over their end of the conversation, and their own behavior. If two parties have tried to come to an agreement, but one party encounters a closed door and lack of flexibility, or an unwillingness to talk about the concerns, a consideration should be made to consider switching care to another clinician.

(a)   (b)

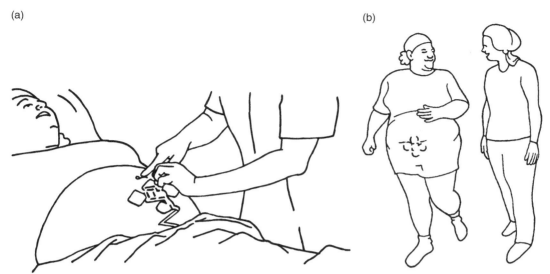

Fig. 2.1a. Placement of Novii monitor.   **Fig. 2.1b.** Pregnant person in larger body
                                                     walking with Novii.

EXPECTATIONS

Giving birth is a rite of passage, and the experience a person envisions around such an important life event matters greatly. Many people have pictured themselves pregnant and giving birth since childhood, and have associated feelings and images with the process. With that birth image comes an expectation. Making assumptions that the person attending you understands your vision and expectations is common. Expectations about a birth experience drive how people will feel about it afterwards.

Passive participation in birth is the norm in many cultures. If a pregnant person is more comfortable being told what to do than determining their own path, their labor and birth will follow the path set forth by the provider, friends, or relatives. The person may find in retrospect that it did not meet their expectations. In some cultural settings, birthing people are not given a choice to speak up or actively participate, or have a person in their lives who makes crucial decisions for them.

Locus of control is the degree to which people believe that they, as opposed to external forces, have control over the outcome of events in their lives. If a person believe that they have control over what happens, then they have what psychologists refer to as an "internal locus of control." Conversely, if a person believes that they have no control over what happens and that external variables are to blame, then they have what is known as an "external locus of control." People with an internal locus of control believe that they are in control of their circumstances. They can take self-blame to an extreme and may beat themselves up over small things that were likely out of their control. People with an external locus of control tend to be more comfortable with concepts like fate and religion, and predestination, when circumstances fit in a construct where a deity, another entity, or a concept such as The Universe destines outcomes.

It can be helpful to understand where a pregnant person is on this spectrum, and it may help both themselves and their providers to have this insight as they develop the skills to have crucial conversations and challenge others, not just as a birthing person, but as a parent. It will also help to know how much they wish to take on as a personal battle. For many people it is easier to leave things to fate and accept an outcome no matter how it unfolds. Not everyone is able or willing to advocate for themselves. Each person is unique in their faiths and beliefs, and all people deserve to be respected and supported no matter how they choose to approach and process a situation.

THE IMPACT OF CULTURE ON THE BIRTH EXPERIENCE

The way people picture their own birthing experience is shaped throughout our lifetime. Images in children's stories, stories from friends and relatives, social media memes and pictures, blogs, scenes from popular movies and depictions of birth in reality television shows all shape expectations. Society has a powerful influence on pregnancy and birth. There is a societally defined role associated with being pregnant. Pregnant people are treated differently the minute they announce their pregnancy. Unsolicited advice, uninvited touching, and being challenged by strangers on their behavior and dress are commonplace in some cultures.[1] During pregnancy, some societies see it as a collective duty to protect the baby from the behavior of its "gestator" (the pregnant person) and cross a boundary that would not be crossed normally.[1] The idea that the baby belongs to the village, and that society can direct behavior, diet, dress, and personal choices is likely rooted in human survival. It does take a village to raise a child, metaphorically in today's world, but in reality in years past. If a person were unable to breastfeed, someone else in the village had to do that for them in order for the child to live. These reciprocal relationships were therefore paramount, and there was a greater tolerance of communal ownership of the baby. There are many myths about pregnancy that are rooted in protection. The village surrounded and protected its pregnant members, which increased the odds of survival.

The unwelcome effects of communal ownership of the baby in today's societies may lead to tremendous amounts of guilt and confusion. In years past, the baby was only accessible to others via the pregnant person's body, and by breaking the boundary of personal touch. In today's high-tech world, the fetus is visible to others via advanced technology, and it does not require touch, which is intensely personal. By incorporating impersonal touch, as with an ultrasound wand, it is easier to not ask permission to do things to a pregnant person. This lays a foundation of implied consent (see section on consent). The baby becomes its own person, its own patient, on the ultrasound screen, and it is easier to dissociate from the person carrying the baby deep within their body. We no longer have to look at or talk to someone in order to examine their baby prenatally. The baby hereby becomes the main patient, rather than the pregnant person.[1] The baby is the product of the gestation, and the more baby is separated from carrier, the less autonomy the birthing person cultivates with the provider. Every bit of guidance and treatment is focused on producing a healthy baby, and the person carrying the baby is expected to comply.

Directive language is sometimes used by healthcare providers.[2,13] In most societies, the healthcare provider rather than the pregnant person is considered the expert on pregnancy. Statements that begin with "you can't," or "you're not allowed to," or "you have to" are examples of directive language, are loaded with implied threat or consequences if the pregnant person does not comply, and are a therefore a red flag to shared decision making. There are many examples of people being fired from care or labeled "bad mothers" or "bad patients" or "non-compliant" if they do not follow guidance during pregnancy, or miss a visit, or decline a test, or do something they were warned against. Nobody likes being chastised or judged, but it becomes particularly difficult to process when the person is pregnant and vulnerable. The fear of abandonment is amplified during pregnancy. In most societies, being labeled a "bad mother" or "bad person" is one of the worst things a person can imagine being called, and they will accept a lot of discomfort and forego questioning a provider on specific recommendations in order to avoid that label. Many providers would be well served to heed the advice to stop equating someone's worth and intrinsic value as a parent or person to their personal healthcare and ethical decision-making.[13] While it takes a lot more time to answer questions, build relationships, listen to concerns, and participate in shared decision making, it is time to insist on this, as birth outcomes and emotional and physical wellbeing are directly tied to it.

TRAUMATIC BIRTHS

Sometimes giving birth is traumatic, and a person may have all the symptoms of PTSD.[14–16] Both clinical and interpersonal factors affect how a person experiences their baby's birth. Much depends on how the individual perceives events, rather than on how others perceive them.[17]

A birthing person is more likely to experience their baby's birth as traumatic if labor pain exceeds their ability to cope with it, if the birth is complicated or premature,[15] involves an emergency cesarean,[18] or if they or their baby suffer bodily damage or injury or when the baby has birth defects, or dies.[15]

While medical interventions, emergencies, and complications may contribute to birth trauma, there are those who experience an essentially normal birth as traumatic due to the loss of control in the situation, perceived threat, or attitudes of the birth care providers. There are three likely pathways to trauma during birth.[19]

- Coercion or Obstetric Violence;
- A classic obstetric emergency, where the person thought they or their baby were in danger of dying;
- Everything else, which may include things that caused confusion, were not aligned with expectation, uncontrolled pain, poor communication, unmet cultural expectations, or wishes that were not honored.

Each of these pathways has the potential to leave a lasting trauma memory and somatic response. There are four trajectories that people recovering from a traumatic birth can follow: resilience, recovery, delayed PTSD, or chronic PTSD. More than three quarters of people who report a traumatic birth do not meet criteria for PTSD by 6 months postpartum.[20]

Research from a variety of countries shows that a person giving birth is also more likely to experience giving birth as traumatic if they perceive the clinical professionals as uncaring, if they feel disrespected or that their dignity has been stripped away,[15] or that they had no control over what was done to them[18] or their baby.[21]

Survivors of sexual trauma are more susceptible to perceiving childbirth events as dangerous, and being retraumatized[14] as a result. Even with pain relief, a childhood sexual abuse survivor may feel violated with their legs separated or in stirrups, private parts being exposed, and people starting at them.[15]

Whether a person has experienced prior trauma or not, a traumatic birth experience adds distress and may take away confidence, at a time when they need all their resources for postpartum recovery and infant care.[17] On the other hand, if a birthing person feels respected, supported, informed, included in decisions, and adequately in control of what is happening to themselves and their baby, they may experience frightening or challenging clinical events without being traumatized. In fact, they may feel that their clinical professionals were especially supportive and skilled. Trauma-informed care supports this type of outcome, and helps prevent trauma responses and PTSD.[14]

TRAUMA SURVIVORS AND PREVENTION OF PTSD

When present prior to pregnancy and childbirth, PTSD can impact pregnancy outcomes and subsequent parenting.[22] Trauma and PTSD may be responsible for the excessive fear and apprehension some people experience around childbirth. PTSD affects approximately 8% of pregnant people, and is gaining recognition as a common perinatal mental health condition.[23]

What defines trauma is how a person's memories are formed. Positive and negative recollections of the birth experiences are related more to feelings and exertion of choice and control than to specific details of the birth experience.[6] The first 4 weeks after experiencing a trauma will determine if this becomes a traumatic memory, or a memory that does not have a lasting impact. Memory can be sharp and detailed moments or even days after an event; people can often remember smells, taste, and sounds, as well as emotions and sensations of the event for a while.[24] Usually, memory fades, and within days an individual will have difficulty recalling the event in great detail. Only the memory of the fact is left, without a physiologic response. Traumatic memory starts off the same way, but over time the somatic, or body response, to the memory does not fade. Trauma is experienced through the 5 senses (sight, sound, smell, taste, and touch) and can be triggered to bring someone back to the moment of trauma in the same way, experiencing the same emotions and body reaction as they did during the original traumatic event.[25] Sometimes the traumatic event is remembered, and at other times people experience a trauma response to an event of which they had no prior conscious memory. The body can respond to an event that is not happening in the present, triggering a fight or flight response that can manifest in different ways.

Often, symptoms of PTSD may not begin until many years after the traumatic event. The National Institute of Mental Health lists the below signs and symptoms of PTSD.[26] For most people, these symptoms disappear within a month of experiencing a trauma. If symptoms persist after that, the diagnosis of PTSD is made.

- Flashbacks—reliving the trauma over and over, including physical symptoms like a racing heart or sweating
- Bad dreams

Respectful Care

2

- Frightening thoughts
- Staying away from places, events, or objects that are reminders of the traumatic experience
- Avoiding thoughts or feelings related to the traumatic event
- Being easily startled
- Feeling tense or "on edge"
- Having difficulty sleeping
- Having angry outbursts
- Trouble remembering key features of the traumatic event
- Negative thoughts about oneself or the world
- Distorted feelings like guilt or blame
- Loss of interest in enjoyable activities

People carry their trauma history in their nervous system. PTSD is sometimes referred to as "somatic time travel."[27] Unaddressed PTSD can impact the way birth is experienced. A look, touch, or behavior that triggers or cues a traumatic memory will lead the body to respond to what happened outside the birth room, not necessarily to what actually happened in the room. If people are aware of their trauma history, and are concerned about their response to birth, they may be able to prepare for their birth.

A clinician or birth provider is walking into a history to which they are not privy. If a person has been unable to share their history for any reason, the provider has no idea that there are specific triggers that may bring them back to a lived trauma. A birthing person is under no obligation to disclose abuse, or to relive a trauma by telling it. All providers should approach the care of birthing people from a place of trauma-informed care (TIC), assuming every human has experienced trauma and approach each situation accordingly.[28]

A trauma-informed provider asks permission, asks questions, listens, positions themselves in a non-threatening way, and honors wishes.[29] Birthing people report that their trauma could have been reduced or prevented by better communication and support by their caregiver or if they themselves had asked for or refused interventions.[30] It is important that someone in the room other than the birthing person understands the potential trauma triggers, and knows what helps bring the person back to the present moment. The people who are not in labor, outside of the moment, can help them, and bring them back to the present. Touch in particular is often a trigger for abuse survivors. If touch of certain parts of the body is identified as a trigger for someone to pull them back to the trauma, it helps for them to be very specific about that, without necessarily having to disclose a trauma history.[29] The person should be clear about their needs and have a fallback plan if they are triggered that their support people know how to enact. In a safe space with safe support system, the birthing person should consider what the triggers are and how to be prepared for them, be aware of the normal things that happen at a birth, and what things are the standard of care in the birth location. People are not shocked by things that they see coming, rather they are shocked by what we were not prepared for. It is easier to experience psychological shock if you did not know it was normal. If something is entertained as a possibility, it is less shocking.

Because trauma is experienced and triggered through the five senses, the five senses are also the way back to the present.[25] Being present and calm are opposites of "fight or flight." The brain is incapable of holding an anxious thought while at the same time being in the present moment. Here are some things that may help someone stay present in the moment[31]:

- Music
- Headphones to drown out conversation or certain noises
- Compassionate eye contact
- Smells that evoke happy memories
- Holding hands or being embraced by someone who makes them feel safe
- Visualization
- A focal point or object
- Affirmations
- Lighting
- Bodily position in the room (not with their back to the door)
- Hydrotherapy

- Distraction
- Rhythm (breathing)
- Ritual (repetitive behaviors or movements, mantras)
- Watching movies
- Dancing
- Aromatherapy
- Massage
- Mindfulness
- Yoga
- Prayer

One exercise taught in Mindfulness is the *5 Senses Exercise*.[25] It helps reduce anxiety, and can help ground trauma survivors to the present. If possible, the clinician can discuss the following steps for the birthing person to use:

- Notice *5 things you can see*. Look at each in turn. You may choose to bring 5 specific things from home.
- Second, notice *4 things you can feel*. Spend some focusing on each of those, choosing touch that does not cause pain or discomfort, such as socks on your feet, or the way a ring feels on a finger.
- Third, notice *3 things you can hear*. Specifically focus on sounds that do not cause anxiety, avoiding things like beeping machines, or loud voices.
- Fourth, notice *2 things you can smell*. You can bring your own scents.
- Finally, notice *1 thing you can taste*. You can bring gum or hard candy, or sip something with a strong flavor.

If the nature of the trauma involved physical suffering or pain, it can be helpful to have an epidural or other effective intervention to minimize or eliminate pain. For some people, it keeps them grounded in the present. Without the repeated trigger of pain, it is then easier to reestablish control. However, for people whose trauma history is based in dissociative behavior, an epidural can be triggering because they cannot move and feel like they have no authority over the body. The epidural itself can trigger dissociation. It is hard for the people in the room to advise someone on pain management, and to know how to help, unless they understand details of trauma. What is triggering to one may be healing to another. Fears are informative in helping make decisions about pain management. It is important for the laboring person to withhold judgment and ask questions. What are expectations placed upon me, by myself, others, and my culture, and what do I fear more? If they find that they are most afraid of suffering, then an epidural is a good option. If they are most afraid of not being in control, it may not be.

Once people know what their triggers are, they can decide:

- How they can stay present,
- What they would like to do about pain management,
- How to communicate their needs to their birth team. This can be done in the form of a written birth plan, or can be done in person, with direct verbal communication.

TRAUMA-INFORMED CARE AS A UNIVERSAL PRECAUTION

Given the large subset of childbearing people who have experienced sexual trauma, many authors suggest that trauma-informed care become a "universal precaution" in perinatal care.[15,32–36] This means working on the assumption that any laboring person may have experienced trauma that is not yet resolved, and treating all with the consideration and respect.

This is because:

- Some people do not disclose their trauma histories to their clinical providers, preferring not to think about trauma during pregnancy. Others do not remember traumatic experiences due to dissociation[34,36–38] or repression of the memory. In either case, they may still be strongly affected by the trauma.
- A satisfying birth experience, as the person defines it, can be healing and empowering when the care given is respectful, kind, and individualized to the person's needs.

- If a person was abused in childhood, trauma-informed care helps reduce the risk that their own children will be abused.[34]
- Trauma-informed care is harmless to those who do not need it. All people tend to appreciate care that is individualized and includes collaborative decision-making.

Birth attendants can routinely make accommodations in three areas to improve the comfort of pregnant people: verbal (always ask before touching and explain procedures to the level desired by the pregnant person), nonverbal (make eye contact as appropriate and sit down when talking with the person whenever possible), and environmental (use soft lights and soothing sounds).

OBSTETRIC VIOLENCE

The World Health Organization (WHO) defines abuse during childbirth as "the mistreatment of women during childbirth in the form of neglect, physical abuse, and/or lack of respect." *Obstetric Violence* (OV) is a term for trauma experienced during childbirth at the hands of others. This may include a violation of rights, inappropriate physical touch, or forced intervention.[39] It can range from disrespect to overt physical harm.[2] Any action by a provider that makes the birthing person acutely uncomfortable can be construed as Obstetric Violence. There are reports of Obstetric Violence from all over the world, and it is a problem that deserves the focus of all agencies seeking to improve the care of childbearing persons.[2] What makes it so challenging to stop Obstetric Violence is the authority position of the person inflicting the trauma, and the normalization of birth-related trauma in various cultures.[40]

In addition to the person positioning themselves as the expert in the room, there may also be a gender imbalance, which adds an additional layer of power over the birthing person. Birthing people place a tremendous amount of trust in their providers, and are conditioned by society to follow their guidance, to be "a good patient" and not to challenge this authority.[1] It often comes as a great shock that the trusted person can become the abuser. Perceptions between providers and patients often differ. When a person complains of feeling abused or coerced, the provider will often say that they followed a standard of care, and that everything they did was in the best interest of the person and their baby. The reality is that providers may be following appropriate standards of care, and following policies, but the things that happened may still feel wrong to the laboring person. While the person giving birth may have felt acutely traumatized, the provider and support people in the room may not even have noticed that their actions were perceived that way, and may have thought that everything went well. Usually there is more than one member of the healthcare team in the room, and if nobody acts shocked by the interaction or intervention that did not feel right to the birthing person, it is likely that no one will question it. The birthing person may believe it is a normal part of the birth experience. This phenomenon is so common that people who are initially very happy with their birth sometimes find themselves confused later on as they try to come to terms with the experience.

It is difficult for people to challenge authority in the moment, and it may be equally difficult to address it afterwards.[2] In some institutions, provider behavior may not be addressed adequately. Trauma perpetuated by medical personnel manifests in different ways for the healthcare consumer, including expressions of inappropriate medical humor and various degrees of insensitivity to pain and emotions. Rather than building sincere relationships with patients and opening themselves up to vulnerability, some healthcare providers may avoid connection. Dissociation from people in their care can translate into overtly directive or coercive care, and a laboring person may be told to "do as I say," and feel powerless to advocate. Pregnant people may hope that the entire healthcare system must revolve around the birthing person, but in reality that laboring person is often seen as a temporary guest in a house with strict rules and rigid beliefs. Well informed health care providers play an important role in helping people navigate the system, and assuring that birthing people's voices are heard.

Obstetric Violence can occur anywhere.[2,39] The actions and beliefs of the people in the birth space have a lasting impact. Talking about the birth afterwards with the birthing person is helpful. Asking questions about the things that were really hard, or were confusing, may help a person process their birth. Knowing more about why things happened the way they did may help them make sense of their birth.

It is helpful for people to know their rights if they encounter a situation where they need to escalate an issue that had a profound impact on their birth experience. A birthing person's physical safety and emotional wellbeing take precedence over everything else, and unprocessed trauma may have a lasting impact on parenting and overall wellbeing. If someone feels they may have been a victim of Obstetric Violence, they have several recourses to address it. All people deserve to be respected and feel heard, and are entitled to answers about their birth.

If a person who gave birth believes they had a bad experience, they were harmed, or have other concerns, they can escalate that to hospital administration if they gave birth in a hospital. Many people are intimidated by the hierarchy and complexity of hospital leadership, but it is important to hospitals that patients are safe and happy with their care. If people are not ready or able to address concerns in the moment, they can still connect with the hospital at any time after they recover. Feedback from patients is taken seriously, and many important initiatives and safety measures have taken place in hospitals because patients spoke up and demanded change. In birth center settings the issue may need to addressed by the director or owner. In homebirth practice settings, the person may need to discuss directly with the midwife, or may report the issue to the state licensing board.

PATIENT RIGHTS

In the United States, *The Patient Bill of Rights* outlines the rights and responsibilities of a patient in a hospital. Most hospitals specifically outline a patient's right to safe, considerate, individualized, and respectful care, provided in a manner consistent with their beliefs, free from abuse or harassment. However, it also outlines that the hospital reserves the right to terminate their relationship with someone if their refusal of recommended care goes against ethical or professional standards. There are federal laws that protect pregnant people from being dismissed from care without immediate access to another provider. Every hospital has to assess a person when they come in with a pregnancy or labor concern. Every laboring person must be given care, and cannot be asked to leave until a proper assessment has been done.

All people have the right to refuse any intervention during their labor. Forced compliance—the alternative to respecting a patient's refusal of treatment—raises profoundly important issues about patient rights, respect for autonomy, violations of bodily integrity, power differentials, and gender equality. Coercive interventions often are discriminatory and act as barriers to needed care.[13]

If the physician or midwife is recommending an intervention to save the life of a baby, the pregnant person still has the right to refuse it. Decision-making in the context of someone's life and beliefs can be challenging, and may require the involvement of an ethics board or a mediator in extreme circumstances. This can happen when a person has lost trust in the team, has specific reasons for the refusal (cultural, religious, personal), is very afraid of the procedure, or does not fully understand the implication. With effective communication, trust building, and understanding barriers to treatment, these situations can be resolved. In rare instances, people refuse absolutely necessary care, and there is a tragic outcome. This is still within their right. Under no circumstances can a birthing person be coerced, forced or bullied into the intervention. Nobody can force a person to do something without their explicit consent. As difficult as it is for the medical teams, people have the right to refuse lifesaving care, including blood transfusions and cesarean sections. People have the right to fire their doctor or midwife from care, and they have the right to ask for a different nurse if the care they are receiving is not optimal.

CONSENT

Consent is permission for something, and that permission can be given in different ways. The form a person signs when they are admitted to a hospital is a written consent that allows the staff to treat the person for the duration of their admission. It is important to remember that this does not negate their right to have things explained to them, or to refuse care. There are usually birth-specific written consents as well, including potentially a vaginal birth consent, a cesarean birth consent, and a consent for blood products. Another type of consent is verbal consent. Someone can say out loud that they accept a certain procedure. This may happen in the case of a sudden change in circumstances, when a quick discussion is all time allows.

The most controversial and unclear type of consent is *implied consent*. Implied consent means that someone assumes the person is consenting by their actions or body language. If a person remains silent, hospital staff may interpret that as consent. If a person opens their legs for an exam for labor progress, it may be interpreted as a consent to break their water, with the provider making assumptions that they can make a decision to change the course of labor based on their medical opinion, without prior discussion or specifically obtaining consent. Implied consent is often used in emergency situations. There is a belief among medical personnel that in the case of imminent danger to the birthing person or baby, decision-making lies with the provider. The reality is that even during emergencies people can ask their providers to stop what they are doing, and ask to have things explained to them, and to be an active partner in the decision-making process. It is important to speak up if something does not feel right, or is painful. If something is really uncomfortable for the person, ask questions about it. And if the birthing person is truly unhappy with the answers, it is acceptable to escalate those concerns up the chain of command. The best prevention of trauma is participating in decision-making.

MATERNAL MORTALITY

Pregnancy and childbirth carry inherent risk to birthing people and babies. In some nations, the risk is very high due to a lack of access to skilled care. There are regions on the planet where help is not available, and where pregnant people have to travel many hours or days to find a skilled labor attendant. Maternal mortality is highest in regions with low and lower-middle income, accounting for 94% of cases, with 86% occurring in sub-Saharan Africa and Southern Asia.[41] In nations where hospitals and skilled care are usually easy to access, maternal mortality is rare. There is a lot to be learned from the data available about maternal mortality, including the cultural and economic hardships that force children into marriage and must be addressed on a global level. Many maternal deaths occur among pregnant people/girls age 10–14.[41]

Most of the complications that develop during pregnancy are preventable or treatable. Some complications may exist before pregnancy but are worsened during pregnancy, especially if not managed as part of the person's care. The major complications that account for nearly 75% of all maternal deaths are[41]:

- severe bleeding (mostly bleeding after childbirth)
- infections (usually after childbirth)
- high blood pressure during pregnancy (pre-eclampsia and eclampsia)
- complications from delivery
- unsafe abortion

In the United States, where 4 million babies are born every year, about 700 deaths occur that can be directly contributed to pregnancy, birth, or postpartum complications. Maternal mortality is on the rise, and disproportionally affects birthing people of color.[42] Up to age 30, maternal mortality rates are the same across all races. Over age 30, the maternal mortality rate for people of color is 3–4 times higher. It is easy to jump to conclusions, and assume there must something different in these populations that make birth more dangerous. Healthcare providers may make assumptions and believe negative birth outcomes are unpreventable because people of color are coming to pregnancy "older, sicker, and fatter."[43] However, skin color does not affect birth outcomes around the world, other than when people lack resources or access to care. What, then, makes birth outcomes so different for birthing people of color in the United States? Education, BMI, insurance, and other factors often blamed for poor obstetric outcomes, however none of these protect black pregnant people. All people of color are equally at a 3–4 fold increased risk of maternal mortality, and are far more likely to have a traumatic birth, or suffer from severe complications.[44] At the root of this alarming discrepancy is racism, and a concept referred to as "weathering."[45] People of color experience racism throughout their lives, both personal and institutional, and are victims of inequity and disparity. The constant stress of racism may lead to premature biological aging. People who experience weathering may have poor health outcomes, and disproportionately high death rates from chronic conditions. Bias can be explicit (conscious) or implicit (unconscious). Levels of bias among healthcare providers are similar to levels of bias in the general population.[46] The constant onslaught of adversity, and of disproportionate hardship and stress associated with living in a society that judges people of color harshly through a lens of generational systemic racism chips away at health, resolve, and resilience, making the birthing person of color inherently more vulnerable in many facets of life. Pregnant people who report racist experiences have three times the likelihood of adverse birth outcomes, including giving birth to low-birthweight or preterm newborns.[40]

Childbearing people of color who present to a hospital often report not feeling heard, having their pain dismissed, and report experiencing abusive encounters with healthcare providers and ancillary hospital staff.

Healthcare providers are overwhelmingly White/Caucasian in the United States, and births are primarily attended by physicians. While 13% of the overall population is Black/African American, this is not proportionally reflected in healthcare, where only 11% of obstetricians and 9% of nurses are Black/African American. There is ample evidence suggesting that when people are cared for by providers from their own culture, outcomes are improved.[46] Culture matters, and individualized care matters. Everyone has certain biases and stereotypical beliefs about others, and both patient and provider come with their own set of beliefs and experiences. If a person is stoic and quiet and reports a lot of pain, someone from a culture that strongly emotes may not believe them. If someone does not sound like the other people around them, perhaps because of a language barrier, or has difficulty communicating for any other reason, there may be a perception that they cannot understand complex information. Self-advocacy is more complicated and less effective when the birthing person belongs to a marginalized population.

REFERENCES

1. Breedlove, et al. (2018) *Nobody Told Me About That: The First Six Weeks*. Printed by the author.
2. Bowser D, Hill K. (2010) Exploring evidence for disrespect and abuse in facility-based childbirth. *Report of a Landscape Analysis*. Harvard: Harvard School of Public Health University Research Co. https://www.hsph.harvard.edu/wp-content/uploads/sites/2413/2014/05/Exploring-Evidence-RMC_Bowser_rep_2010.pdf
3. Bohren MA, Vogel JP, Hunter EC, Lutsiv O, Makh SK, et al. (2015) The mistreatment of women during childbirth in health facilities globally: A mixed-methods systematic review. *PLOS Medicine* 12(6), e1001847. doi: 10.1371/journal.pmed.1001847
4. Price A. (2016) *Original Lecture: Respectful Maternity Care of the Obese Intrapartum Patient*.
5. Bhatia MS, Jhanjee A. (2012) Tokophobia: A dread of pregnancy. *Industrial Psychiatry Journal* 21(2), 158–159. doi: 10.4103/0972-6748.119649
6. Cook K, Loomis C. (2012) The impact of choice and control on women's childbirth experiences. *The Journal of Perinatal Education* 21(3), 158–168. doi: 10.1891/1058-1243.21.3.158
7. WHO. (2016) *FAQ on health and sexual diversity: The basics*. Geneva: World Health Organization. https://www.who.int/gender-equity-rights/news/20160517-faq-on-health-and-sexual-diversity.pdf (accessed January 9, 2022).
8. Rönnedal D. (2014) The golden rule and the platinum rule. *The Journal of Value Inquiry* 49(1–2). doi: 10.1007/s10790-014-9471-8
9. Johnson J, Clifton RG, Roberts JM, et al. (2013) Pregnancy outcomes with weight gain above or below the 2009 Institute of Medicine guidelines. *Obstetrics & Gynecology* 121(5), 969–975. doi: 10.1097/AOG.0b013e31828aea03
10. Bradford H, DePalma K, Mole K, Olsen S. (2020) Weight stigma and fatphobia in healthcare. Are we practicing evidence based care? *ACNM 65th Annual Meeting & Exhibition*. Retrieved from: www.midwife.org
11. Begley K, Daly D, Panda S, Begley C. (2019 Dec) Shared decision-making in maternity care: Acknowledging and overcoming epistemic defeaters. *Journal of Evaluation in Clinical Practice* 25(6), 1113–1120. doi: 10.1111/jep.13243. Epub 2019 Jul 23. PMID: 31338953; PMCID: PMC6899916.
12. Patterson K, Grenny J, McMillan R, Switzler A. (2002) *Crucial Conversations*. McGraw-Hill Contemporary.
13. American College of Obstetricians and Gynecologists. (2016) *ACOG Committee Opinion on Refusal of Medically Recommended Treatment during Pregnancy*. Washington, DC: American College of Obstetricians and Gynecologists.
14. Poote A, McKenzie-McHarg K. (2015) The experience of post-traumatic stress disorder following childbirth. *Journal of Health Visiting* 3(2), 92–98.
15. Beck CT, Driscoll J, Watson S. (2013) *Traumatic Childbirth*. New York, NY: Routledge.
16. James S. (2015) Women's experiences of symptoms of post-traumatic stress disorder after traumatic childbirth: A review and critical appraisal. *Archives of Women's Mental Health* 18(6), 761–771. doi: 10.1007/s00737-015-0560-x
17. Beck CT. (2004) Birth trauma: In the eye of the beholder. *Nursing Research* 53(1), 28–35.
18. Kendall-Tackett K. (2005) Trauma associated with perinatal events: Birth experience, prematurity, and childbearing loss. In: K Kendall-Tackett (ed), *Women, Stress, and Trauma*. New York, NY: Brunner-Routledge. 53–75.
19. Dancy K. (2021 June 30) Personal communication [Interview].
20. Dikmen-Yildiz P, Ayers, S, Phillips, L. (2018) Longitudinal trajectories of post-traumatic stress disorder (PTSD) after birth and associated risk factors. *Journal of Affective Disorders* 229, 377–385. doi: 10.1016/j.jad.2017.12.074

21. U.S. National Institute of Mental Health. Post traumatic stress disorder (PTSD)(publication No. 08 6388). Washington, DC: NIMH. Available from: http://www.nimh.nih.gov/health/publications/post-traumatic-stress-disorder-basics/ptsd-etr-web_38054.pdf (retrieved October 20, 2016).

22. Gerber MR. (2019) Trauma-informed maternity care. In: M Gerber (ed), *Trauma-Informed Healthcare Approaches*. Cham: Springer. doi: 10.1007/978-3-030-04342-1_8

23. Seng JS, Sperlich, M, Low, LK, Ronis, DL, Muzik, M, Liberzon, I. (2013 Jan-Feb) Childhood abuse history, posttraumatic stress disorder, postpartum mental health, and bonding: A prospective cohort study. *Journal Midwifery Women's Health* 58(1), 57–68. doi: 10.1111/j.1542-2011.2012.00237.x. PMID: 23374491; PMCID: PMC3564506.

24. Iyadurai L, Visser RM, Lau-Zhu A, Porcheret K, Horsch A, Holmes EA, James EL. (2019) Intrusive memories of trauma: A target for research bridging cognitive science and its clinical application. *Clinical Psychology Review* 69, 67–82. doi: 10.1016/j.cpr.2018.08.005

25. Bank Lees A. (2020 Oct 28) 7 tools for managing traumatic stress. *National Alliance on Mental Illness*. https://www.nami.org/Blogs/NAMI-Blog/October-2020/7-Tools-for-Managing-Traumatic-Stress

26. U.S. Department of Health and Human Services, National Institutes of Health, National Institute of Mental Health. (2019) Post-Traumatic stress disorder. Retrieved from https://www.nimh.nih.gov/health/topics/post-traumatic-stress-disorder-ptsd

27. Blix I, Brennen T. (2011) Mental time travel after trauma: The specificity and temporal distribution of autobiographical memories and future-directed thoughts. *Memory (Hove, England)* 19, 956–967. doi: 10.1080/09658211.2011.618500

28. Hall S, White A, Ballas J, Saxton SN, Dempsey A, Saxer K. (2021) Education in Trauma-informed care in maternity settings can promote mental health during the COVID-19 Pandemic. *Journal of Obstetric, Gynecologic, and Neonatal Nursing: JOGNN* 50(3), 340–351. doi: 10.1016/j.jogn.2020.12.005

29. Sperlich M, Seng JS, Li Y, Taylor J, Bradbury-Jones C. (2017) Integrating trauma-informed care into maternity care practice: Conceptual and practical issues. *Journal Midwifery Women's Health* 62(6), 661–672.

30. Hollander MH, van Hastenberg E, van Dillen J, van Pampus MG, de Miranda E, Stramrood C. (2017) Preventing traumatic childbirth experiences: 2192 women's perceptions and views. *Archives of Women's Mental Health* 20(4), 515–523. doi: 10.1007/s00737-017-0729-6It

31. Mosley E, Lanning, R. (2020) Evidence and guidelines for trauma-informed doula care. *Midwifery* 83, 102643. doi: 10.1016/j.midw.2020.102643

32. Substance Abuse and Mental Health Services Administration. (2014) SAMHSA's concept of trauma and guidance for a trauma-informed approach. HHS publication No. (SMA) 14-4884. Rockville, MD: SAMHSA. Retrieved from http://store.samhsa.gov/shin/content/SMA14-4884/SMA14-4884.pdf

33. Behrendt A, Moritz, S. (2005) Posttraumatic stress disorder and memory problems after female genital mutilation. *American Journal of Psychiatry* 162(5), 1000–1002.

34. Simkin P, Klaus, P. (2004) *When Survivors Give Birth: Understanding and Healing the Effects of Early Sexual Abuse on Childbearing Women*. Seattle, WA: Classic Day Publishing.

35. Seng J, Taylor J. (2015) *Trauma Informed Care in the Perinatal Period: Protecting Children and Young People*. Edinburgh: Dunedin Academic Press.

36. Raja S, Hasnain, S, Masnain, M, Hoersch, M, Grove-Yin, S, Rajagopalan, C. (2015) Trauma informed care in medicine: Current knowledge and future research directions. *Family and Community Health* 38(3), 216–226. doi: 10.1097/FCH.0000000000000071

37. White AA. (2014) Responding to prenatal disclosure of past sexual abuse. *Obstetrics & Gynecology* 123(6), 1344–1347. doi: 10.1097/AOG.0000000000000266

38. Seng JS, Sperlich M, Low LK. (2008) Mental health, demographic, and risk behavior profiles of pregnant survivors of childhood and adult abuse. *Journal of Midwifery and Women's Health* 53(6), 511–521. doi: 10.1016/j.jwwh.2008.04.013

39. Sadler M, Santos MJDS, Ruiz-Berdún D, Gonzalo LR, Skoko E, Gillen P, Clausen JA. (2016) Moving beyond disrespect and abuse: Addressing the structural dimensions of obstetric violence. *Reproductive Health Matters* 24(47), 47–55. doi: 10.1016/j.rhm.2016.04.002

40. Weinstein A. (2019 May 31). *Trauma-informed care needed to address obstetric violence*. Psychology Today. https://www.psychologytoday.com/us/blog/the-beginning/201903/trauma-informed-care-needed-address-obstetric-violence

41. UNFPA, World Health Organization, UNICEF, World Bank Group, the United Nations Population Division. (2019) Trends in maternal mortality: 2000 to 2017: Estimates by WHO, UNICEF, UNFPA, World Bank Group and the United Nations Population Division. Geneva: World Health Organization.

42. Scott KA, MD, MPH, Britton L, PhD, RN, McLemore MR, PhD, MPH, RN. (2019 April/June) The ethics of perinatal care for black women. *The Journal of Perinatal & Neonatal Nursing* 33(2), 108–115. doi: 10.1097/JPN.0000000000000394.

43. Pregnant women of color described stressful interactions with all levels of health care staff, McLemore M, Altman M, Cooper N, Williams S, Rand, L, Franck L. (2018) Health care experiences of pregnant, birthing and postnatal women of color at risk for preterm birth. *Social Science and Medicine* 201, 127–135. doi: 10.1016/j.socscimed.2018.02.013

44. Petersen E, Davis N, Goodman D, Cox S, Syverson C, Seed K, Barfield W. (2019) Racial/ethnic disparities in pregnancy-related deaths—United States, 2007–2016. *Morbidity and Mortality Weekly Report* 68(35), 762–765. doi: 10.15585/mmwr.mm6835a3

45. Geronimus AT, Hicken M, Keene D, Bound J. (2006 May) "Weathering" and age patterns of allostatic load scores among blacks and whites in the United States. *American Journal of Public Health* 96(5), 826–833. doi: 10.2105/AJPH.2004.060749. Epub 2005 Dec 27. PMID: 16380565; PMCID: PMC1470581.

46. Greenwood BN, et al. (2020) Physician–patient racial concordance and disparities in birthing mortality for newborns. *Proceedings of the National Academy of Sciences* 117(35), 21194–21200.

Chapter 3

Normal Labor and Labor Dystocia: General Considerations

Lisa Hanson, PhD, CNM, FACNM, FAAN, Venus Standard, MSN, CNM, LCCE, FACNM, and Penny Simkin, BA, PT, CCE, CD(DONA)

WHAT IS NORMAL LABOR?

Normal labors vary in length, and degree of pain. A normal labor may take place in a hospital, birth center, or at home.

Numerous professional organizations and working groups of care providers (midwives; obstetricians; family physicians) in North America and Europe have defined normal labor.[1–5] These definitions are summarized in Table 3.1.

The WHO criteria for normal labor have not changed since 1997, when they were first published. The problem is that normalcy is defined in retrospect, after the birth has occurred. This uncertainty can lead to management of all labors as high risk until proven otherwise after the births. WHO estimates that "between 70 and 80% of all pregnant [people] may be considered low-risk at the start of labor."[6] WHO stated, "In normal birth there should be a valid reason to interfere with the normal process."[6] However, assessments of risk must continue throughout pregnancy and labor: "At any moment early complications may become apparent and induce the decision to refer the [person] to a higher level of care."[6] Therefore, the practice of supporting normalcy but continuing vigilant assessments is recommended to limit unnecessary intervention and support normal labor and birth. In 2017, the Royal College of Midwives abandoned its normal birth campaign in favor of an evidence-based "better birth" initiative.

Simkin's Labor Progress Handbook: Early Interventions to Prevent and Treat Dystocia, Fifth Edition. Edited by Lisa Hanson, Emily Malloy, and Penny Simkin.
© 2024 John Wiley & Sons Ltd. Published 2024 by John Wiley & Sons Ltd.

Table 3.1. Definitions of Normal Labor and the Ability of the Birthgiver to Cope.

Defining organization or individual	Definition	Comments
World Health Organization (WHO), 1997[6]	"Spontaneous in onset, low-risk at the start of labor and remaining so throughout labor and delivery. The infant is born spontaneously in the vertex position between 37 and 42 completed weeks of pregnancy. After birth mother and baby are in good condition."	This **retrospective definition** of normal labor is based on healthy outcomes. Normal labor can only be diagnosed in retrospect
Society of Obstetricians and Gynecologists of Canada (SOGC); Association of Women's Health, Obstetric and Neonatal Nursing of Canada (AWHONN); Canadian Association of Midwives (CAM), College of Family Physicians of Canada (CFPC); and Society of Rural Physicians of Canada (SRPC)[5]	Same as WHO, above, plus: "**Normal birth includes** the opportunity for skin-to-skin holding and breastfeeding in the first hour after the birth. **A normal birth does not preclude possible complications** such as postpartum hemorrhage, perineal trauma and repair, and admission to the neonatal intensive care unit. **Normal birth may also include evidence-based interventions** in appropriate circumstances to facilitate labor progress and normal vaginal delivery; for example: • Augmentation of labor and artificial rupture of the membranes (ARM) if it is not part of medical induction of labor • Non-pharmacologic and pharmacologic pain relief (nitrous oxide, opioids and/or epidural) • Managed third stage of labor • Intermittent fetal auscultation **A normal birth does not include:** • Elective induction of labor prior to 41 + 0 weeks • Spinal analgesia, general anesthetic • Instrumental delivery • Cesarean delivery • Routine episiotomy • Continuous electronic fetal monitoring for low-risk birth • Fetal malpresentation	• This is a **prospective process-based definition of normal labor**. With this definition, one may have a normal labor, but a poor outcome. The group advocates:Spontaneous labor onset • Freedom to move throughout • Continuous labor support • No routine intervention • Spontaneous pushing in position the laboring person prefers • Fetal surveillance by auscultation • Good information for laboring people • Education on normal birth for childbirth educators and care providers

(Continued)

Table 3.1. *(Continued)*

Defining organization or individual	Definition	Comments
UK Maternity Care Working Party [MCWP],[8] including the Royal College of Midwives [RCM], Royal College of Obstetricians and Gynecologists (RCOG), and National Childbirth Trust (NCT)[7] and Australian College of Midwives, National midwifery guidelines for consultation and referral,[2]	**The "normal delivery" group includes:** Person whose labor starts spontaneously, progresses spontaneously without drugs, and who gives birth spontaneously; **AND** those who experience any of the following, provided they do not meet the exclusion criteria (see below): <ul><li>augmentation of labor, artificial rupture of the membranes (ARM) if not part of medical induction of labor,</li><li>nitrous oxide/oxygen,</li><li>opioids,</li><li>electronic fetal monitoring,</li><li>managed third stage of labor,</li><li>antenatal, intrapartum, or postnatal complications (postpartum hemorrhage, perineal tear, repair of perineal trauma, admission to SCBU or NICU).</li></ul> **The "normal delivery" group excludes:** Pregnant people who experience any one or more of the following: <ul><li>induction of labor (with prostaglandins, oxytocics or ARM),</li><li>epidural or spinal, general anesthetic,</li><li>forceps or vacuum,</li><li>cesarean section, or episiotomy.</li></ul> *"Some MCWP members would like the Information Centre definition tightened in future to also exclude procedures like augmentation of labor, use of opioid drugs, artificial rupture of membranes or managed third stage. This would depend on the necessary statistics being routinely collected. Alternatively, a tighter definition could lead to the establishment of a separate definition of 'physiological' or 'natural' birth."*	Similar to SOGC definition above, this is another *Prospective Process-based definition* except it does not include epidural, and does include electronic fetal monitoring in the definition of "normal."

American College of Nurse-Midwives, Midwives Alliance of North America, National Association of Certified Professional Midwives (NACPM),[1]	"A normal physiological labor and birth is one that is powered by the innate human capacity of the pregnant person and fetus" "Normal physiologic childbirth (NPC)" • is characterized by spontaneous onset and progression of labor; • includes biologic and psychologic conditions that promote effective labor; • results in the vaginal birth of the infant and placenta; • results in physiologic blood loss; • facilitates optimal newborn transition through skin-to-skin contact and keeping the mother and infant together during the postpartum period; and • supports early initiation of breastfeeding. The document names factors that influence Normal Physiologic Childbirth (NPC), including: • for the new parent—good health, autonomy, knowledge, and confidence about the value of NPC, shared decision-making, and access to this type of care; • for the clinician—education, competence, skill, confidence in supporting NPC and helping the laboring person cope with pain; commitment to enhancing their confidence and diminishing their fear, and sharing decision-making; • and a commitment to provide a birth setting and environment that fosters the elements required for success of NPC.	Includes prescriptive physiologic care practices and normal healthy outcomes in the definition of NPC
Debbie Gould, British midwife[3]	WHO definition, plus: • labor and birth involves strenuous physical work by mother; • includes movement by mother (seeking comfort and progress); and • movement by fetus through the birth canal. • "Movement and the notion of hard work are crucial to a midwifery understanding of normal labor" (ref. 6, p. 424) PLUS psychosocial outcomes: • A healthy parent and baby who are ready to adjust together to their new roles. • Empowerment of the woman. • Sense of achievement resulting from their own productive efforts and their ACTIVE control (rather than passive) role in the birth.	This *holistic definition* includes references to the birthing person and fetus's physical effort and emphasizes their shared roles in accomplishing the birth and postpartum adjustment together. With this definition, normal birth also includes psychological benefits for the mother[6]

WHAT IS LABOR DYSTOCIA?

The term "labor dystocia" is a catch-all term that means difficult labor and refers to protracted or arrested progress in cervical dilation during the active phase of labor, or protracted or arrested descent during the second stage. Numerous other terms, such as "dysfunctional labor," "uterine inertia," "persistent malposition," "cephalo-pelvic disproportion," "failure to progress," "protracted labor," have been used to refer to labor dystocia. Diagnosis and management of labor dystocia vary, depending on the philosophy of the care provider.

What is normal labor progress and what practices promote it?

Although none of the definitions of normal birth in Table 3.1 specify rates of labor progress, numerous authors consider adequate labor progress to be a defining characteristic of normality and a major focus of intrapartum care, along with the wellbeing of birthing person and fetus. A historical perspective of the scientific knowledge of labor progress is presented to offer perspective since the evidence has changed substantially.

Historically, Friedman's graphic analyses of labor progress, published between the mid-1950s and the 1970s, have profoundly influenced obstetrics in America and elsewhere for decades. He defined labor dystocia as a rate of dilation less than 1.2 cm/h in nulliparas and less than 1.5 cm/h in multiparas during the active phase of labor, which he defined as dilation from 3 to 10 cm.[9] Laboring people experienced frequent vaginal examinations with the expectation of cervical change every two hours. This definition of labor progress is no longer considered valid. The duration of normal labor has been studied for decades. Contemporary researchers have found labor to be longer that described by Friedman[10] and it is clear that strict adherence to arbitrary limits for low-risk laboring people contribute to the rising cesarean rate.

In 2018, WHO published Intrapartum Care for Positive Birth Experiences.[10] This document presented a comprehensive summary of the evidence on labor duration and labor care practices. The following statements from this document summarize the scientific evidence on labor duration and care practices including which are recommended and not recommended for low-risk laboring people:

- **Latent labor**
  - Standard duration has not been established
  - Duration varies widely
  - Interventions to accelerate the rate of dilation latent labor are not recommended before 5 cm status of the birthing person and fetus are reassuring.

- **Active labor**
  - Begins at 5–6 cm dilation (*Note: ACOG/SMFM states 6 cm)
  - Duration is typically, not more than 12 hours in primigravida and 10 hours in multiparas
  - The cervical dilation threshold of 1cm/hour is unrealistic and inaccurate and does not predict adverse outcomes; this threshold is not recommended as an indication for intervention or prediction of adverse outcomes.
  - These specific routines are ***not recommended***:
    - Clinical pelvimetry on admission
    - Fetal monitoring tracing (cardiotocography) on admission
    - Continuous electronic fetal monitoring for low-risk laboring people
    - Pubic shaving
    - Chlorhexidine vaginal cleansing
    - Strategies to prevent labor delays for low-risk people (***not recommended***):
      - Enemas
      - Intravenous fluids
      - Active management of labor (package)
      - Amniotomy alone
      - Early amniotomy with oxytocin

- These specific routines are ***recommended*** for low-risk laboring people:
  - Assessment of fetal well-being using Doppler or Pinard fetal stethoscope on admission and intermittently through labor
  - Oral intake of food and fluids
  - Encouragement of movement and upright positions
  - Digital vaginal examination at 4-hour intervals during active labor
  - If requested, pain relief based on laboring person's preference
    - Relaxation techniques (e.g. breathing, mindfulness etc.)
    - Manual techniques (e.g. massage, warm compresses)
    - Intravenous (parenteral) opioids
    - Epidural anesthesia
- **Second Stage Labor**
  - Duration is variable
  - These strategies are ***recommended***:
    - Upright positions and those preferred by the laboring person with and without an epidural
    - Support of spontaneous bearing down
    - Laboring down (delayed) pushing with an epidural for 1–2 hours (when fetal assessment and fetal monitoring allow)
    - Perineal management techniques based on laboring person's preference
      - Perineal massage
      - Warm compresses
      - "Hands on"
  - These interventions are ***not recommended***
    - Routine episiotomy
    - Fundal pressure
    - Routine suctioning of the neonatal oral and nasopharynx
- **Third Stage Labor**
  - These strategies are ***recommended***:
    - Delayed cord clamping (at least one minute, longer as clinically appropriate)
  - Uterotonics to prevent postpartum hemorrhage are recommended for all births
    - Oxytocin is a recommended uterotonic
    - If oxytocin is not available, the use of other uterotonics is recommended
  - When skilled birth attendants are available, controlled cord traction (may result in slightly smaller blood loss and shorted third stage duration)
  - These interventions are ***not recommended***
    - Sustained uterine massage to prevent hemorrhage in people who received prophylactic oxytocin.
- **Fourth Stage Labor**
  - For a healthy newborn, immediate skin-to-skin contact with parent for the first hour after birth
  - Immediate breastfeeding when clinically stable
  - Administration of Vitamin K after birth
  - Delay bathing for 24 hours. If this is not possible, delay bathing for at least 6 hours
  - Avoid separation of the parent and the baby
  - Assess uterine tone for early identification of atony
  - For 24 hours conduct regular assessment of vaginal bleeding, fundal height, and vital signs
  - For those who birth in a hospital or birth center, provide facility care for 24 hours after birth
- These interventions are ***not recommended***
  - Routine antibiotics for uncomplicated vaginal birth or episiotomy.

The Chapters of Simkin's Labor Progress Handbook are intended to assist readers to apply scientific evidence to practice and to apply a variety of strategies to promote progress and enhance coping.

WHY DOES LABOR PROGRESS, SLOW OR STOP?

Most cases of dystocia are caused by one or a combination of factors, as listed in Table 3.2. Some of these etiologies disappear with changes in labor management. Others are corrected with skilled diagnosis and appropriate treatments based on the diagnosis. With time, patience, and trial and error, some will self-correct while others will not respond and will require obstetric interventions as indicated.

Labor progress and prevention of dystocia depend on harmonious inter-actions among a variety of psycho-emotional, interpersonal, physical, and physiologic factors. Progress is facilitated when a laboring person feels safe, respected, and cared for by expert caregivers; when they can remain active, mobile, and upright; and when their pain is adequately and safely managed. Their sense of wellbeing is enhanced by a caring, attentive partner or loved ones; competent, confident, compassionate caregivers and doulas; and a calm comfortable, and well-equipped birthplace. If these are not available, the laboring person may feel ashamed, embarrassed, inhibited, alone, judged, unsafe, restricted, disrespected, ignored, or insignificant.[11] Such feelings may elicit a psychobiological reaction that interferes with efficient progress in labor.

Table 3.2.   Etiologies and risk factors for labor dystocia.

Etiology	Description	Comments
Cervical qualities	Posterior unripe cervix at labor onset, scarred, fibrous cervix or "rigid os," "tense cervix," or thick lower uterine segment	Unripe cervix may prolong latent phase. Surgical scarring, damage from disease, or structural abnormality may increase cervical resistance
Emotional stressors	Distress, fear, exhaustion, or severe pain	Increased catecholamine production may compete with oxytocin effects and inhibit contractions
Fetal characteristics	Malposition, asynclitism, large or deflexed head, lack of engagement	Pendulous abdomen, size and shape of pelvis or fetal head may predispose fetus to malposition
Iatrogenic events	Misdiagnosis of labor onset, active labor, second stage, or "protracted" labor; elective induction, inappropriate, oxytocin use, maternal immobility, drugs, dehydration, disturbance	Misdiagnosis or unneeded interventions or restrictions can slow or interfere with labor progress
Pelvic characteristics	Bony pelvis structures such as a flat or narrow pubic arch, prominent ischial spines, and childhood conditions such as rickets	Birthing person movement, and upright squatting, forward-leaning, or asymmetrical positions increase pelvic dimensions
Uterine factors	Hypotonic contractions (Inadequate and or inefficient), hypertonic uterus	May be secondary to fear, fasting, dehydration, supine position, cephalopelvic disproportion, lactic acidosis in myometrium, or structural abnormalities
Soft tissue characteristics (uterine, cervical, pelvic and spinal ligaments, muscles, and fascia).[12,13] See Box below (Spinning Babies®)	Imbalance of tone or tension, due to laboring person's habitual posture or injury, may negatively influence flexibility and symmetry of pelvic structures, uterine activity, and fetal position	May reduce mobility of spine and pelvic joints, causing torque or other uneven pressures on the uterus, and impairing optimal fetal positions

The Spinning Babies® approach: prevention and resolution of labor dystocia

Spinning Babies® approaches birth preparation and the childbirth process from the perspective of fetal rotation, hence "spinning." This approach is based on the knowledge of soft tissue influences, pelvic mobility, fetal rotation, and descent. Spinning Babies® borrows the architectural concept of "tensegrity" (tension integrity) to explain the play of forces among the soft tissues and bones[12,13] and how they support the birth process.

The Spinning Babies® three principles of **Balance, Gravity, and Movement** ease birth by restoring Balance before or along with the widely used techniques that utilize Gravity and Movement to facilitate labor progress. For example, getting a laboring person up and moving does not always advance labor as desired. The problem may be that some soft tissues—muscles, ligaments, or connective tissue—may be too tight, too loose, or torqued. This can cause resistance, pain, and even reduction in the pelvic diameters. The intention of Spinning Babies® is to correct this problem.

Spinning Babies® recommends activities during pregnancy designed to release muscles, ligaments, and connective tissue to promote pelvic flexibility. Currently, intrapartum care focuses on cervical dilation, baby's size, and pelvic size as factors in labor progress. Spinning Babies®, however, addresses pelvic station and fetal position to select solutions for labor dystocia or options in pain management.

Specific progress techniques are matched to the level (high, middle, or low) of the pelvis where the baby's progress stalls. In addition to its potential mechanical benefits, this approach empowers the birthing person instead of stirring fears about malposition.

The Questions We Ask Lead Us to the Solutions We Seek: Current questions

Current Questions	Spinning Babies Questions
How far is the cervix dilated?	Where is the baby in the pelvis?
Is the baby too big?	Can fetal head flexion and/or rotation create more space?
Is the pelvis too small?	Can we maximize the pelvic space by increasing flexibility of the pelvic joints? Can we mobilize the sacrum?
Can we avoid interventions by giving more time?	Is this labor pattern reflecting a truly obstructed labor or will it resolve with Balance, Gravity and Movement?

PROSTAGLANDINS AND HORMONAL INFLUENCES ON EMOTIONS AND LABOR PROGRESS

The neurobiological processes that result in the onset and progress of labor and birth are referred to as the hormonal physiology of labor. This involves complex interactions between several hormonal systems: oxytocin, beta-endorphins, and stress hormones such as epinephrine, norepinephrine. These processes have evolved over millions of years to optimize birth outcomes and are shared by all mammals.[14,15]

Besides being influenced by the factors listed in Table 3.2, the labor process is influenced by a complex interplay of a variety of hormones. The major hormones that contribute to pregnancy, labor, birth and postpartum physiology are described in Table 3.3 based on a synthesis of work of several prominent experts.[16–18] Each of these hormones has specific functions, which may either facilitate or inhibit the effects of the others. It is the balance of hormones that determines the net effects on labor progress, postpartum mental health, parent–infant interaction, and the initiation of breastfeeding.

Table 3.3. Major hormones of pregnancy, labor, birth, and postpartum.

Prostaglandins	Promotes cervical ripening making it softer and more elastic.[14]
Oxytocin	Known as the hormone of "calm and connection," "closeness," or the "love" hormone. Contributes to uterine contractions, the urge to push, including the Ferguson Reflex also called the "fetus ejection reflex,"[18] Causes the "letdown" of breastmilk, maternal behavior, and feelings of wellbeing and love[19]. It reduces both pain perception and memory of aversive experiences.[14] It has effects opposite to those of catecholamines, as described later.

Table 3.3.   *(Continued)*

Endorphins	These morphine-like hormones increase with pain, exertion, stress, and fear and tend to counteract associated unpleasant feelings. During labor, they are instrumental in creating an altered, trance-like state of consciousness (withdrawn, dreamy, and instinctual behavior) characteristic of people in active labor. They contribute to the "high" feelings that many unmedicated birthing people have after birth. Once the stress or pain ends, the birthgiver has the leftover euphoric effects of the endorphins.
Catecholamines	These stress hormones—adrenaline (epinephrine), noradrenaline (norepinephrine), cortisol, and others—are secreted when a woman is frightened or angry, is in danger, or feels that she or her baby is in danger. These are the hormones of "fight-or-flight." Their physiologic effects enable the person's body to endure, defend against, or flee a dangerous situation. High levels of catecholamines tend to counteract the effects of oxytocin and endorphins during labor. During most of the first stage, excessively high levels of circulating catecholamines cause maternal blood to be shunted from the uterus, placenta, and other organs that are not essential for immediate survival, to the heart, lungs, brain, and skeletal muscle—the organs essential to fight-or-flight. The resulting decrease in blood supply to the uterus and placenta slows uterine contractions[20] and decreases the availability of oxygen to the fetus.[21] Psychological effects on the laboring person include muscle tension, hyper alertness, fear, help-seeking, and protectiveness of their unborn child. The term "fight- or-flight" accurately describes the physiologic response to danger of all mammals, as well as the behavioral response of males. Studies of female behavior when in fear or danger have shown that female behavior is often better described as "tend-and-befriend"—that is, protecting their offspring and reaching out for support.[22] See below for further discussion of "tend-and-befriend." In the second stage of labor, a surge of catecholamines is physiologic and helps mobilize the strength, effort, and alertness needed to push out the baby.[18]
Prolactin	This "nesting hormone" prepares the breasts for breastfeeding during pregnancy and after birth, promotes the synthesis of milk, and has mood-elevating and calming effects on the birthing person. It seems to play a role in the altruistic behavior of a new mother—the ability to put the baby's needs before their own.

DISRUPTIONS TO THE HORMONAL PHYSIOLOGY OF LABOR

The delicate interplay between the hormonal systems is an important consideration in prolonged labor. For example, endogenous oxytocin is required for uterine contractions but also decreases fear, anxiety, and pain. When events or stimuli occur that cause fear, anxiety and increased pain, stress hormones are over-produced. This decreases oxytocin and can disrupt labor, and in turn reduces the protective effects of oxytocin's role in decreasing fear, anxiety, and pain which can further increase stress hormone production and decrease oxytocin. Overstimulation of the neocortex is also theorized to inhibit the "primitive" part of the brain which is responsible for the cascade of hormones required for effective labor.[23]

Environmental factors that may disrupt the hormonal physiology of labor:

- noise
- bright lights
- lack of privacy
- interaction with strangers
- painful procedures (IV insertions, vaginal exams)
- restricted activity
- food and drink restrictions
- lack of support
- conversation
- asking the laboring person too many questions
- a hectic environment[23]

Hormonal responses and gender

The research conducted on hormonal influences and emotions on labor progress has been conducted with cisgender women and men. To be most clear in explaining this research, we have elected to leave the gendered language in this table and section. Research on hormonal influences of trans and nonbinary birthing people is greatly needed to broaden our understanding of hormonal responses.

"Fight-or-flight" and "tend-and-befriend" responses to distress and fear during labor

When hospitals had separate "labor" and "delivery" rooms, laboring people were moved during late first stage (multiparas) or at complete dilation (primiparas) to prepare for the birth of the baby. These environments had bright lights, lots of equipment, and tables that had stirrups for feet and/or legs. Laboring people were admonished not to touch the sterile drapes or their perineum that had just been sanitized with a soap scrub. It was quite common for contractions to completely stop for a time after the laboring person was moved, repositioned, and "prepped" for birth.

The well-known "fight-or-flight" response, a physiologic process that promotes survival of the endangered or frightened animal or human, is initiated by the outpouring of catecholamines, or stress hormones. Triggered by physical danger, fear, anxiety, or other forms of distress, the fight-or-flight response has the potential of slowing labor progress (Fig. 3.1). During most of the first stage of labor, excessively high levels of circulating catecholamines cause blood to be shunted from the uterus, placenta, and other organs not essential for immediate survival to the heart, lungs, brain, and skeletal muscle—the organs essential to fight-or-flight. The resulting decrease in blood supply to the uterus and placenta slows uterine contractions[20] and decreases the availability of oxygen to the fetus.[21]

Although the physiology of the fight-or-flight response is similar in men and women, behavioral differences exist between the sexes.[22] While fight-or-flight may characterize the primary physiologic responses to stress, behaviorally, male responses are more likely to follow the fight-or-flight pattern (fight to protect self, family, village, or country against dangerous attackers, or flee from danger if the odds against success are too and reaching out for help or affiliating with others to reduce the risks to themselves and their offspring).

A woman's protectiveness toward their child is evident when they are told by a respected caregiver that their baby is in danger. They will quickly agree to what-ever treatment is suggested, even if it does not fit with her prior

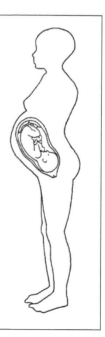

Effects of Anxiety in Labor

Excessive catecholamine levels during first stage of labor
Physiologic response in laboring person: decreased blood flow to uterus, suppression of oxytocin effects, decreased uterine contractions, increased duration of first stage of labor, decreased blood flow to placenta

Psychological response: increased negative or pessimistic perception of events and the words of others, increased need for reassurance and support, protectiveness toward fetus

Physiologic response in fetus: increased fetal production of catecholamines, fetal conservation of oxygen, fetal heart rate decelerations

High catecholamine levels in second stage labor
Maternal effects: Alertness, renewed energy, strength
Fetal effects: same as listed above

Fig. 3.1.   Physiological and psychological effects of anxiety on laboring person and fetus.

preferences for her birth. In doing this, she is "tending" her baby. (On the other hand, if she does not trust the caregiver, she may try to protect her child by resisting the suggested treatments.)

Women want and need supportive people around them during labor, that is, to be "befriended" when stressed or fearful. In fact, the absence of this kind of support is one of the most frequently mentioned reasons for later dissatisfaction with childbirth (22) and is commonly associated with posttraumatic stress disorder (PTSD) after childbirth.[24–27]

Fear or anxiety may cause the pregnant people to perceive labor events or caregivers' words as threatening or dangerous, when a non-fearful person might have no such reaction. As a result, they may remain vigilant or hyper-alert, to protect herself against the perceived danger.[28,29] Fear and anxiety may also interfere with the laboring person's ability to absorb and retain information that is being provided. High levels of catecholamines during labor suppress the usual endorphin effects that would otherwise alter the person's state of consciousness, and help them enter an instinctual mental state, sometimes referred to as the "zone."

Avoiding or reducing psychological distress appears to facilitate both the physiologic labor process and the sense of wellbeing that allows the person to enter this instinctual, almost trance-like state. It is worth noting that even when a person in is in this state, they are aware, allow themselves to remain there, and are fully capable of becoming alert and making decisions when necessary. Interestingly, as they near the second stage of labor, which requires alertness and great physical effort, an outpouring of catecholamines normally occurs and has the beneficial effect of speeding the birth by causing the Fergeson Reflex also known as the "fetal ejection reflex."[18] Some birth givers exhibit fear, anger, or even euphoria—typical catecholamine responses—just before and just after the birth.[16,17]

Optimizing the environment for birth

For many people, the birth of their first child is the reason for their first hospital admission. This means few or none of the usual sights, sounds, and smells of the birth environment are familiar to them. Most hospitals address safety issues for parents and babies with uniform care protocols and a large assortment of diagnostic and therapeutic interventions managed by skilled clinical professionals, in a working environment designed for efficiency and the safety of the clinical staff.

Michel Odent, MD a well-known advocate of normal birth, identified when the neocortex or the "newer," more uniquely human part of the brain—the thinking, reasoning part—is over- stimulated, the birth process is inhibited. When people labor in hospitals, the neocortex is constantly stimulated with bright lights, strangers, many questions, unfamiliar sights and sounds, and other disturbances, that may inhibit primitive brain function and the release of oxytocin and endorphins, while increasing the release of labor-inhibiting catecholamines, which contribute to dystocia in first stage labor. He suggested that instead humans, like other mammals, need privacy in a comfortable, cozy, quiet space and dim light for labor and birth to proceed undisturbed. The primitive parts of the brain work to balance the hormones and uterine functioning allowing instinctual physiologic labor and birth can unfold.[16,17]

People chose to give birth at home for a variety of reasons, including familiarity with the environment, comfort, and desire for normalcy. There is emerging evidence that people of birth may shape the microbiome of the neonate, with significant changes between hospital and home born neonates.[30,31] Birth settings modified to optimize privacy and the sensory environment are often referred to as "alternative settings." Birth centers are example of an alternative setting. A 2012 Cochrane Review of ten trials involving almost 12,000 women reported: "When compared to conventional institutional settings, alternative settings were associated with reduced likelihood of medical interventions, increased likelihood of spontaneous vaginal birth, increased maternal satisfaction, and greater likelihood of continued breastfeeding at one to two months postpartum, with no apparent risks to mother or baby."[32] One large, retrospective observational study of over 16,000 North American planned home births for low risk laboring people found low rates of intervention and high rates of normal births, with no increase in adverse events for the neonate or birthing person.[33] Understanding what makes laboring people vulnerable to disruptions of the hormonal physiology of labor allows caregivers to counteract these factors and create an environment optimal for the necessary hormonal milieu.[34]

Strategies to optimize oxytocin, beta-endorphins and minimize stress hormone production

- touch
- support
- privacy
- small spaces
- low lighting
- quiet
- calm demeanor of caregivers and others present
- unrestricted activity
- warm water immersion

THE PSYCHO-EMOTIONAL STATE OF THE PREGNANT PERSON: WELLBEING OR DISTRESS?

Pain versus suffering

Wellbeing in labor is associated with numerous factors, among which survival of a healthy laboring person and baby are unquestionably the most important. Much of this book is devoted to safe practices to achieve optimal outcomes. Besides safety, labor pain, and the fear of that pain and associated damage are among the next greatest concerns of both laboring people and their caregivers.

The distinction between pain and suffering is crucial to our understanding of laboring person's emotional wellbeing in labor. For our purposes, the pain of labor might be defined as an intensely unpleasant bodily sensation, associated with contractions that one wishes to avoid or relieve. *Suffering*, however, is a distressing psychological state that includes feelings of helplessness, fear, panic, loss of control, and aloneness. Suffering may or may not be associated with pain, and pain may or may not be associated with suffering.[35]

We postulate that it is not pain, but an inability to cope with pain that is at the root of the concern. In fact, in our discussions with pregnant people, it is not the pain of labor itself that worries them as much as how the pain will affect their behavior (losing control, crying out, writhing, struggling, showing weakness, or behaving shamefully) and whether they will find themselves in a state of helplessness, or isolation, not knowing how long the pain will go on and being unable to do anything to reduce it. In other words, they are afraid of suffering. Suffering is similar in definition to trauma and can lead to emotional distress (even post-traumatic stress disorder) that sometimes continues long after the birth.[35]

There are two main approaches to pain management:

Avoidance—using medication to modify or remove the sensation of pain; and acceptance—resolving to use non-pharmacologic methods to keep the pain manageable, with the primary goal being the prevention of suffering, not removal of the sensation of pain.

Following are measures a caregiver may use to assess labor pain versus suffering, and suggestions to enhance the laboring person's feelings of security and trust, with the goal of reducing the likelihood of suffering, fear, and anxiety.

Assessment of pain and coping

The hospital requirement for regular assessments of pain in acute care settings has led to widespread intrapartum use of a numeric rating scale (NRS); the 1–10 visual analog scale describes zero as no pain and 10 indicating the worst possible pain. This approach is based on a pharmacologic philosophy where the minimization or elimination of pain is the primary goal. Using the NRS, pain can be objectively measured before and after administration of analgesia or anesthesia. The use of the NRS has several limitations. Labor pain represents a combination of physiological, social, emotional, and cultural experiences uniquely felt by each person. Laboring people who wish to delay, reduce, or eliminate the need for pharmacologic pain management benefit from a multidimensional assessment of coping.[36] Coping is a complex stress-specific phenomenon where cognition, emotions, perceptions, and behaviors are engaged in by the individual and continually adapt.[37,38] There are two pathways to the Coping Algorithm: Coping (Fig. 3.2) and Not Coping (Fig. 3.3). The Not Coping pathway presents a list of options to consider in assisting the laboring person to return to the coping pathway.

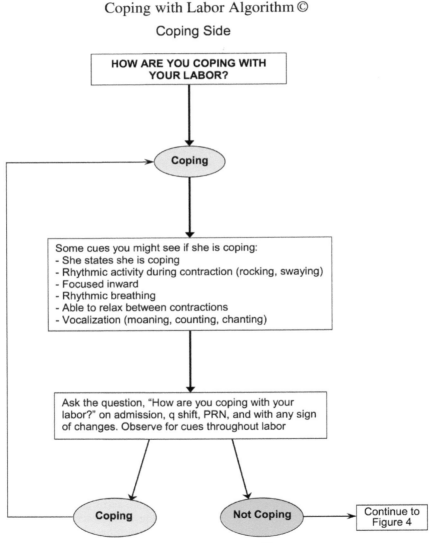

Fig. 3.2.   Coping from Roberts et al., 2010 / with permission of Elsevier.[36]

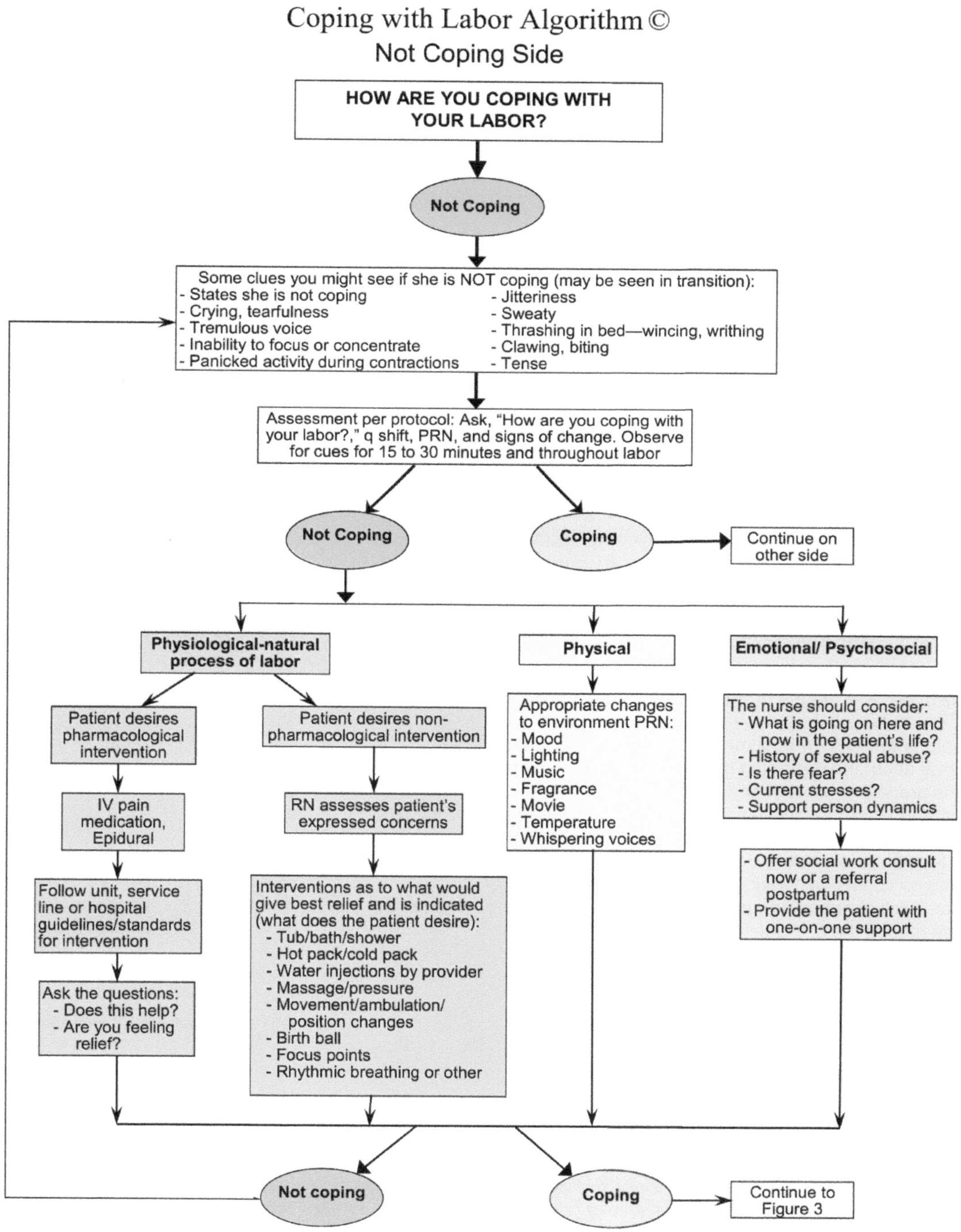

Coping with Labor Algorithm ©
Not Coping Side

HOW ARE YOU COPING WITH YOUR LABOR?

Not Coping

Some clues you might see if she is NOT coping (may be seen in transition):
- States she is not coping
- Crying, tearfulness
- Tremulous voice
- Inability to focus or concentrate
- Panicked activity during contractions
- Jitteriness
- Sweaty
- Thrashing in bed—wincing, writhing
- Clawing, biting
- Tense

Assessment per protocol: Ask, "How are you coping with your labor?," q shift, PRN, and signs of change. Observe for cues for 15 to 30 minutes and throughout labor

Not Coping

Coping → Continue on other side

Physiological-natural process of labor

Patient desires pharmacological intervention

IV pain medication, Epidural

Follow unit, service line or hospital guidelines/standards for intervention

Ask the questions:
- Does this help?
- Are you feeling relief?

Patient desires non-pharmacological intervention

RN assesses patient's expressed concerns

Interventions as to what would give best relief and is indicated (what does the patient desire):
- Tub/bath/shower
- Hot pack/cold pack
- Water injections by provider
- Massage/pressure
- Movement/ambulation/ position changes
- Birth ball
- Focus points
- Rhythmic breathing or other

Physical

Appropriate changes to environment PRN:
- Mood
- Lighting
- Music
- Fragrance
- Movie
- Temperature
- Whispering voices

Emotional/ Psychosocial

The nurse should consider:
- What is going on here and now in the patient's life?
- History of sexual abuse?
- Is there fear?
- Current stresses?
- Support person dynamics

- Offer social work consult now or a referral postpartum
- Provide the patient with one-on-one support

Not coping

Coping → Continue to Figure 3

Fig. 3.3. Not coping from Roberts et al., 2010 / with permission of Elsevier.[36]

Emotional dystocia

Some caregivers use the term "emotional dystocias" to denote an increase in fear, anxiety or other emotions that disrupts labor. This can be caused by environmental factors such as those listed above, but theoretically can also result from pre-existing factors that contribute to the laboring person's emotional state. Emotional dystocia can occur in latent, active, or second stage labor.

Psycho-emotional measures to reduce suffering, fear, and anxiety

Before labor, what the caregiver can do

Before birth, the caregiver should check the laboring person's psychosocial history to detect any emotional or mental health issues that might become problematic during labor.

In childbirth classes, and in prenatal conversations, each expectant parent should be encouraged to think about comforting things they might have available during labor, for example, a doula, favorite music, pictures, loved ones, their own clothing to wear during labor, visualizations, aromatherapy, massage, or relaxation techniques. Such things contribute to the laboring person's comfort in the environment. Of course, most of these are easily available in a home birth or birth center and may be possible with some advanced planning and/ or packing for a hospital birth.

Encourage parents to write a letter or birth plan to the staff, introducing themselves and describing their concerns, fears, preferences, and choices regarding their care.[39] Caregivers can ask to review and discuss the birth plan with the parents during a prenatal appointment. This provides an opportunity to communicate as equals, identify and clear up misunderstandings, and establish trust. If the nurse, midwife and/or physician are strangers to the client, they should check the chart for the client's psychosocial history, birth plan, and clinical notes.

See Box: The birth plan—a means to promote shared decision-making.

The birth plan—a means to promote shared decision-making

Birth plans are written documents[39] prepared by parents to introduce themselves, reveal their major priorities and concerns about the upcoming birth, and describe their preferences among the options for their and their infants' care. Parents are asked to learn and prioritize their options, and discuss them with their care provider, childbirth educator, and others. Then they finalize it and it will be included in their chart, with the intention that all those involved in the person's care will read it and respect it. Benefits of a written birth plan are that all involved in the client's care can consult it instead of expecting the parents to make decisions and explain their preferences during labor when they are focusing on coping with their contractions. Birthing parents can make truly informed decisions while free of the stress of labor. Such collaboration promotes satisfaction. Flexibility in the birth plan allows for modifications should circumstances require them. Studies indicate that preferences (especially for approaches to care, if not all elements of care) are more likely to be honored when there is a birth plan. First choices cannot always be honored, but if parents are informed of why the change in plan is deemed necessary, and they participate in the decision, they are more likely to be satisfied with their care.[40–42]

While the concept of Birth Plans is quite popular, especially in North America, the plans are not always well received by hospital staff. In fact, they are sometimes perceived by caregivers to result in worse outcomes than having no birth plan. In one survey, approximately 55–65% of medical personnel versus 3–10% of patients believed that people have worse outcomes with a birth plan than without (including cesarean deliveries, and an increased rate of chorioamnionitis).[43] These beliefs may influence the relationship between client and caregiver, and the care given. We suggest that a long birth plan written in negative terms is usually a symptom of anxiety and fear that, if not addressed prenatally, is likely to interfere with labor progress.

This situation demonstrates the benefit of midwives and physicians discussing pregnant people's birth plans during prenatal care. An unhurried conversation about a person's fears and concerns, and how specific events would be handled during labor, will often reduce those fears. One useful strategy is to discuss the caregiver's usual practices first. Next, a detailed discussion of risks, benefits, and alternatives for various approaches and interventions can be discussed. This would include rationales or indications for interventions. These discussions can be spread over several prenatal appointments. Using graphical decision aids will assist clients to understand quantitative information and put risks and benefits in context.[44] In addition to alleviating fears, these discussions have the potential to increase mutual trust and respect between the person and their care providers.

Rather than a checklist of options (which requires little thought or knowledge), we recommend that the birth plan be a brief but thoughtful description of the parents' priorities, issues, and concerns; their preferences regarding labor and birth management, care, and feeding of their newborn; and other options that are personally meaningful to them. The plans should include acknowledgement that flexibility is sometimes necessary to accommodate other-than-normal situations.[36] Caregivers and hospitals who support birth plans recognize that there are many safe options in maternity care, and that parents differ in their values and needs. Birth plans can guide the staff in the kind of support and labor management that will ultimately result in parents' satisfaction with their birth experiences and the care they received.[42] These measures create an atmosphere in which the laboring person feels well cared for, with the added advantages of taking little time and costing next to nothing.

During labor: tips for caregivers and doulas, especially if meeting the laboring client for the first time in labor

- Introduce yourself by name, and call the client by name. Greet them and their support people and orient them to the unit (room, lighting, use of bed, bath or shower, call buttons, temperature control, kitchen, nurses' station, lounge). Try to convey a sense of hospitality and friendliness, along with safety and competence.
- Verify the birthing and support person's pronouns (e.g. she, he, they).
- Ask about their plans and preferences. Try to be supportive of their wishes. Do they have a birth plan or preference list? If some of their wishes are unrealistic, discuss these items kindly and respectfully, offering the choices you can provide.[45] Because a detailed or negative birth plan may reflect fear and mistrust of staff, try to be reassuring and use the birth plan discussion as an opportunity to establish rapport.
- Encourage an atmosphere of privacy, comfort, and intimacy:

  ○ knock before entering and keep the door closed;
  ○ do not leave the laboring person's body exposed;
  ○ tell them what comfort devices you have available (ice pack, hot pack, warm blankets, birth ball, peanut ball, beanbag chair, bath, shower, squatting bar, birth stool, music players, beverages, snacks, others);
  ○ encourage cuddling, hugging, "slow dancing" with their partner;
  ○ reassure the laboring person and try to remain with them as much as they wishes and as much as your other responsibilities allow.

- Explain any clinical procedures or tests. Share the results. When the test results, vital signs, and labor progress are normal, be sure to tell them so, to reassure her. (Laboring people sometimes worry that their babies are in danger after staff members discuss a fetal monitor strip in their presence, without explaining it to them.) If problems are developing, do not be falsely reassuring, and do not exaggerate the seriousness.
- Share the signs of labor progress as you identify them.
- Suggest comfort measures that help people cope with labor.
- Ask the person if there are any cultural or religious practices that should be honored or incorporated.
- Reassure the laboring person, not only with words, but also, as culturally appropriate, with praise, smiles, touch, hand-holding, or gestures of kindness and respect.

The measures described in this section allow one to bathe and change positions to prevent problems commonly associated with EFM (i.e., fetal malposition, slower progress, and excessive pain).[46]

CONCLUSION

This chapter differentiates between normal labor progress and labor dystocia. It describes practices that tend to prevent dystocia, with particular emphasis on minimizing maternal emotional distress, promoting physiologic measures that maintain progress, and encouraging movement and position changes by the laboring person.

REFERENCES

1. American College of Nurse-Midwives, Midwives Alliance of North America, & National Association of Certified Professional Midwives (2012) Supporting healthy and normal physiologic childbirth: A consensus statement by the American College of Nurse-Midwives, Midwives Alliance of North America, and the National Association of Certified Professional Midwives. *Journal of Midwifery & Women's Health* 57(5), 529–532. doi: 10.1111/j.1542-2011.2012.00218.x
2. Australian College of Midwives. (2008) *National Midwifery Guidelines for Consultation and Referral*, 2nd edn. Canberra: Australian College of Midwives.
3. Gould D. (2000) Normal labour: A concept analysis. *Journal of Advanced Nursing* 31(2), 418–427. doi: 10.1046/j.1365-2648.2000.01281.x
4. Royal College of Midwives (RCM). (2008) Birth environment. In: *Evidence-Based Guidelines for Midwifery-Led Care in Labour*. London: RCM, p. 2.
5. Society of Obstetricians & Gynecologists of Canada, Association of Women's Health, Obstetric and Neonatal Nursing of Canada, Canadian Association of Midwives, College of Family Physicians of Canada, Society of Rural Physicians of Canada. (2008) Joint policy statement on normal childbirth. *Journal of Obstetrics and Gynaecology Canada* 30, 1163–1165. Retrieved from: http://sogc.org/guidelines/joint-policy-statement-on-normal-childbirth-policy-statement
6. World Health Organization. (1997 Jun) Care in normal birth: a practical guide. Technical Working Group, World Health Organization. *Birth* 24(2), 121–123. PMID: 9271979.
7. Nursing Times News Desk. (2019, Aug 5) 'Normal birth' campaign abandoned by Royal College. *Nursing Times*. (retrieved February 21, 2022) from https://www.nursingtimes.net/news/policies-and-guidance/normal-birth-campaign-abandoned-by-royal-college-14-08-2017
8. UK Maternity Care Working Party including the Royal College of Midwives, Royal College of Obstetricians & Gynecologists, and National Childbirth Trust. (2007) Making normal birth a reality: Consensus statement from the Maternity Care Working Party. Retrieved from: https://www.rcog.org.uk/en/guidelines-research-services/guidelines/making-normal-birth-a-reality (accessed September 2, 2016).
9. Friedman E. (1978) *Labor: Clinical Evaluation and Management*, 2nd edn. New York: Appleton-Century-Crofts.
10. World Health Organization. (2018) *WHO Recommendations on Intrapartum Care for a Positive Childbirth Experience*. World Health Organization.
11. Hodnett ED. (2002) Pain and women's satisfaction with the experience of childbirth: A systematic review. *American Journal of Obstetrics and Gynecology* 186(5 Suppl Nature), S160–S172. doi: 10.1067/mob.2002.121141
12. Myers T. (2014) *Anatomy Trains: Myofascial Meridians for Manual and Movement Therapists*, 3rd edn. Edinburgh: Churchill Livingston Elsevier
13. Tully G, Holt, L. (2016) Personal communication: The spinning babies approach to labor progress. February 29, 2016.
14. Buckley SJ. (2015) Executive summary of hormonal physiology of childbearing: Evidence and implications for women, babies, and maternity care. *The Journal of Perinatal Education* 24(3), 145–153.
15. Olza I, Uvnas-Moberg K, Ekström-Bergström A, Leahy-Warren P, Karlsdottir SI, Nieuwenhuijze M, Villarmea S, Hadjigeorgiou E, Kazmierczak M, Spyridou A, Buckley S. (2020 Jul) Birth as a neuro-psycho-social event: An integrative model of maternal experiences and their relation to neurohormonal events during childbirth. *PLoS One*.
16. Moberg KU. (2014) *Oxytocin: The Biological Guide to Motherhood*. Praeclarus Press, LLC.
17. Moberg KU. (2019) *Why Oxytocin Matters* (Vol. 16). Pinter & Martin Ltd.
18. Johnson MH. (2018) *Essential Reproduction*. John Wiley & Sons.
19. Moberg KU. (2013) *The Hormone of Closeness: The Role of Oxytocin in Relationships*. Pinter & Martin Limited.
20. Lederman RP, Lederman E, Work BA Jr, McCann DS. (1979 Mar-Apr) Relationship of psychological factors in pregnancy to progress in labor. *Nursing Research* 28(2), 94–97. PMID: 254068.

21. Lederman E, Lederman RP, Work BA Jr, McCann DS. (1981 Apr 15) Maternal psychological and physiologic correlates of fetal-newborn health status. *American Journal of Obstetrics and Gynecology.* 139(8), 956–958. doi: 10.1016/0002-9378(81)90967-4. PMID: 7223798.

22. Taylor SE. (2006) Tend and befriend: Biobehavioral bases of affiliation under stress. *Current Directions in Psychological Science* 15(6), 273–277. doi: 10.1111/j.1467-8721.2006.00451.x

23. Odent M. (1999) *The Scientification of Love.* London: Free Association Books.

24. Ayers S. (2017) Birth trauma and post-traumatic stress disorder: The importance of risk and resilience. *Journal of Reproductive and Infant Psychology* 35(5), 427–430.

25. Beck CT, Driscoll JW, Watson S. (2013) *Traumatic Childbirth.* Routledge.

26. Garthus-Niegel S, Knoph C, von Soest T, Nielsen CS, Eberhard-Gran M. (2014) The role of labor pain and overall birth experience in the development of posttraumatic stress symptoms: A longitudinal cohort study. *Birth* 41(1), 108–115.

27. Horsch A, Garthus-Niegel S. (2019) Posttraumatic stress disorder following childbirth. In: *Childbirth, Vulnerability and Law.* Routledge, pp. 49–66. 36. Ayers S. (2007) Thoughts and emotions during traumatic birth: A qualitative study. *Birth (Berkeley, Calif.)* 34(3), 253–263. doi: 10.1111/j.1523-536X.2007.00178.x.

28. Lerner JS, Keltner, D. (2001) Fear, anger, and risk. *Journal of Personality and Social Psychology* 81(1), 146–159. doi: 10.1037//0022-3514.81.1.146

29. Schacter CL, Stalker CA, Teram E, Lasiuk GC, Danilkewich A. (2008) Handbook on sensitive practice for health care practitioners: Lessons from adult survivors of childhood sexual abuse [originally published by the Public Health Agency of Canada]. Retrieved from: http://www.integration.samhsa.gov/clinical-practice/handbook-sensitivve-practices4healthcare.pdf

30. Combellick JL, Shin H, Shin D, Cai Y, Hagan H, Lacher C, … Dominguez-Bello, MG. (2018a) Differences in the fecal microbiota of neonates born at home or in the hospital. *Scientific Reports* 8(1), 1–9.

31. Combellick JL Shin H, Shin D, Cai Y, Hagan H, Lacher C, Lin DL, McCauley K, Lynch SV, Dominguez-Bello MG. (2018b) Differences in the fecal microbiota of neonates born at home or in the hospital. *Scientific Reports* 8(1), 15660. doi: 10.1038/s41598-018-33995-7

32. Hodnett ED, Downe S, Walsh D (2012) Alternative versus conventional institutional settings for birth. *The Cochrane Database of Systematic Reviews* 2012(8), CD000012. doi: 10.1002/14651858.CD000012.pub4

33. Cheyney M, Bovbjerg M, Everson C, Gordon W, Hannibal D, Vedam S. (2014) Outcomes of care for 16,924 planned home births in the United States: The Midwives Alliance of North America Statistics Project, 2004 to 2009. *Journal of Midwifery & Women's Health* 59(1), 17–27.

34. Jenkinson B, Josey N, Kruske S. (2014) BirthSpace: An evidence-based guide to birth environment design.

35. Simkin P. (2011) Pain, suffering, and trauma in labor and prevention of subsequent posttraumatic stress disorder. *The Journal of Perinatal Education* 20(3), 166–176. doi: 10.1891/1058-1243.20.3.166

36. Roberts L, Gullivar B, Fisher J, Cloyes KG. (2010a) The coping with labor algorithm: An alternative pain assessment tool for the laboring women. *Journal of Midwifery and Women's Health* 55(2), 107–116. https://rdcu.be/bE5EM

37. Abushaikha LA. (2007) Methods of coping with labor pain used by Jordanian women. *Journal of Transcultural Nursing: Official Journal of the Transcultural Nursing Society* 18(1), 35–40. doi: 10.1177/1043659606294194

38. Beutler LE, Moos RH. (2003) Coping and coping styles in personality and treatment planning: Introduction to the special series. *Journal of Clinical Psychology* 59(10), 1045–1047. doi: 10.1002/jclp.10196

39. Simkin P, Whalley J, Keppler A, et al. (2016) *Pregnancy, Childbirth and the Newborn*, 5th edn. Deephaven, MN: Meadowbrook Press.

40. Lothian J. (2006) Birth plans: The good, the bad, and the future. *Journal of Obstetric, Gynecologic, and Neonatal Nursing: JOGNN* 35(2), 295–303. doi: 10.1111/j.1552-6909.2006.00042.x

41. Pennell A, Salo-Coombs V, Herring A, Spielman F, Fecho K. (2011) Anesthesia and analgesia–related preferences and outcomes of women who have birth plans. *Journal of Midwifery & Women's Health* 56(4), 376–381.

42. Penny Simkin P. (2007) Birth plans: After 25 years, women still want to be heard. *Birth (Berkeley, Calif.)* 34(1), 49–51. doi: 10.1111/j.1523-536X.2006.00126.x

43. Farahat AH, Mohamed HES, Elkader SA, El-Nemer A. (2015) Effect of implementing a birth plan on womens' childbirth experiences and maternal & neonatal outcomes. *Journal of Education and Practice* 6(6), 24–31.

44. Anderson CM, Monardo R, Soon R, Lum J, Tschann M, Kaneshiro B. (2017) Patient communication, satisfaction, and trust before and after use of a standardized birth plan. *Hawai'i Journal of Medicine & Public Health* 76(11), 305.

45. (2014, Mar) Obstetric care consensus no. 1: Safe prevention of the primary cesarean delivery. *Obstetrics and Gynecology* 123(3), 693–711. doi: 10.1097/01.AOG.0000444441.04111.1d. PMID: 24553167.

46. Zhang J, Landy HJ, Ware Branch D, Burkman R, Haberman S, Gregory KD, Hatjis CG, Ramirez MM, Bailit JL, Gonzalez-Quintero VH, Hibbard JU, Hoffman MK, Kominiarek M, Learman LA, Van Veldhuisen P, Troendle J, Reddy UM, & Consortium on Safe Labor. (2010) Contemporary patterns of spontaneous labor with normal neonatal outcomes. *Obstetrics and Gynecology* 116(6), 1281–1287. doi: 10.1097/AOG.0b013e3181fdef6e

Chapter 4

Assessing Progress in Labor

Wendy Gordon, DM, MPH, CPM, LM, with contributions by Gail Tully, BS, CPM, and Lisa Hanson, PhD, CNM, FACNM, FAAN

Simkin's Labor Progress Handbook: Early Interventions to Prevent and Treat Dystocia, Fifth Edition. Edited by Lisa Hanson, Emily Malloy, and Penny Simkin.
© 2024 John Wiley & Sons Ltd. Published 2024 by John Wiley & Sons Ltd.

Many important assessments help determine when labor is progressing normally and when it is not. These assessments inform and guide clinicians in promoting normal labor progress, recognizing dysfunctional labors, and treating dystocia appropriately when it occurs. While training and practice are required to master these assessment skills, this chapter will provide descriptions, rationales, and practical tips.

Those who do not have professional training in perinatal care and who do not have clinical responsibility for the health of pregnant or laboring individuals do not use these hands-on assessment techniques because they are outside their scope of practice. Doulas and childbirth educators may, however, find this chapter helpful in understanding the reasons for and meanings of these assessments.

This chapter focuses on assessment of labor progress with a full-term singleton fetus in a longitudinal lie (aligned vertically in the gestational parent's torso) and a cephalic presentation (with head lying over the pelvic inlet).

BEFORE LABOR BEGINS

Fetal presentation and position

The presentation of the fetus (cephalic, breech, or shoulder) should be assessed in the last two months of pregnancy. A fetus in a breech presentation may be coaxed into a cephalic presentation using various evidence-based methods, and this is desirable for those wishing to have a vaginal birth. A fetus in a transverse lie must also be moved into a longitudinal lie, as a transverse fetus cannot be born vaginally (https://www.breechwithoutborders.org). In many countries, such as the USA, the majority of persistently breech fetuses are born by cesarean. In other countries, such as Canada and England, the option of a planned vaginal breech birth is offered to some pregnant people based on specific criteria such as a normally growing fetus.[1]

Pregnant parents are often interested in the fetal positions that correspond to the fetal movements that they feel. The skilled practitioner may be able to assess the fetal presentation and position at prenatal visits in late pregnancy (see figures in Table 4.1). These prenatal assessments offer clues to the location and orientation of the fetal back, although this may not necessarily correlate with the position of the fetal head in the gestational parent's pelvis.

The assessments include:

1. Observing the contour of the gestational parent's abdomen.
2. Locating the point of maximum intensity (PMI) of the fetal heart tones via auscultation.
3. Performing abdominal palpation using Leopold's maneuvers.

Although many experienced midwives believe in the utility of these assessments as indicators of fetal position, no well-designed studies have ever assessed the reliability of the abdominal contour or the PMI of the fetal heart tones for this purpose.

Abdominal contour

When the fetus is lying with the back anterior as in Fig. 4.4, the parent's abdominal wall looks convex and the umbilicus may appear "popped out." The pregnant individual reports fetal movement predominantly in the upper quadrant opposite from the fetal back.

When the fetal back is oriented more posteriorly as shown in Fig. 4.5, the parent's abdomen may appear concave, especially depressed in the region of the umbilicus or below, in a peanut shape. The parent may report feeling fetal movement in the midline, or "everywhere." These observations may not be apparent for all pregnant individuals.

Location of the point of maximum intensity (PMI) of the fetal heart tones via auscultation

In most fetuses near term, the loudest sounds of the fetal heart are typically heard through the fetal back, at approximately the level of the fetal shoulder blades. Locating this PMI of the fetal heart tones may help determine the orientation of the fetal back. The best tool for this purpose is a fetoscope (such as the Leff or DeLee-Hillis fetoscope or the Pinard Horn), which allows for direct auscultation of the fetal heart (Fig. 4.6), rather than a

Table 4.1.   Fetal positions—abdominal views. Fetal position is described by the location of the occiput (the back of the fetal head) in relation to the gestational parent's left or right, and to the front (anterior) or back (posterior) of the pelvis.

Fig. 4.1. A fetus in the left occiput anterior (LOA) position has his occiput on his gestational parent's left and in the front of the pelvis.	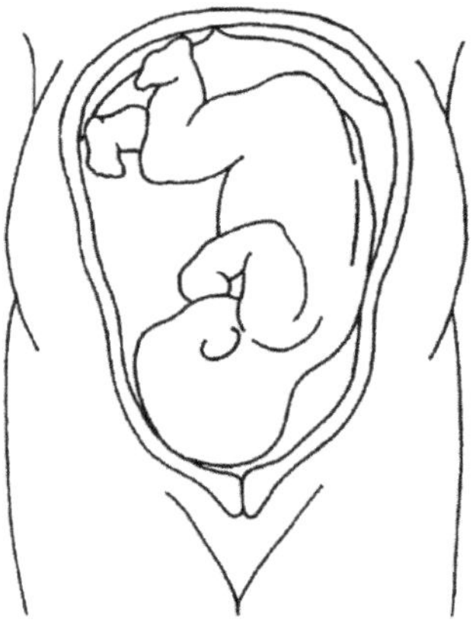
Fig. 4.2. A fetus in the right occiput posterior (ROP) position has his occiput on his gestational parent's right and in the back of the pelvis.	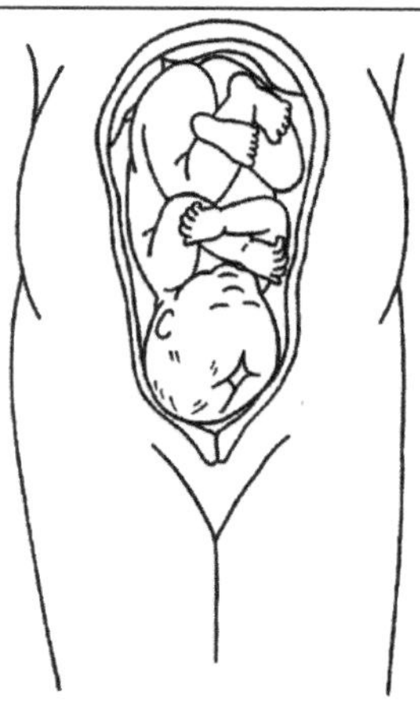
Fig. 4.3. A fetus in the left occiput transverse (LOT) position has his occiput on his gestational parent's left side and is looking straight across at the other side.	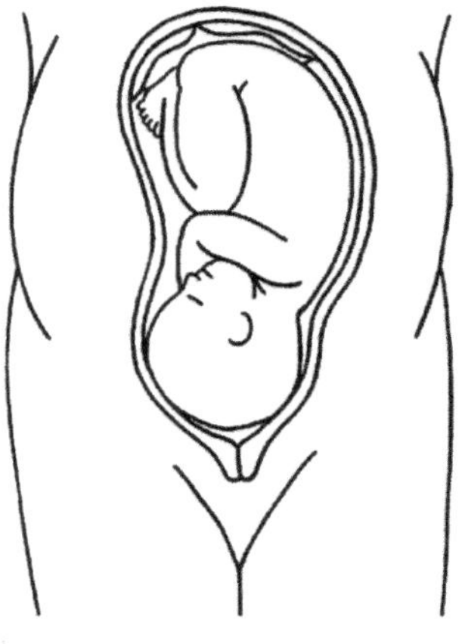

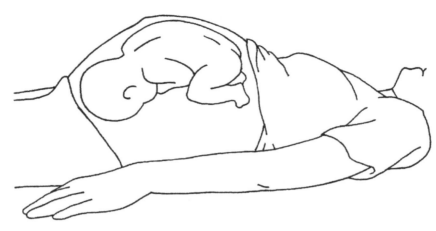

Fig. 4.4. Abdominal contour with fetal back anterior.

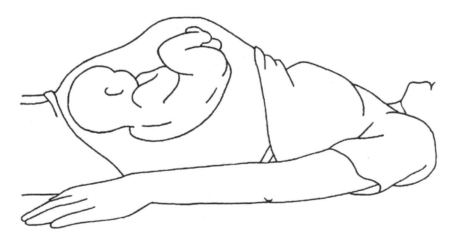

Fig. 4.5. Abdominal contour with fetal back posterior.

Doppler device. (Dopplers use ultrasound to create an artificial sound, the volume of which can be affected by the angle of the probe or the volume dial on the device rather than proximity to the heart valves.)

When a cephalic fetus near term is oriented with its curved back toward the gestational parent's front (spine anterior), the heart tones are crisp and clear and are easily heard on the side of the parent's abdomen where the fetal back lies, several centimeters below the parent's umbilicus and may be to the left or right of midline, shown in Fig. 4.7. When the fetus is oriented with its curved back next to the gestational parent's spine (spine posterior), the PMI may be in the right or left lateral area of the parent's abdomen as shown in Fig. 4.7.[2]

Does knowing the location of the fetal back, however, predict the position of the fetal head? The answer appears to be "not necessarily." Peregrine et al.[3] found that the position of the fetal spine can differ from the position of the fetal head in the pelvis. For example, when the fetal spine is positioned along the gestational parent's right side, the fetus may be looking at the left hip (occiput transverse), forward to the pubic bone (occiput posterior), or back to the sacrum (occiput anterior).

4

(a)

(b)

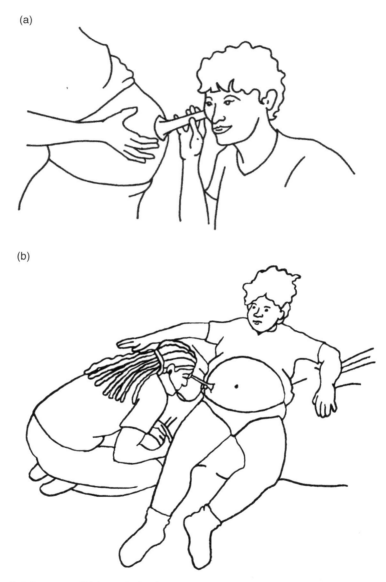

Fig. 4.6. (**a**) Using a Pinard stethoscope. (**b**) Auscultating fetal heart tones with a fetoscope.

This finding also holds during labor. Several researchers have found that fetuses who were positioned with their spines in a transverse or anterior position but their heads in an OP position were more likely to rotate their heads to OA before delivery, while those whose spines and heads were both in a posterior position were more likely to deliver in an OP position.[4,5]

It appears that knowing the location of the fetal back in relation to the position of the occiput may be useful in the management of the fetus with an OP position during labor.

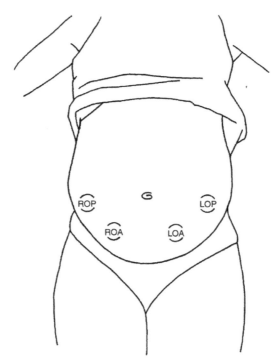

Fig. 4.7.   Location of fetal heart tones with fetus in right occiput posterior (ROP), right occiput anterior (ROA), left occiput anterior (LOA), and left occiput posterior (LOP).

Leopold's maneuvers for identifying fetal presentation and position

Many studies have examined the accuracy of Leopold's maneuvers for determining fetal presentation, with similar results over decades. Clinicians are generally able to identify fetuses in a cephalic presentation with 94–95% accuracy (when compared to ultrasound).[6–10] However, clinician skills vary widely regarding the ability to identify fetuses who are not head-down. In general, clinicians correctly identify only about 30% of breech fetuses using Leopold's maneuvers.[7] Experience of the clinician may improve this accuracy,[6,9] with experienced nurse-midwives demonstrating the highest breech detection accuracy in the research literature at 88%.[8] Factors that may influence accuracy of Leopold's maneuvers include an anterior placenta, abdominal adipose tissue,[6] and a large fetus.[10] Abdominal palpation by experienced clinicians may serve as an adequate screen for identifying malpresentations, but confirmation with ultrasound should be undertaken before taking action or making decisions about mode of birth or setting.

Much less is known about the accuracy of detecting fetal head position with Leopold's maneuvers. In one study,[6] 20 clinicians assessed 131 women with fetuses in a cephalic presentation as determined by ultrasound. Clinicians accurately identified the location of the fetal back in 84% of the cases, but their assessments of the fetal head position were correct in only 60%. In assessing fetal position, neither experience of the examiner nor increasing gestational age improved the accuracy, although higher pre-pregnancy weight decreased it.

Details regarding the maneuvers follow.

Abdominal palpation using Leopold's maneuvers

Leopold's maneuvers are a systematic four-step method for palpating the uterus to determine fetal lie, presentation, position, and engagement in the pelvis. Other information, such as uterine tone and estimated fetal weight, is also obtained by careful abdominal palpation in late pregnancy or during labor.

The technique. The gestational parent should empty their bladder and then recline on a comfortable, firm surface, with the abdomen exposed. They should be helped to relax their abdominal muscles by bending their knees slightly or resting them on a pillow. The clinician should warm their hands, explain the procedure, and ask the parent to provide feedback if anything causes them discomfort. Generally, the clinical provider stands or kneels beside the examination surface—right-handed people on the pregnant individual's right, left-handed people on their left. Leopold's maneuvers should be paused during Braxton Hicks contractions.

The four steps. The order in which the following maneuvers are performed is not important.

1. The first maneuver (Fig. 4.8) helps identify what part of the fetus is in the fundus (the top of the uterus). Facing the pregnant person's head, the clinician places both hands on the person's upper abdomen and, using steady, firm pressure, feels the fundus and the height, shape, size, and consistency of the fetal parts in that area. When the fetal lie is longitudinal and the presentation is cephalic, the breech is palpated in the fundus. It may feel bony and relatively large but is differentiated from the head by feeling continuous with the spine and moving with it. In contrast, when the head is in the fundus (breech presentation), it usually feels ballotable—it "bounces" between the palpating hands because it can be moved independently from the fetal back. When the lie is transverse, neither a head nor a breech can be palpated in the fundus.

2. The second maneuver (Fig. 4.9) helps determine the location of the fetal back. Still facing the pregnant person's head, the clinician places their hands, palm down, on either side of the person's abdomen. By keeping both hands in contact with the abdomen and alternating pressure from one hand to the other, the caregiver can palpate the shape and bulk of fetal parts on either side of the parent's torso and around toward their spine. With this maneuver, the clinician may differentiate the feel of the smooth fetal back from knobby limbs ("small parts") and amniotic fluid from fetal body parts.

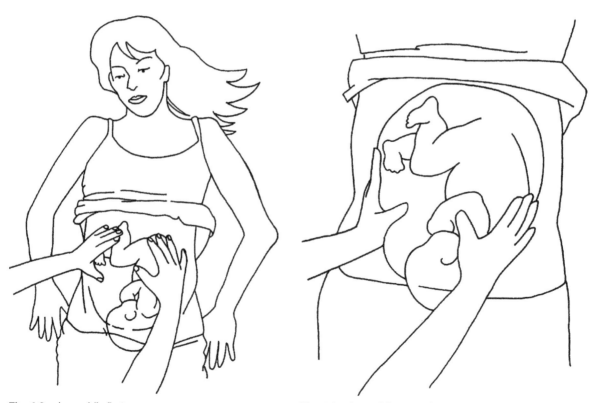

Fig. 4.8. Leopold's first maneuver.   **Fig. 4.9.** Leopold's second maneuver.

When the lie is transverse, the head or breech may be palpated on one or the other side of the parent's torso. The final two Leopold's maneuvers are used to confirm the fetal presentation and lie and to assess the presenting part and its descent into the pelvis.

3. For the third maneuver (Fig. 4.10), the clinician uses the thumb and forefinger of their dominant hand to palpate the lower pole of the uterus, just above the symphysis pubis. The non-dominant hand may be used to grasp the fundus at the same time. If the fetal lie is longitudinal and presenting part is cephalic, the examiner should feel the large bony skull, which is often mobile if not yet deeply engaged in the pelvis. If the presenting part is the breech, although it may feel bony, it is much smaller than the head and does not move independent of the body. When the lie is transverse, the lower pole, like the fundus, feels empty of fetal parts.

4. For the fourth maneuver (Fig. 4.11), the clinician turns to face the pregnant person's feet and places one hand on each side of their abdomen. With the fingers pointing toward the parent's feet, the clinician presses the fingertips gradually and firmly toward the parent's spine and around the presenting part.

A fetal head that is floating above the pelvic brim at term is easily palpated. It feels round, large, and mobile. As the head descends into the bowl of the pelvic inlet, it becomes more difficult to palpate. When the fetal head is deeply engaged prior to labor, it may be nearly impossible to feel with external palpation and sometimes requires internal assessment or ultrasound to confirm a cephalic presentation.

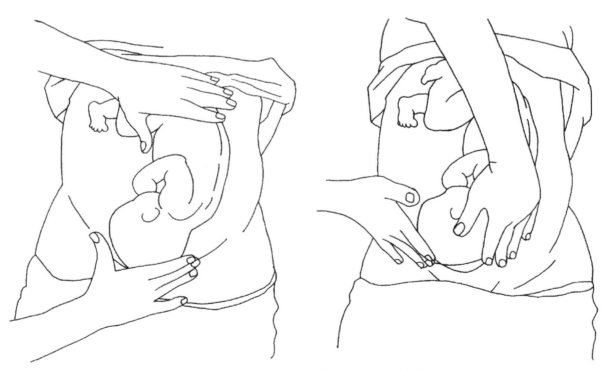

Fig. 4.10. Leopold's third maneuver.   **Fig. 4.11.** Leopold's fourth maneuver.

Estimating engagement: The rule of fifths

To assess engagement of the fetal head by abdominal palpation, the clinician mentally divides the fetal head into five horizontal sections, each about the width of one of their fingers. Here are some examples of how this system is used:

- When the entire fetal head is above the pubic symphysis, as in Fig. 4.12a, it can be palpated with all five fingers and is said to be "five fifths" palpable (5/5)—see Fig. 4.12b. (At this height, the head is mobile.)
- When the head can only be felt with two fingers above the symphysis, it is said to be "two fifths" palpable (2/5), as shown in Fig. 4.12c.
- When the head is entirely below the symphysis, it is said to be "zero fifths" palpable (0/5).

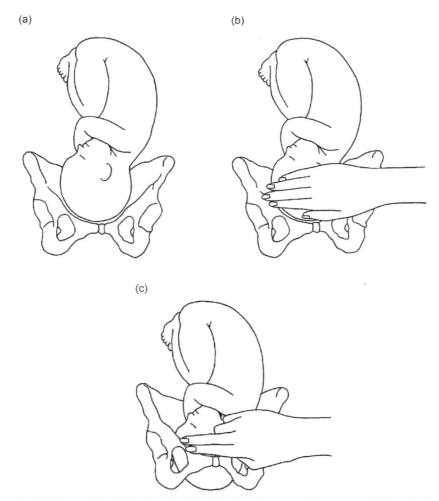

(a)

(b)

(c)

Fig. 4.12. Assessing fetal descent by abdominal palpation. Fetal head above pubic symphysis (**a**), palpating fetal head at 5/5 (**b**), and palpating fetal head at 2/5 (**c**). (Source: Adapted from[11]).

4

Table 4.2 describes the Belly Mapping® Method as another way of determining fetal position.

Table 4.2. Belly Mapping® Method as another way of determining fetal position.

Belly Mapping® Method is a three-step process conceived by Gail Tully to identify fetal position, integrating pregnant person's observations, palpation, and auscultation of the fetal heart. Belly Mapping® Method was originally designed as a way for pregnant people themselves to record the approximate fetal position. Midwives, doctors, and nurses may find it helpful to combine Tully's process [or Tully's method, or Tully's approach] with Leopold's maneuvers to involve pregnant people in their care and enhance communications. We include here a description of this process, condensed from Tully's 2010 book, The Belly Mapping Workbook: How Kicks and Wiggles Reveal Your Baby's Position.[12]

Step 1: Make a pie

Belly Mapping® Method involves mentally dividing the pregnant abdomen into quadrants ("pie pieces") and drawing it on paper as shown in Fig. 4.B1. The pregnant person can often contribute much of the information needed to identify the position of their fetus, including:

- Which side, if either, of their belly is firm
- Where they feel the "big bulge" of the fetal buttocks or head
- Where they feel stronger kicks (fetal feet or knees)
- Where they feel stretching from fetal leg movements
- Where they feel smaller movements (hands, elbows)

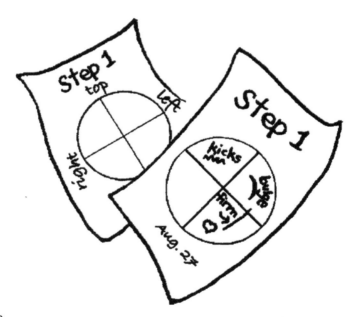

Fig. 4.B1. "Pie" map form.

Figure 4.B2 shows a pregnant person's experiences and how the map they create represents their findings. The midwife, doctor, or nurse uses clinical skills (Leopold's maneuvers, auscultation, and possibly ultrasound) to confirm and/or add to their subjective information on fetal position and marks all this in more detail on their paper map. (The "heart" represents where fetal heart tones are heard using a fetoscope or Pinard Horn. Because Doppler ultrasound fetoscopes can detect fetal heart tones farther from their point of maximum intensity, they are not as useful for this purpose.)

Table 4.2. *(Continued)*

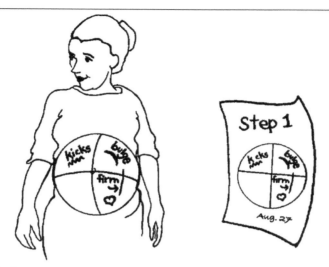

Fig. 4.B2.   Example of a belly map.

Step 2: Visualize the baby

Putting all the information together, the clinician gets a good picture of the baby in the womb. When they are certain of the fetal position, some providers actually draw an outline of the fetus on the pregnant person's abdomen with a non-toxic marker or face paints so that they can visualize how the fetus is positioned in their womb. Another option is to position a fetal doll over the pregnant person's abdomen to show them how the fetus is positioned (Fig. 4.B3).

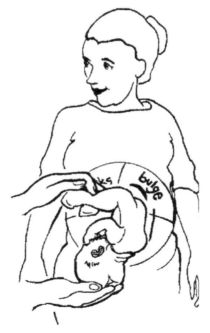

Fig. 4.B3.   Using a doll to explain the position.

(Continued)

Assessing Progress in Labor

4

Table 4.2.   *(Continued)*

Step 3: Name the position

Both the pregnant person and their clinician will gain a clear picture of the fetus's position and will be able to discuss it. Figures 4.B4 and 4.B5 show the correlation between belly maps, see-through views, and fetus-in-the-pelvis views for fetuses in LOA and ROP.

(a)   (b)   (c)

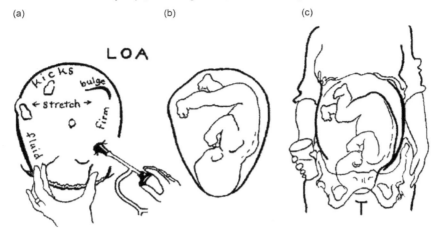

Fig. 4.B4.   Left occiput anterior (LOA) depiction [or drawing] showing pregnant person's experience and clinician's findings (**a**), LOA fetus (**b**), and LOA fetus in the pelvis (**c**).

(a)   (b)   (c)

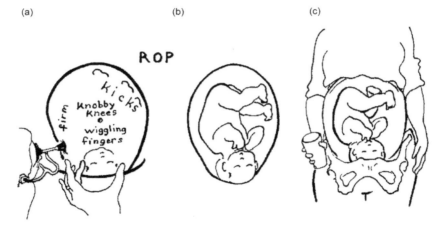

Fig. 4.B5.   Right occiput posterior (ROP) drawing showing pregnant person's experience and clinician's findings (**a**), ROP fetus (**b**), and ROP fetus in the pelvis (**c**).

If the provider identifies an unfavorable position in late pregnancy, the pregnant person may be able to use maternal positioning and body balancing activities to reposition the fetus before labor. These may be more successful if they can be done in the last weeks of pregnancy before the fetal head is engaged. Sutton and Scott[13] devised an approach, "optimal fetal positioning" (OFP), that combines late pregnancy and intrapartum positions to facilitate and maintain favorable fetal positions. This approach should be studied scientifically for its effectiveness. Tully's Spinning Babies® approach[14] goes further to release tension or torsion with specific other positions to create subtle movements, and stretches that have been learned from traditional midwives, physical therapists, chiropractors, and from her own original discoveries while working with laboring people.

Source: Adapted from Tully 2010.[12] Reproduced with permission of Gail Tully.
Belly Mapping Workbook is being rereleased as Belly Mapping® Method in 2022.

Malposition

A primary cause of dysfunctional labor is fetal malposition, and occiput posterior (OP) is the most common. It is estimated that 25–30% of cephalic fetuses are in an OP position prior to labor at term, although about 90% of them will rotate to a more favorable position during labor.[15] However, for some, this can be accompanied by hours of painful, exhausting, and slowly progressing labor.

Persistent OP fetal positioning can produce a prolonged and/or arrested labor, creating a higher risk for interventions such as augmentation, instrumental delivery, and cesarean birth.[16–18] Neonates born in a persistent OP position are more likely to have an Apgar score below 7, blood gases indicative of acidosis, meconium-stained amniotic fluid, and birth trauma.[19] It follows that providers and parents would be interested in avoiding malposition during labor if possible. This begs the question: Can we influence fetal position prior to the onset of labor?

Simkin[20] performed a review of the literature on the OP position and found only two published trials that examined whether the OP position could be changed by prenatal maneuvers. These small and methodologically weak studies showed that although maternal positioning could change the fetus from OP to OA for short periods, there was no evidence that these changes were maintained throughout labor and birth. Additional studies on this topic are needed.

Indeed, many fetuses change position during labor. In a prospective multicenter trial,[15] 89% of OP fetuses rotated to an OA position at some point during labor; only 11% remained persistently OP. The mechanisms of labor and descent require fetuses to be active navigators of their course. These requirements are not present in the prenatal period, which may explain the ambiguity in Simkin's findings.[20]

Other assessments prior to labor

Estimating fetal weight

At term, approximately 3% of US infants are born at a low birth weight (<2500 g) and 7.5% are macrosomic (>4000 g).[21] The ability to accurately estimate fetal weight may help the family and provider to be most prepared for complications that are more common at the ends of the weight spectrum. When the fetus is large, problems associated with malposition may be compounded. Although most people with large babies deliver them without difficulty, macrosomia can complicate labor and birth for both the gestational parent and the fetus.[22] Small fetuses may deliver quickly while others may not tolerate labor well, and newborns of low birth weight are more prone to morbidity and mortality.[23]

Methods of estimating fetal weight at term include the gestational parent's estimate, measurement of fundal height, clinical palpation, ultrasound measurement, and magnetic resonance imaging (MRI), all of which are quite inaccurate when compared with actual birth weight. Fundal height measurement, ultrasound assessments, and abdominal palpation have similarly poor accuracy, detecting only 36–55% of too-small and too-large fetuses.[24]

Ultrasound has the advantage over abdominal palpation for estimating fetal weight in overweight pregnant people but is still over a full pound off from actual birth weight nearly 10% of the time.[25] The multipara's prediction of their baby's birth weight is on par with the accuracy of clinical palpation and ultrasound measurement.[26] MRI has been shown to have a higher sensitivity and specificity for large fetuses,[27] although this technology is quite expensive and impractical in many settings. Estimates of fetal weight should be used with extreme caution, as a prediction of fetal macrosomia has been shown to be an independent factor in the diagnosis of labor dysfunction, leading to cesarean delivery.[28]

To summarize, the value of estimating fetal weight is questionable because all current methods of predicting birth weight are unreliable, the impact of macrosomia is variable, and it is not possible to reverse excessive fetal weight at or near term. Nonetheless, when labor progress is poor, caregivers may use an estimation of fetal weight as just that: an estimation and one of many variables factored into the complex problem-solving needed to help resolve dysfunctional labors.

Assessing Progress in Labor

4

Assessing the cervix prior to labor

During pregnancy, the cervix is composed of dense collagen fibers providing a firm tubular structure that helps keep the uterine contents safely contained. In labor, the role of the cervix is reversed. It must become elastic enough for the muscular activity of the uterus to open it. To accomplish this, hormonal changes cause alterations in the composition of the cervical tissue. Collagen fibers break down; elastin fibers in the internal os provide stretch; and the water content of the connective tissue increases, making the cervix soft and stretchy. These changes, called cervical ripening, begin weeks before labor's onset and are caused by hormonal influences distinct from the mechanisms of effacement and dilation.[29] Some labor problems, both preterm labors and prolonged labors at term, may be the result of cervical dysfunction, rather than uterine dysfunction, when the cervix undergoes these changes too soon or does not complete them.[30]

The Bishop scoring system. In 1964, Bishop[31] published a 13-point scoring system for predicting the onset of spontaneous labor in multiparas based on five factors: cervical dilation, effacement, consistency, position in the vagina, and station of the head (Table 4.3). Bishop proposed that elective induction could be safe and successful with a score of 9 or higher on this scale, although provided no data to support this. Other models and modifications have been proposed,[32] including simplifying the assessment by reducing the number of assessments from five to three (omitting cervical consistency and position, which were found not to improve the predictability of a successful vaginal birth).[33] A different method of measuring cervical effacement was proposed by Malapati et al.[34] Rather than Bishop's original technique of estimating the percentage of thinning that has taken place, they propose measuring the length of the remaining cervix in centimeters (either digitally or by transvaginal ultrasound). The original Bishop score, however, remains the most widely used pre-induction assessment tool,[35] despite systematic reviews and a meta-analysis that demonstrated that cervical favorability does not predict success of labor induction.[35–37] The Bishop score is also commonly used today to assess the need for pre-induction cervical ripening agents.

Some clinicians use Bishop's five variables to evaluate cervical ripeness in individuals who are not necessarily candidates for induction, sometimes with weekly routine cervical examinations in the last month of pregnancy. How useful are these examinations? Assessing the prelabor cervix at term may help identify those more likely to experience short or prolonged latent phases[38] but should not be used to predict when labor will begin.

Many clinicians agree that, especially in nulliparas, people who begin labor with a cervix that is long, firm, closed, and posterior are more likely to experience prolonged latent phases, while those whose cervix is thin, stretchy, and partially dilated are likely to progress more rapidly to the active phase. However, the value of cervical assessments done before labor in predicting the onset of labor or active phase disorders is not substantiated in any research literature.[39]

It may be tempting to tell a person whose cervix is soft, thin, anterior, and 2 centimeters dilated that they will surely be in labor soon, or to tell a person with a closed, uneffaced cervix that they will have a long wait. However, the condition of the cervix late in pregnancy does not predict when labor will begin or how it will progress, and these statements are inaccurate often enough to cause laboring people unnecessary distress. The decision to

Table 4.3. The original Bishop Score,[32] adapted to include cervical length as a measure of effacement.[35]

SCORE	0	1	2	3
Dilation of cervix	Closed	1–2 cm	3–4 cm	5 cm
Effacement (%) OR	0–30%	40–50%	60–70%	80% +
Cervical length (cm)	*(>4 cm)*	*(3–4 cm)*	*(1–2 cm)*	*(0 cm)*
Station of head	−3	−2	−1, 0	+1, +2
Consistency of cervix	Firm	Medium	Soft	–
Position of cervix	Posterior	Midline	Anterior	–

Source:[31,32] Reproduced with permission of the American College of Obstetricians and Gynecologists.

examine the cervix before the onset of labor should be based on a balanced assessment of the value of the information provided and client preference.

Assessing prelabor

While labor for some people can begin with a short latent phase, or prelabor, latent labor for others can be difficult to distinguish from active labor, especially for nulliparas. Contractions may be occurring in a regular or irregular pattern, and for those who have not experienced labor contractions before, "intensity" is a relative term that can sometimes only be assessed in hindsight. With prelabor contractions, the laboring person can usually talk without difficulty while having a contraction. However, the contractions may be of such a frequency and intensity that the individual is not able to sleep well.

Although prelabor contractions can signal the beginning of the process of labor, it is impossible to predict how long the latent phase will last for an individual. Furthermore, definitions vary regarding when exactly the onset of the active phase of labor occurs. However, for many people, this can be the longest phase of labor. Current estimates suggest that this phase lasts an average of 6 hours for first-time birthgivers, although 16–20 hours is not abnormal.[40]

People experiencing prelabor contractions may experience excitement, confusion or fear. As the latent phase continues, this can turn to frustration. It is important to provide information to help them assess their own sensations and contraction patterns as they move slowly toward the active phase of labor. Because the duration of prelabor is unpredictable, the greatest threat is exhaustion of the laboring person if they are not supported to rest as much as possible.

Six ways to progress

Simkin[41] described six ways to progress, similar to the Bishop score, based on changes in the cervix (position moves from posterior to anterior, ripens/softens, effaces, and dilates) and the fetal head (descent, flexion, and rotation). The timing and order of these changes varies greatly from person to person, and many of them must occur before active labor can begin. Simkin's "Six Ways to Progress" can help to reassure the birthing person that although dilation may not be occurring yet, they are making progress in other necessary ways toward labor.

ASSESSMENTS DURING LABOR

It is important to assess labor progress holistically, taking into account the many complex factors and their interactions that influence labor progress. For most labors, a systematic assessment may be performed, starting with visual and verbal assessments, then moving to hands-on external evaluations and finally, internal assessments as needed. A rapidly progressing labor or one in which the laboring person is not coping well may necessitate spending more or less time in each stage of assessment.

Visual and verbal assessments

Trained clinicians assess many factors that pertain to a laboring person's condition. Progress may be positively or negatively affected by the degree to which the birthgiver's physical and emotional wellbeing are supported. The perceptive care provider is able to enter the birth room unobtrusively and gather information visually and with a few well-placed questions between contractions.

Hydration and nourishment

Laboring individuals require approximately 50 to 100 kcal/hour to maintain adequate muscle function.[42] Scientific literature supports the free use of oral intake—both fluids and solids—during labor.[43] In some hospital settings healthy laboring people receive clear liquids but commonly do not receive solid foods, while in other settings both are standard. Given access, some laboring individuals will naturally take in the necessary calories and nutrients to sustain them during labor, but some may need to be reminded. Prolonged labor may be both a cause and an effect of dehydration and insufficient caloric intake.[44] Therefore, the care provider should focus on prevention. Having non-acidic, easy-to-digest carbohydrate snacks and drinks available (broth, electrolyte-balanced sports drinks, fruit, honey, toast, etc.), offering beverages to the laboring parent, and encouraging them to drink according to their thirst represent an effective strategy to prevent both hyponatremia (loss of sodium), which may cause prolonged labor due to overhydration from forced oral fluids, and exhaustion caused by dehydration and poor caloric intake. Assessment of adequate hydration and nourishment includes:

Urine: The laboring person should void at least every 2 hours and produce light yellow urine. Dark, concentrated, or scant urine suggests inadequate fluid intake.

Ketonuria: Ketosis, the accumulation of ketones as a result of metabolizing stored fat in the absence of adequate carbohydrate availability, occurs normally in response to both exertion and fasting. Controversy exists about whether the presence of ketone bodies in urine during labor is a sign of compromise in the laboring person.[45]

Emesis: Vomiting is common in labor. However, when it is prolonged or persistent, dehydration may result. Replacing fluids lost in this way requires additional intake, either oral or intravenous.

Fluid loss through perspiration: People who are laboring in warm conditions, especially those in warm water baths, need additional fluids. They should be reminded to drink to satisfy their thirst. Offering, but not pushing, liquids after each contraction or two is preferable to asking if they want a drink.

Emotional distress: Laboring individuals who become seriously compromised due to inadequate intake may feel anxious, exhausted, and sick. Severe dehydration can exacerbate nausea and vomiting. Intravenous rehydration may be necessary.

Psychology

Much has been written about the positive effects of confidence and wellbeing and the adverse effects of psychological distress on the progress of labor.[46] The laboring person's psychology works synergistically with the physical and hormonal parameters of labor.[29] Poor labor progress can be caused by psychological distress, and psychological distress can be a result of a long and difficult labor. When there are no apparent physical reasons for poor labor progress, a psychological source should be considered.

The clinician and support people's ability to communicate with the laboring person is essential. Establishing a trusting and supportive relationship provides the foundation for positive communication. This is easier when there has been a prenatal relationship, but many skilled intrapartum providers are able to establish good rapport quickly with people they have never previously met.

The importance of minimizing psychological stress for laboring people, including information about creating a supportive labor environment, assessing a person's emotional state, and building trust through good communication, is addressed in elsewhere in this book.

Quality of contractions

Normal labor is characterized by uterine contractions that increase in frequency, duration, and intensity over time. A contraction can be visualized as a bell-shaped curve consisting of three phases: the increment, as the intensity builds; the acme, or peak; and the decrement, or relaxation as the intensity diminishes.

Normal coordination of the uterine muscles during labor causes the uterus to differentiate into a thick, muscular upper segment and a thinning, stretchy lower segment. Retraction, the continual shortening of the vertical muscle fibers, enables the uterus to decrease intrauterine space, thus opening the cervix and pushing the fetus down and out. When labor is dysfunctional, it is important to evaluate uterine contractions. Ineffective contractions can be a primary cause of dysfunctional labor, or it may be an effect of some other problem, such as infection,[47] dehydration,[48] or a malpositioned fetus.[16] When the fetus does not fit well through the pelvis, uterine contractions often diminish in response to this relative obstruction.[49]

The following features of contractions may be assessed through observation of the laboring person:

Frequency is measured from the start of one contraction to the start of the next. Some providers note this as the interval in minutes from onset to onset, that is, "every 5 minutes." Others record the number of contractions in a 10-minute period. Contractions of active labor are characterized by a frequency of two to five contractions in 10 minutes. Concerns arise when contractions are more frequent than five contractions in 10 minutes (tachysystole). Because placental blood flow is markedly diminished during the most intense contractions of labor, a minimum rest of 30 seconds between contractions is essential for adequate fetal oxygenation. When there are more than five contractions in 10 minutes (uterine tachysystole), the fetus may not have adequate time between them to recover. This is rarely a problem in spontaneous labor but must be considered when labor is induced or augmented, particularly with high doses of misoprostol, and, in fact, is a potential risk with any uterine stimulant.[50]

Duration is assessed as the time from the start of a contraction to its end. This varies considerably depending on the stage or phase of labor. Early labor is characterized by contractions that may last only 20 to 30 seconds, and active labor by contractions lasting 60 to 90 seconds.

Resting time is calculated by subtracting the duration from the frequency. For example, if the contractions occur every 3 minutes and last 80 seconds, there is a 100-second rest from the end of one contraction until another contraction begins. Frequency, duration, and resting time can be assessed subjectively by observing the laboring individual's affect or by palpating the abdomen, or measured objectively by electronic monitoring using either a tocodynamometer (external pressure sensitive device) or an intrauterine pressure catheter.

Intensity is defined as the rise in intrauterine pressure above the resting tone with each contraction. Because pain perception is highly variable from person to person, this alone is a poor indicator of contraction quality. However, the birthgiver is able to report whether contractions are becoming more intense over time, a feature of normally progressing active phase labor. Dysfunctional labor may be characterized by contractions becoming less frequent, shorter in duration, or feeling less intense.

Many expectant parents now use downloadable apps on their smartphones or computers to keep track of frequency and duration of contractions. They only need to touch the screen at the beginning and end of contractions; the app does the calculations. Intensity cannot be tracked in a similar way, but parents can record relevant notes on the perceived intensity of the contractions, as well as presence of bloody show, loss of amniotic fluid, and much more. An Internet search reveals the many available apps.

Additional information regarding the quality of contractions may be gathered through a careful palpation of the abdomen during and between contractions. Using a watch with a second hand and firm pressure of the fingers on the fundus, the examiner assesses intensity, frequency, duration, and resting time.

The onset of the contraction may be palpated before the laboring person feels it. At the peak of an adequate contraction, the fundus is not able to be indented with the fingers and feels firm. One guide to aid the inexperienced practitioner in assessing uterine contraction intensity is the "nose, chin, forehead" analogy. If, at the peak of a contraction, the uterus feels like one's nose when pressed, the intensity is mild; like one's chin, it is moderate; like one's forehead, it is strong. With practice, the care provider can learn to detect differences in contraction quality.

The examiner may detect the relaxation phase and the end of the contraction before the laboring person's pain sensation abates. This is because they still perceive the stimulation of nerve fibers in the cervix and lower uterine segment. Resting tone is an important assessment that can also be assessed via palpation. Between contractions, the fundus should feel soft and relaxed. It may be more difficult to assess resting tone in people with substantial adipose tissue over the uterine wall. Although resting tone and intensity can be assessed with external palpation, precise measurements are only possible using an intrauterine pressure catheter (IUPC).

Vital signs

After the care provider has gathered information from visual assessments and sensitive questioning of the laboring person, additional determination of the birthgiver's wellbeing can be assessed by monitoring vital signs.

Vital signs should be assessed at regular intervals throughout labor; evaluations should be done between contractions. The presence of elevated blood pressure, pulse, or abnormal respiration rate must be noted and addressed. A slight rise in temperature is normal during labor, but if elevated more than 0.5 °C or 1°F and labor has been prolonged, it may signal dehydration. Also, a slight temperature rise is associated with an increase in occiput posterior positions in the second stage of labor.[51] Hyperthermia is a rather common side effect of epidural analgesia. A significant increase in temperature (above 38 °C or 100.4°F), especially in the presence of ruptured membranes, may signal infection, a serious intrapartum complication. When the laboring person's vital signs are normal and their fetus has normal fetal heart rate, there is more leeway for patience.

Purple line

Several small research reports in the midwifery literature regarding the "purple line" have described the appearance of a reddish/purple discoloration in the gluteal cleft of the laboring person that begins near the anus and extends upward between the buttocks as dilation and descent progress. Byrne & Edwards (1990)[52] were the first to report this in an article in *The Lancet*, even going so far as to correlate the length of the line with cervical dilation. Research that has been done since then has found rather low accuracy when trying to predict the centimeters of cervical dilation based on length of the purple line.[53] However, several researchers have found a fairly strong correlation between *progress* in first or second stage and a growing length of the purple line.[53–58] Not all laboring individuals produce a purple line in labor; studies range from 56%[54] to 86%[53] in both nullips and multips. Of those who do produce a purple line, it is not always present at the start of labor; it may appear at some point later.[53] Studies have shown independent correlations of the length of the purple line with progress in first stage (increasing dilation)[53–55, 58] and progress in second stage (descent of the fetal head).[53,57,58]

Assessing the fetus

Most of the time, the term fetus of the otherwise healthy parent tolerates prolonged or dysfunctional labor well. When the information about fetal wellbeing is reassuring, caregivers and parents can focus on the challenges of coping with and resolving the dysfunction. Conversely, when signs of fetal compromise are present, attention to resolving the distress becomes paramount. Most parents are keenly aware of the potential for fetal compromise during labor and appreciate accurate information from caregivers when concern about the baby arises.

Elements of fetal assessment discussed here are fetal movements, the gestational age, the presence or absence of meconium in the amniotic fluid, and the fetal heart rate.

Fetal movements

Detection of normal fetal movement as felt by the examiner and/or by the laboring person is assumed by many midwives to be a reassuring sign of fetal oxygenation.[59] Lack of fetal movement in labor is not necessarily an ominous finding, as fetal sleep cycles continue during labor. Sudden frantic fetal movements followed by a cessation of movement should be noted in the chart and immediately assessed as it may be a sign of severe fetal hypoxia.[60] Some fetuses can also be visualized abdominally as they change positions during labor.

Gestational age

Both preterm (<37 completed weeks) and post-term (>42 completed weeks) fetuses are more vulnerable to the stress of labor than term fetuses. Preterm fetuses may experience additional risks related to the cause of preterm labor (i.e., infection or placental abruption). With post-term fetuses, there are increased risks of oligohydramnios, meconium staining, meconium aspiration syndrome, and cord compression.[61] There is an increased likelihood of macrosomia, with its attendant labor risks such as cephalopelvic disproportion, malposition, shoulder dystocia, and interventions such as instrumental and surgical delivery.[61] Finally, there is increased risk for placental insufficiency in post-term pregnancies, resulting in growth restriction and higher rates of stillbirth.[61]

Meconium

The fetus may pass meconium in utero when there is a brief episode of hypoxia that causes relaxation of the anal sphincter. Most often it is a normal maturational event, occurring more frequently as gestational age reaches or exceeds 40 weeks. Meconium should be considered a sign of fetal compromise if it is associated with a non-reassuring fetal heart rate pattern, fever in the laboring parent or other signs of infection, or if it is thick, or particulate (containing discrete pieces or chunks).

Fetal heart rate (FHR)

The primary sources of information about fetal wellbeing during labor are the FHR, indicating the fetus's response to contractions. For this reason, clinicians receive training and continuing education on interpreting FHR patterns according to the current guidelines of their countries' professional bodies or of the International Federation of Gynecology and Obstetrics (FIGO) and the World Health Organization (WHO). Current US guidelines adhere to the 2008 guidelines of the National Institute of Child Health and Human Development (NICHD).[62] This overview is based largely on guidelines provided by American obstetric, nursing, and midwifery organizations.[63–65] While there are similarities among the guidelines provided in Canada,[66] the United Kingdom,[67] and the International Federation of Gynecology & Obstetrics (FIGO),[68] readers should consult the specific guidelines that apply to their own country.

Intermittent auscultation

Intermittent auscultation requires frequent one-to-one assessments. Intermittent auscultation (IA) is the method of fetal assessment used in home and free-standing birth center settings. In many hospital birth settings, intermittent auscultation is underutilized, despite the evidence proving it to be a reliable method of monitoring fetal wellbeing for low-risk labors.[69,70] The findings of numerous clinical trials have led the professional organizations of obstetricians in the United States (American College of Obstetricians and Gynecologists),[71] Canada (Society of Obstetricians and Gynecologists [SOGC]),[72] and the United Kingdom (Royal College of Obstetricians and Gynecologists [RCOG] and the National Institute for Care Excellence),[67] to support or promote intermittent auscultation as either equal to or preferred over EFM, for low-risk laboring people with healthy pregnancies. The organizations describe similar specific protocols for intermittent auscultation and offer strict guidelines on circumstances that require continuous EFM. The SOGC stated that intermittent auscultation is preferable for normal labor.

The following recommendations are derived from published IA guidelines of the American College of Nurse-Midwives,[65] American College of Obstetricians and Gynecologists,[63] the Association of Women's Health, Obstetric and Neonatal Nurses,[64] and the Society of Obstetricians and Gynecologists of Canada.[66] These organizations publish updated guidelines periodically.

Appropriate candidates for intermittent auscultation[73]:

* Healthy full-term pregnancy with the absence of medical or obstetric risk factors.
* Absence of medical interventions such as oxytocin and/or epidural anesthesia.
* Presence of care provider(s) skilled in the use of IA.

General principles of intermittent auscultation

Frequency of auscultation: There is limited evidence regarding the frequency of IA during the latent phase of labor. However, it is prudent to monitor the fetus at the time of assessments, approximately every hour during latent labor.[65] During active first stage labor, IA should be accomplished every 15 to 30 minutes.[62–65] During second stage, auscultation should occur every 15 minutes prior to expulsive pushing[62–64] and every 5 minutes with active bearing down.[64,65] If an abnormality is detected, more frequent auscultation should be performed.

Timing of auscultation: Contractions should be palpated, and auscultation to establish a FHR baseline should be done between contractions when the fetus is not moving.[63,64] The baseline rate should be reassessed in this way periodically throughout labor. To detect increases or decreases in the FHR with contractions, there is no clear consensus in the guidelines regarding the best time to auscultate in relation to the contraction. Some recommend listening after a contraction,[62,65] from the peak of the contraction until a short time afterward,[64] or before, during, and after the contraction.[63]

Method of counting: Counting the FHR for a full 60–120 seconds provides the most accurate baseline rate.[65] Assessments made during or after contractions may use 30- or 60-second counts, although a 60-second count has been shown to be more reliable.[65] When an audible increase or decrease in the rate occurs, the FHR may be counted in 5- or 15-second increments to more accurately describe to peak or nadir of the FHR.[63,64] The laboring person's pulse should be evaluated periodically to ensure that the rate being counted is fetal and not maternal. This distinction should be documented in the laboring person's medical record.

The technique for IA, widely used by midwives, especially in home and birth center settings[65] is described here in detail.

How to perform intermittent auscultation: A handheld Doppler devise, fetal stethoscope or Pinard Stethoscope (Figure 4.13) may be used. Ultrasound detects motion of the heart valves and converts this into a manufactured sound that replicates the fetal heartbeat. The fetal stethoscope is specially designed to use the bone conduction of the examiner's skull to transmit the subtle sounds of fetal cardiac activity through the earpieces. It generally requires more practice than the Doppler to use correctly.

Intermittent auscultation technique:[64]

- Use Leopold's maneuvers to locate the fetal back, the point of maximal ability to auscultate the FHR.
- Palpate for contractions.
- Palpate the laboring person's pulse.
- Place the fetal stethoscope or Doppler over the fetal back at the point of maximal intensity (PMI).
- Determine the FHR baseline by listening for 60 seconds between contractions.
- Record findings including any accelerations or decelerations.

Reassuring signs of fetal wellbeing that can be assessed without continuous electronic fetal monitoring (CEFM):

- Normal baseline FHR
- Absence of decelerations
- Absence of FHR arrhythmia
- Accelerations of the FHR with or without fetal scalp or vibroacoustic stimulation[73]
- Fetal movement reported by the birth giver or palpated by the examiner
- Clear amniotic fluid

The Doppler offers these advantages over the fetal stethoscope:

- allows easier auscultation in a variety of positions
- allows easier auscultation during contractions
- enables parents and others to hear the FHR
- does not require pressure on the laboring parent's abdomen, so it is more comfortable
- can be adapted for use in water (requires special waterproof probe)

The fetal stethoscope (fetoscope) offers these advantages over the Doppler:

- detects true sounds of the fetal heart, including dysrhythmias, avoiding risks of artifact or detecting laboring parent's pulse in error
- requires no battery or mechanical parts that can malfunction
- can also be used to help verify fetal position, as discussed earlier in this chapter

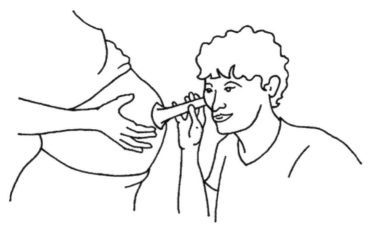

Fig. 4.13.   Using the Pinard stethoscope to assess fetal heart tones.

Continuous Electronic Fetal Monitoring (CEFM)

While recommendations and policies on the selection criteria for the use of CEFM vary among countries,[61,65–67] CEFM is widely used for people with risk factors or fetuses with non-reassuring fetal heart rate patterns. When using CEFM, it is critical to establish and maintain vigilance that it is the fetal heart rate, not the laboring person's, that is being recorded on the tracing.[74] In 2008, the National Institute of Child Health and Human Development (NICHD) published revised guidelines that provide "specific recommendation for FHR pattern classification and intrapartum management actions."[62] These guidelines include the "three-tiered fetal heart rate interpretation system"[62] that allows more standardized interpretation of fetal status during labor as well as recommendations for interventions. The following are the NICHD definitions of these components of FHR interpretation. While the NICHD guidelines are specific to CEFM, most also apply to IA (except for those relating to variability and types of decelerations, which require visual graphic renditions for interpretation).

Baseline FHR definitions:

- Normal FHR baseline rate is 110 to 160 beats per minute (bpm).
- Tachycardia is a baseline rate that exceeds 160 bpm.
- Bradycardia is a baseline rate that is less than 110 bpm.

Variability defined:

- Defined as "fluctuations in the baseline FHR that are irregular in amplitude and frequency."[62] This can only be assessed with CEFM, not through the use of IA.[66]
- Classifications of variability:[62]
  ○ Absent: no variability detectable
  ○ Minimal: less than 5 bpm
  ○ Moderate: 6 to 25 bpm
  ○ Marked: greater than 25 bpm.

Accelerations defined:

- According to the NICHD guidelines, an acceleration is a visually apparent, abrupt increase in FHR of 15 or more beats for 15 seconds or longer.[62] In the preterm fetus (<37 weeks gestation), accelerations are defined as 10 or more beats for 10 seconds or longer.[62]
- Accelerations are considered a sign of fetal wellbeing.

- To determine the presence of accelerations, the FHR can be counted for segments of 5- to 15-second duration. The rates between the segments can be compared for the presence of an increase that would indicate an acceleration.[64] Accelerations can and should be listened for and documented during IA.

Decelerations defined:

- Decelerations are periodic changes in the FHR that fall below the baseline and are defined by their time of onset, timing, and shape on the CEFM tracing. The types of deceleration are not well distinguished by the use of IA.
- *Early decelerations* are considered a normal finding during labor. They are symmetrical, gradual declines in FHR with the lowest point of the deceleration occurring less than 30 seconds from onset of the contraction.[62] The onset and recovery to baseline are both early compared to the start and end of the contraction. Early decelerations mirror the shape of the contraction. Early decelerations are associated with compression of the fetal head that leads to vagal nerve stimulation. Therefore, early decelerations are most common in late active and second stage labor.
- *Variable decelerations* are V-shaped, irregularly timed, abrupt decelerations with the lowest point of the deceleration occurring less than 30 seconds from the onset to nadir. The decrease is greater than 15 beats per minute, lasting more than 15 seconds and less than two minutes. Variable decelerations indicate mechanical compression of the umbilical cord that may lead to fetal compromise. Changing the laboring person's position often reduces pressure on the umbilical cord and is the first step in appropriate care. The significance of variable decelerations depends on the entire context of the CEFM tracing according to the three-tiered categorization system.[62]
- *Late decelerations* are gradual uniform declines in the FHR with the lowest point of the deceleration occurring more than 30 seconds from the onset of the contraction.[62] A defining characteristic is their timing, because they begin late in the contraction and return to baseline following the end of the contraction. They are considered an indication of potential uteroplacental insufficiency (diminished blood and oxygen flow to the baby). The significance of late decelerations depends on the entire context of the CEFM tracing according to the three-tiered categorization system.[62]

The three-tiered fetal heart rate interpretation system. The three-tiered FHR interpretation system is described in Table 4.4. This system was developed to improve CEFM interpretations, communication of findings and increase interventions to improve fetal status. It is incumbent on care providers to have skill in using this system for assessment and documentation of fetal status. This system can be applied to intermittent auscultation.

King (2019) presented a schema of how to interpret intermittent auscultation (IA) findings in relation to the three-tiered system (Table 4.5). It is notable that only Categories I and II are interpretable with IA. Category III fetal heart tones (Fig 4.13) are not included in this table because the absence of variability cannot be detected using IA.

Admission fetal heart rate tracing. A brief, often 20 min fetal heart rate tracing has been adopted in numerous hospital settings as a screening test for fetal wellbeing. Devane, et al.[69] systematically reviewed the four clinical trials that included 13,000 low risk laboring study participants. The authors found no evidence to support that the admission FHR tracing improved outcomes. Rather, the admission FHR tracing was associated with increased use of CEFM and a 20% increase in the cesarean rate.

Intermittent electronic fetal monitoring. Some caregivers do not trust their skills in auscultation with the handheld Doppler but do feel comfortable with Intermittent Electronic Fetal Monitoring (IEFM). The clinician or nurse can merely hold the EFM ultrasound transducer on the laboring person's abdomen for a minute or more at the recommended intervals. The heart rate tracing will appear on the monitor and/or computer screen and may be printed if necessary. IEFM may be easier to interpret for those who prefer a visual printout, along with the auditory transmission. This may also allow for the use of the three-tiered interpretation system.

Table 4.4. Three-tiered fetal heart rate (FHR) interpretation system.

Features	Implications
Category I	
Baseline: 110–160 bpm Baseline FHR variability (BLV): moderate Accelerations: present or absent Decelerations: • Early decelerations: present or absent • Late or variable decelerations: absent	• Normal • Strongly predictive of normal fetal acid–base status at the time of observation • No specific action is required
Category II (these include all FHR tracings that are not Category I or III. Examples below)	
Baseline variability: • Minimal variability • Absent variability not accompanied by recurrent decelerations • Marked variability Accelerations: • Absence of induced accelerations after fetal stimulation Periodic or episodic decelerations: • Recurrent variable decelerations with minimal or moderate BLV • Prolonged deceleration (>2 minutes but <10 minutes) • Recurrent late decelerations with moderate BLV • Variable decelerations with other characteristics, such as slow return to baseline, "overshoots," or "shoulders"	• Indeterminate • Not predictive of abnormal fetal acid–base status • Requires evaluation, continued surveillance, and re-evaluation • Take into account the entire associated clinical circumstance
Category III	

Baseline variability:
Absent BLV
AND
Any of the following:
• Decelerations:
  ○ Recurrent late decelerations
  ○ Recurrent variable decelerations
• Bradycardia
• Sinusoidal pattern:
  ○ Smooth, sine wave-like, undulating pattern of the FHR baseline
  ○ of regular frequency of 3–5 cycles per minute
  ○ that persists for >20 minutes
	• Predicts abnormal fetal acid–base status
	• Requires prompt evaluation
	• Warrants efforts to expeditiously resolve the abnormal FHR pattern including but not limited to intrauterine resuscitation:
	  ○ Provide oxygen to the mother
	  ○ Change maternal position
	  ○ Discontinue labor stimulation
	  ○ Treat hypotension

Source: Adapted from Macones 2008.[62] Reproduced with permission of Elsevier.

Table 4.5. Interpretation of auscultation findings relative to NICHD 3-tier categories.

Category I FHR Characteristics by Auscultation	Category II FHR Characteristics by Auscultation
FHR baseline between 110 and 160 bpm with regular rhythm	Tachycardia (baseline > 160 bpm) or bradycardia (baseline < 110 bpm)
No FHR decelerations from the baseline	
FHR increases (accelerations) of 15 seconds in duration and amplitude from the baseline may or may not be present, but should be assessed for and documented if present	Audible irregular rhythm Presence of FHR decreases or decelerations from the baseline

Abbreviations: FHR, fetal heart rate; NICHD, National Institute of Child Health and Human Development.

Comparing intermittent auscultation and continuous EFM

There is a tradeoff between the advantages of maternal mobility versus continuous electronic fetal monitoring (CEFM), which usually requires the laboring person to remain lying in bed or semi-sitting. This tradeoff can be resolved in a variety of ways. One way is to discontinue the routine practice of continuous EFM. In a Cochrane Review Alfirevic and colleagues[70] compared the effectiveness and safety of CEFM for fetal wellbeing during labor to intermittent auscultation. Thirteen trials with 3700 laboring people as participants were included in the meta-analysis. Compared with intermittent auscultation, CEFM did not reduce cerebral palsy or neonatal death rates, but significantly increased cesarean and instrumental deliveries. Continuous EFM offers a small advantage in that it lowers the rate of neonatal seizures from approximately 1 in 500 to 1 in 250. This means that continuous EFM must be used during 661 labors, to prevent one case of neonatal seizure (95% CI 484–1667).[70] Other disadvantages of EFM are considerable inter-observer and intra-observer variability in interpretation, and inconsistent terminology.[71]

Despite the notable endorsements of intermittent auscultation, and the lack of scientific evidence of benefit of CEFM, the latter remains well established in many hospitals in the United States, United Kingdom, Canada, and other countries. Continuous CEFM remains a common feature of "usual care," even with low-risk clients. Many physicians, nurses, and midwives who were trained in reading electronic monitor tracings remain uneasy with auscultation. Furthermore, many people labor in institutions where policies require continuous CEFM, and despite doctrines of informed consent and informed choice they are not offered the option of IA. Oxytocin induction or augmentation is a prevalent indication for CEFM. There are numerous high-risk indications for CEFM.

Maintaining movement when using CEFM

The laboring person does not have to remain in a single position or in bed when CEFM is used. They may lie on their side, sit up, kneel and lean forward, get out of bed and rock in a chair, stand and lean over the bed or a birth ball on the bed, sway or "slow dance" (Fig. 4.14) with their partner beside the monitor, lunge, or even sit in the bath. Even if the fetal heart rate is easier to detect in one position, the laboring person should maintain mobility for comfort and to promote progress. The laboring person's support person may hold the transducer in place (Fig. 4.15) when they are standing, on hands-and-knees, or in another position.

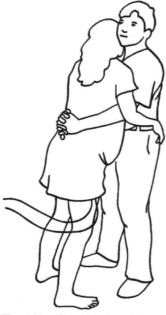

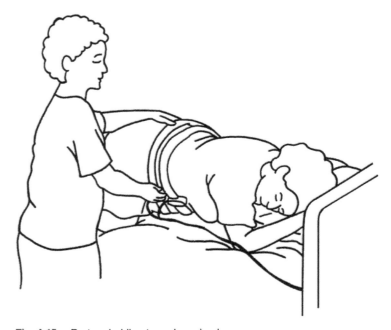

Fig. 4.14.   Slow dancing with electronic fetal monitoring (EFM).

Fig. 4.15.   Partner holding transducer in place.

An internal scalp electrode usually has the advantage over an external ultrasound transducer in that it is more likely to stay in place when the person rolls over, kneels, or squats. It also is less likely to lose the signal when the fetus moves. However, it is more invasive and requires ruptured membranes with all the accompanying risks (vertical transmission of infectious organisms, cord compression, and persistent fetal malposition). The ultrasound transducer should be repositioned when the signal is unclear, or the fetus moves. A broken or unclear fetal monitoring tracing defeats the purpose of CEFM and decreases the accuracy of interpretation while increasing safety and liability concerns.

Intrauterine pressure catheters (IUPC) are used to accurately assess the intensity of contractions for specific clinical indications, such as with augmentation or induction of labor and for situations of when the timing of fetal heart rate decelerations (early vs late) in relationship to the uterine contractions cannot be determined by use of an external toco transducer. The person laboring with an IUPC may use upright positions, but it usually requires an adjustment or "zeroing" of the pressure gauge when they change positions, in order to maintain accurate baseline and peak pressure readings.

Monitoring during water immersion. For laboring individuals who prefer to spend part of their labor in the bath (Fig. 4.16), there are waterproof handheld Dopplers. If these are not available in the hospital, the ultrasound transducer that comes with the CEFM can also be used while the person is immersed in water (only if confirmed as waterproof by the monitor manufacturer). Another option if no waterproof monitoring equipment is available is to ask the laboring person to rise out of the water intermittently to facilitate fetal monitoring with a fetoscope, doppler, or ultrasound transducer (Fig. 4.17).

Wireless telemetry. Considering the documented benefits of free movement and various positions[75] and hydrotherapy[76] in speeding slow progress and reducing pain, telemetry may be the optimal choice of monitoring methods when CEFM is called for. The laboring person may walk in or outside the labor room (Fig. 4.18a) or sit in the bath (Fig. 4.19) or shower (Fig. 4.20). Within wireless telemetry units, both the ultrasound transducer and the contraction sensor have built-in radio transmitters, which are secured on the laboring person's trunk with the

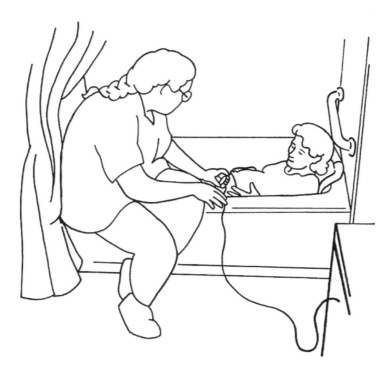

Fig. 4.16. Monitoring with a waterproof hand-held Doppler.

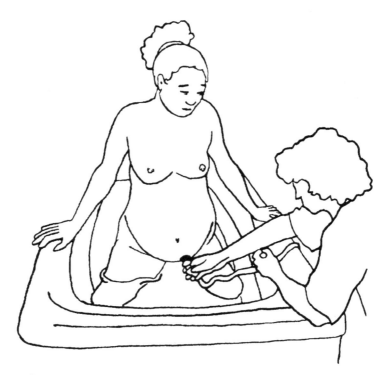

Fig. 4.17.   Monitoring out of water.

(a)   (b)

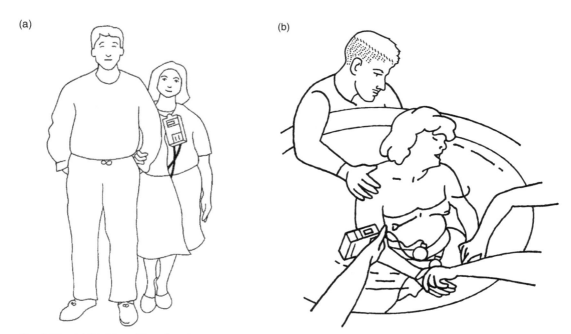

Fig. 4.18.   (**a**) Walking with radio telemetry monitor. (**b**) Using radio telemetry in bath.

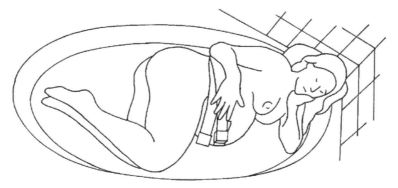

Fig. 4.19. Using wireless telemetry in bath.

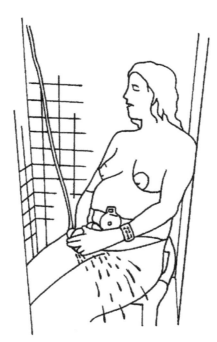

Fig. 4.20. Using wireless telemetry in shower.

elastic belts. Waterproof ultrasound transducers can be used in the bath, and water resistant ones can be used in the shower, as shown in Figs. 4.19 and 4.20.

Fig. 4.18. Internal assessments

In some labors, visual and external assessments may be all that are needed to make an accurate assessment of progress in labor. However, it may be necessary to perform an internal assessment to gather more information or to confirm findings from external evaluations. Cervical change, along with fetal rotation and descent, are the definitive signs of progress in labor, whereas external signs may provide only indirect clues to what is happening.

Vaginal examinations: indications and timing

Vaginal assessment of the laboring person should be individualized. This means that rather than being done in all labors at a predetermined time interval, vaginal examinations should be done as the need for information about the cervix and fetus arises, and with the laboring person's understanding and consent. Clinicians should take time to establish rapport before performing a vaginal examination and ask for consent prior to the exam since it is intrusive. Vaginal examinations should not be performed on a laboring person who is bleeding unless the location of the placenta is known (rule out placenta previa).

Indications for vaginal examinations during labor include:

- At the beginning of care in labor, to verify the fetal presenting part and establish a baseline of dilation, efface-ment and station so that future progress or lack of progress can be better assessed.
- When a period of time in active labor has elapsed, usually more than 3 hours, and the labor pattern does not seem to be progressing (contractions are not becoming longer, more frequent, or more intense) or when there are no other outward signs of progress (laboring person's affect, spontaneous bearing down efforts, etc.), and a decision must be made about interventions to correct a dysfunctional labor.
- After an intervention has been implemented for some time (for example, a period of stair climbing to aid in rotation of the fetal head or time in the bath), to assess whether the desired effect has been achieved.
- When the laboring person requests an assessment of progress or expresses discouragement or a desire for anal-gesia or anesthesia.
- When there is a spontaneous urge to push without other signs of fetal descent.
- When there are non-reassuring fetal heart-rate (FHR) changes or any other concerning signs.
- When an internal monitor (scalp electrode or intrauterine pressure catheter) is indicated.

Performing a vaginal examination during labor

Preparing for the examination. Prior to a vaginal exam, ask the laboring person to empty their bladder. After explaining the procedure and asking for consent, the laboring person should lie down on a firm, comfortable sur-face, preferably on their back with their head supported by a pillow, as shown in Fig. 4.21a. The laboring person's legs should be well supported, with knees flexed and wide apart, and the soles of their either together or flat on the surface of the bed. If lying on the back is too uncomfortable, they can rest in a supported semi-prone position with a pillow wedged under one hip with their upper knee and hip flexed and supported (Fig. 4.21b). Some experi-enced practitioners perform vaginal exams with the laboring person in other positions (on hands and knees, standing, sitting, or squatting). This allows them to assess the cervical dilation and effacement. However, it is dif-ficult to gain more detailed information, such as station and the position of the presenting part, with the laboring person in non-supine positions. When detailed information is needed, it is better to ask the laboring person to lie down briefly than to have to repeat the exam.

The person's ability to relax during this exam is important if the provider is to obtain the necessary information and is also a quality of care issue. Good care is defined as being both sensitive to the laboring person's needs and effective in obtaining the needed data. Some people experience fear during vaginal exams and may not be able to tolerate them, especially when performed by unfamiliar people or done without consideration of their discomfort. Often, these are people who have experienced previous trauma (i.e., sexual abuse or rough and inconsiderate vag-inal exams). In order to be examined, they need patience, gentleness, and understanding from their providers and a sense of being in control over whether, when, by whom, and how the exam will be done.[77]

Beginning the vaginal examination. The clinical care provider washes and warms their hands and asks the pregnant person's permission to begin the vaginal exam. Of course, if permission is not granted, the caregiver does not perform the procedure. Between contractions, the examiner inserts first one (the forefinger) and then two fin-gers (adding the middle finger) into the vagina, putting firm but gentle pressure on the posterior vaginal wall and avoiding pressure on the urethra. At the same time, the examiner asks the pregnant person to relax the vaginal muscles. Without the pregnant person's cooperation and active relaxation, this exam may be uncomfortable, and accurate assessment may be difficult or impossible.

(a)

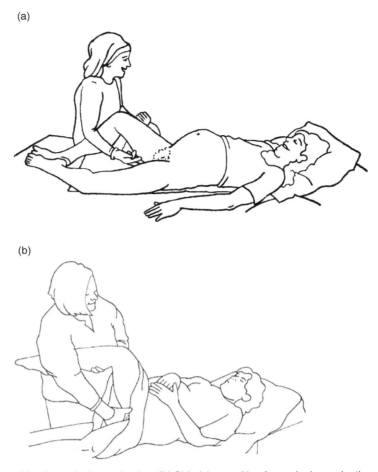

(b)

Fig. 4.21. (**a**) Supine position for vaginal examination. (**b**) Side-lying position for vaginal examination.

When the fingers are inserted with the pads down, to about 3 to 4 cm within the vagina, the examiner explains that they will rotate the fingers so that the wrist is face up. This position allows for better assessment of the cervix, the presenting part, the vagina, and the pelvis.

Assessing the cervix

Position: Is the os anterior, posterior, or midline? When the cervical os is posterior, sometimes it is just barely possible to reach it, but not enough to assess dilation. In this case, the caregiver may be able to reach the os by applying gentle, steady pressure and manually pulling it forward. Another aid is to ask the pregnant person to place a fist under each buttock or use a bedpan with a towel over it to help tilt the pelvis. This should bring the cervix into a more "reachable" position.

Consistency: Is the cervical tissue and the os stretchy and soft or firm? As labor progresses, the cervix should become softer and more yielding. A thick, rigid cervix is abnormal in labor.

Effacement: How long is the cervical canal? It is difficult, if not impossible, to assess effacement digitally without being able to insert at least one finger into the cervix. Since the length of the cervix prior to labor varies from 1 to 4 cm, effacement is best expressed in terms of the remaining length of the cervical canal, in centimeters or fractions of centimeters. Another option is to report effacement as a percentage.[77,78] Using centimeters versus a percentage will depend on the convention of the birth setting. A completely effaced cervix is very thin.

Dilation: How open is the cervix, measured in centimeters, without manual stretching? The first 6 to 7 centimeters are assessed by evaluating how open the cervix is. It takes practice to know the approximate number of fingerbreadths, or the distance between fingers, and the corresponding dilation. Practice tools include plastic models made for this purpose, as well as household objects, such as jars with various sized mouths. The last 3 centimeters of dilation (from 7 centimeters to fully dilated) are easier to assess, because they are measured by evaluating how much of the cervix remains on one side, between the open edge of the os and where the cervix meets the lower uterine segment. Although "10 centimeters" has been used to express complete dilation, measurable full dilation could vary between 9 and 12 centimeters depending on the size of the fetal head. Also note whether the cervix is unevenly dilated and if so where and how much. This detail can offer clues as to the position and angle of the fetal head.

Membranes: Are they intact or ruptured? A large bulging forebag is easy to feel and may make assessment of fetal position difficult. When there is no bulging bag of fluid presenting, the examiner should learn to discern the feel of the slippery membrane over the head compared to the way the scalp feels when membranes are ruptured.

Contraction strength: If the provider suspects that contractions are not intense enough to dilate the cervix, examining the cervix during a contraction can help evaluate contraction strength. This examination is much more uncomfortable for the laboring person than a cervical assessment done between contractions, so it is important to explain the rationale and obtain permission. The examiner holds the fingertips against the cervix. With the onset of an effective contraction, the edges of the cervical os stretch, and the head descends, pressing against the cervix. If there is a forebag with intact membranes, it becomes tight and full. Inadequate contractions are not strong enough to produce these changes, and little stretch is palpated. The cervix may have the "empty sleeve" feel because the head is not brought into contact with it.

Unusual cervical findings:

- The "zipper" cervix: While the cervix is quite effaced, the os is adherent and closed. Sometimes, after nearly complete effacement is achieved, this can be overcome by inserting one or two fingers and massaging the os open during a contraction. As the adhesion releases, the os opens like a zipper, sometimes dilating from 1 to 3 or 4 centimeters in one contraction! Expect bloody show as capillaries rupture with stretching.
- The rigid os: The cervix may be partially dilated but has thickness and lacks a feeling of elasticity. It does not yield easily with contractions. This may be a sign of primary cervical dysfunction,[79] or a consequence of edema in the cervix caused by a poorly fitting head or uneven pressure on the cervix during contractions. With primary dysfunction, the cervix never softens and effaces. When edema is present, the cervix may be thinned and dilated during the latent phase or early active phase but becomes swollen in late active phase.
- Persistent anterior cervical "lip": This occurs when most of the cervix has retracted behind the head (no rim of cervix is palpated around the lateral or posterior aspects of the head) but the anterior portion of the cervix is caught between the head and the symphysis pubis. Position changes, time, and patience usually resolve the situation. If the tissue feels stretchy, it may be reduced manually.

Assessing the presenting part

Is it a head? It is important to consider that the presenting part may not be a head; otherwise, one risks missing an undiagnosed breech presentation. Exam findings with a frank breech may mimic those with an extremely malpositioned head: no sutures or fontanelles are felt, and the leading part feels soft and spongy, as with a caput. One way to clarify this situation, short of ultrasound, is to perform a sterile speculum examination. The presence of hair confirms a cephalic presentation.

What is the fetal station? Stations of descent are expressed in centimeters above or below the level of the ischial spines, which is designated as zero station (Fig. 4.22). When the head has not yet entered the pelvis, the leading edge is said to be "floating."

To assess station by vaginal examination, the examiner first finds the approximate location of one ischial spine. It is easiest to do this by reaching with one's dominant hand diagonally across the pregnant person's pelvis (so a

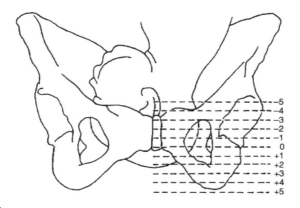

Fig. 4.22. Stations of descent.

right-handed provider will palpate the right maternal spine). In most pregnant people, the spine will be blunt and not easily palpated, so approximating its location takes practice. It helps to find the sacrospinous ligament and follow it with two fingers from the midline to the place of insertion on the sidewall as shown in Fig. 4.23. Because this insertion point is also the location of the pudendal nerve, the person may report an achy "funny bone" sensation when the examiner's fingers press there.

Next, the examiner compares the level of the leading edge of the head with the level of the ischial spines by placing the middle finger on the ischial spine and reaching out with the index finger to the lowest part of the fetal head. It is imperative to use enough pressure to feel the bone, to avoid mistaking a large spongy caput for a head at a lower station. A significant and growing amount of caput may indicate true cephalopelvic disproportion; descent may need to be assessed via careful abdominal palpation (see Fig. 4.12).

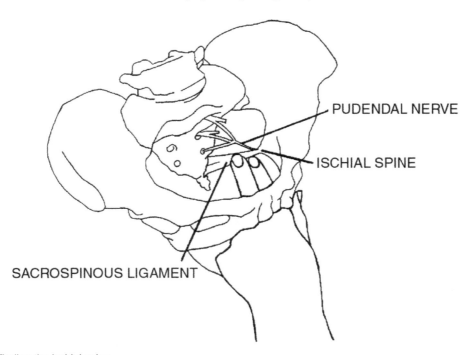

Fig. 4.23. Finding the ischial spine.

A less precise measure, but one that is useful when learning to assess station, is how deeply the examiner's fingers may be inserted before reaching the head.[34] Assuming average-sized fingers:

- If the station is floating, the fingers will be inserted completely into the vagina and not reach the leading edge of the head (Fig. 4.24a).
- With station −4 to −2, the examiner's fingers will be inserted completely and will be able to palpate the head with the tips of the fingers.
- At zero station, or the level of the ischial spines, the fingers easily reach the head (Fig. 4.24b), and at lower stations, the fingers are only inserted half-way or less into the vagina (Fig. 4.24c).

Assessment of station, like many other internal examinations in labor, is not precise and varies from examiner to examiner. In a slow second stage, progress may be incremental, in millimeters, rather than in centimeters. When progress is in question, sequential evaluation by the same examiner is helpful, when possible. A high station in active phase, especially in nulliparas, may suggest malposition or true cephalopelvic disproportion (CPD).

Evaluating fetal position: Identifying fetal position is perhaps the single most difficult assessment to make during intrapartum vaginal examinations. It is commonly ascertained by the examiner palpating bony landmarks on the fetal head through a reasonably dilated cervix, to determine the location of the occiput in relation to the maternal pelvis.

What is known about the accuracy of these digital examinations in labor? Simkin[20] reviewed studies comparing digital assessments of fetal position with ultrasound assessments and concluded that digital assessment of position was often impossible, especially in the first stage. In one study, digital assessment was accurate only 54% of the time when the occiput was posterior or lateral.[80] This research suggests that digital examination is useless for

(a) Floating, or well above spines

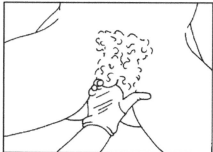

(b) At level of spines – 0 station

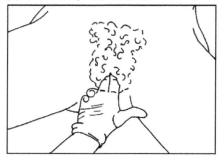

(c) Below the spines

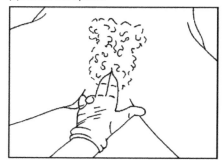

Fig. 4.24. Vaginal examinations to assess descent. (**a**) Floating, or well above spines. (**b**) At level of spines—0 station. (**c**) Below the spines.

determining fetal position in labor and advocates for ultrasound as the "gold standard." However, Akmal et al[81]: found that in about 10% of intrapartum ultrasound examinations, all performed by expert sonographers, the scans were "uninterpretable," raising the question of whether this technology, used by maternity care providers who are not ultrasound experts, would be as useful. Furthermore, though studies have consistently shown a lack of accuracy among maternity professionals in assessing fetal position, there may be care providers who are expert in digital assessment. In the end, however, the 10% error rate found with the use of ultrasound is still far better than the error rates with digital assessment of fetal position.

The lack of demonstrable benefit of digital assessments of fetal position may be difficult for experienced midwives, nurses, and doctors to accept. Simkin[20] suggests that care providers compare some of their digital assessments with ultrasound results to confirm their accuracy or inaccuracy and also use ultrasound comparisons to refine and improve their skills. Misdiagnosis of fetal position may cause more harm than no diagnosis, due to the use of inappropriate action resulting from the misdiagnosis.

With that caveat, and despite the negative findings regarding accuracy, we offer a description of the technique as taught to midwives in a leading midwifery school in the United States. We offer it here in hopes that those who are reluctant to accept the findings reported here will use this careful and methodical approach to digital assessment, with a healthy skepticism and an open mind to the very real possibility that their assessments will be wrong. They should maintain a willingness to question their findings, seek ultrasound confirmation if possible, and resort to trial and error if and when their corrective actions do not result in improved labor progress.

Here is the step-by-step approach to digital assessment of position of the fetal skull:

- The first step is to find the most easily palpated landmark—the sagittal suture. Some degree of asynclitism is normal as the head comes into the pelvic brim in early labor. But with a well-positioned head, throughout most of labor the sagittal suture is usually in the right or left oblique diameter and roughly in the middle of the pelvis (Fig. 4.25). It may also be in a transverse diameter. During the second stage of labor when internal rotation normally occurs, it rotates 45 to 90 degrees to the anterior-posterior diameter of the pelvis.
    - If the sagittal suture is palpated just below the pubic arch, it indicates asynclitism (Fig. 4.26).
    - If the sagittal suture cannot be felt at all, there probably is significant asynclitism, usually posterior, with the posterior parietal bone (i.e., the parietal bone next to the laboring person's back) leading and the sagittal suture tucked under the symphysis pubis.
- Next, the fontanelles are assessed by following the sagittal suture line in both directions from the midline. The posterior fontanelle is smaller and has three points. It does not actually feel like a triangular space as much as the joining of three suture lines. The anterior fontanelle is much larger; it has four points and is shaped like a diamond. See Table 4.6, including Figures 4.27a–f.

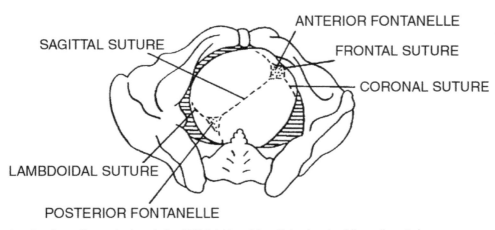

Fig. 4.25.   Landmarks on the occiput posterior (OP) fetal head (sagittal suture in oblique diameter).

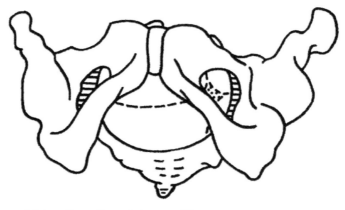

Fig. 4.26. Occiput transverse fetal position with posterior asynclitism.

Table 4.6. Fetal positions viewed from below and from front of pelvis.

Position	Vaginal view	Front view of fetus in pelvis
LOA	Fig. 4.27a	Fig. 4.27b
ROP	Fig. 4.27c	Fig. 4.27d
LOT	Fig. 4.27e	Fig. 4.27f

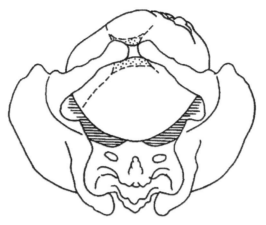

Fig. 4.28. Asynclitic fetus in right occiput posterior (ROP).

Even when it is not possible to accurately locate fontanelles, malposition can often be detected. It is important to notice whether the head fits more or less symmetrically. When the fetal head is malpositioned, it does not fill the pelvis. On examination, the head feels tight in the front of the pelvis, as if it is sitting over the pubic symphysis, while there is room in the back of the pelvis (Fig. 4.28).

Identifying those fetuses likely to persist in an OP position throughout labor

Acknowledging that most fetuses in an OP position will eventually rotate in labor[15] and that outcomes are worst for those that do not rotate,[16–19] is it possible to make predictions about which ones are or are not likely to rotate?

One study[15] found that descent of the fetal head into the pelvis may somewhat reduce the chances of rotation from OP to OA. Eighty-nine percent of OP fetuses that were just beginning to enter the pelvis in labor (-2 station or higher) rotated to OA for delivery at some point on their journey. Fetuses that were in an OP position in the mid-pelvis (-2 to 0 station) had somewhat lower rates of rotation at 74%, and for those in the pelvic outlet (at or below 0 station), 63% rotated to OA. A similar study with only nulliparous birthgivers observed this trend as well, with 77% of fetuses who were OP at a high station eventually rotating, 55% of mid-pelvis OP babies, and 40% who were OP at +1 station or lower.[82] Although station may play a role, many fetuses can and will rotate at any point along the way out.

Several studies have found that the position of the fetal spine is an important factor in predicting which OP fetuses are likely to persist in an OP position until delivery.[3–5] When the fetal spine is positioned anywhere along the birthgiver's front or side, the head is far more likely to turn to an occiput anterior position by delivery. When the fetal spine is positioned along the birthgiver's back, the head is more likely to remain occiput posterior.[5] The latter group are significantly more likely to be managed via operative vaginal delivery or cesarean birth than OP fetuses with their spines in any other position.

Evaluating flexion of the fetal head: With a well-flexed head in the OA position, the small posterior fontanelle is palpable in the right or left oblique diameter of the pelvis while the anterior fontanelle is not. When a large fontanelle is easily palpated, the fetus is usually in a posterior, deflexed position.

Evaluating the presence of molding: Molding is the overlapping of the bones of the fetal head along the suture lines and is a normal response to pressure during labor. Molding of the cranial bones permits the fetal head to better accommodate the tight fit through the pelvis. Molding is often necessary for fetal descent and rotation around the symphysis pubis. However, if excessive molding occurs early in labor, it may be a sign of difficulty.[83] Evaluating the degree of molding, together with the stage of labor, the station, estimated fetal size, and other variables, can aid in the assessment of dysfunctional labor. Molding obscures fontanelles and makes sutures feel more prominent. Magnetic resonance imaging (MRI) technology has been used to quantify the extent of fetal head molding during the second stage of labor.[84]

Evaluating caput: Caput formation, the accumulation of fluid in the tissue of the scalp, is also a result of pressure on the fetal head. It normally occurs in second stage labor with active descent but may be present in the active phase of the first stage if the membranes have ruptured. The finding of "caput formation" with a high station could actually represent an undiagnosed breech (soft and spongy) rather than caput! It might also signify OP position or disproportion. An extensive caput also makes it more difficult to assess position and station and is sometimes mistaken for descent. As the caput forms, the swelling expands lower in the pelvis, but the fetal skull may not have descended at all.[83]

Evaluating the application of the head to the cervix: Is the head well applied to the cervix, or does the cervix feel like an "empty sleeve?" With a malpositioned head, it is common to find that the cervix is soft and stretchy but that, during contractions, the head does not press against it. This gives the impression of a poor fit, rather than a "rigid" cervix.

The vagina and bony pelvis

The vaginal muscles should feel soft and stretchy, not tight or unyielding. Any obvious bony abnormalities (i.e., flat sacrum, short diagonal conjugate, prominent ischial spines, narrow pubic arch, or rigid, prominent coccyx) should be noted. When all of these factors seem normal, it is reassuring to the care provider.

PUTTING IT ALL TOGETHER

Assessing progress in the first stage

Different criteria should be used to assess labor progress for latent phase than for active phase. The *latent phase* is characterized by persistent contractions that do effect change, albeit slow and sometimes subtle. *Active phase* is defined as the time when contractions are more intense and frequent and the rate of change becomes more accelerated.

Features of normal latent phase

* The cervix softens and effaces slowly but progressively.
* Fetal station may or may not change.
* Dilation is slow up to 6 cm.[40]
* Contractions may be regular or irregular, with varying frequency and duration, but are usually mild to moderate in intensity.
* Normal duration is up to 20 to 24 hours.[79] This is the longest phase of labor for most nulliparas. The laboring person may be distractible during contractions and carry on "normal" activities between contractions.
* Laboring person does not become exhausted.

Features of normal active phase

* Cervical effacement completes.
* The rate of cervical change increases over time, although progress may not be uniform from hour to hour.
* Dilation progresses over time to full dilation, but the rate of dilation varies tremendously between people.
* The fetal head engages, particularly in the nullipara.
* The fetal head descends to lower stations, especially toward the completion of first stage.
* The laboring person's behavior becomes serious and focused, both during and between contractions. Coping behaviors may become more dramatic.

- If there is back pain, the place that hurts moves downward over time.
- Normal symptoms during rapid dilation may include an increase in bloody show, nausea, vomiting, shaking, irritability, anger, or feelings of desperation.
- This phase lasts longer for nulliparas than for multiparas.

Assessing progress in the second stage

There is often a latent phase after full dilation and before the fetus descends enough to trigger a pushing urge. If the active phase of second stage is defined to include full dilation and spontaneous active pushing efforts, active second stage progress is assessed by linear descent of the head and concludes with the birth of the baby.

Features of normal second stage

- The laboring person has spontaneous pushing urges (unless they have regional anesthesia or analgesia).
- Contractions increase or remain strong and intense, though they may be shorter or less frequent than those in late first stage.
- The fetal head may rotate, mold, and form a caput.
- All of the mechanisms of labor are accomplished: descent, flexion, internal rotation, birth of the head, restitution, external rotation, and birth of the shoulders and body of the fetus.
- Upper limits of normal duration vary but are longer for nulliparas than for multiparas.

CONCLUSION

This chapter has covered methods of assessment of the laboring person and fetus that are relevant to diagnosis and management of dystocia. These techniques enable the clinical care provider not only to identify dystocia but also its specific etiology.

REFERENCES

1. Kotaska A, Menticoglou S (2019) No. 384: Management of breech presentation at term. *Journal of Obstetrics and Gynaecology of Canada: JOGC = Journal D'obstetrique et Gynecologie du Canada: JOGC* 41(8), 1193–1205. doi: 10.1016/j.jogc.2018.12.018
2. King TL, Jevitt CM. (2019). Appendix 21A: Abdominal examination during pregnancy. In: TL King, MC Brucker, K Osborne, CM Jevitt (eds.), *Varney's Midwifery*, 6th edn. Burlington, MA: Jones & Bartlett Learning, pp. 741–748.
3. Peregrine E, O'Brien P, Jauniaux E. (2007) Impact on delivery outcome of ultrasonographic fetal head position prior to induction of labor. *Obstetrics and Gynecology* 109(3), 618–625. doi: 10.1097/01.AOG.0000255972.48257.83
4. Gizzo S, Andrisani A, Noventa M, Burul G, Di Gangi S, Anis O, Ancona E, D'Antona D, Nardelli GB, Ambrosini G. (2014) Intrapartum ultrasound assessment of fetal spine position. *BioMed Research International* 2014, 783598. doi: 10.1155/2014/783598
5. Svelato A, Ragusa A, Alimondi P, Di Tommaso M, Marci R, Barbagallo V, Alampi RD, Calagna G, Perino A. (2017) Occiput-spine relationship: Shoulders are more important than head. *European Review for Medical and Pharmacological Sciences* 21(6), 1178–1183.
6. McFarlin BL, Engstrom JL, Sampson MB, Cattledge F. (1985) Concurrent validity of Leopold's maneuvers in determining fetal presentation and position. *Journal of Nurse-Midwifery* 30(5), 280–284. doi: 10.1016/0091-2182(85)90043-6
7. Thorp JM, Jr, Jenkins T, Watson W (1991) Utility of Leopold maneuvers in screening for malpresentation. *Obstetrics and Gynecology* 78(3 Pt 1), 394–396.
8. Lydon-Rochelle M, Albers L, Gorwoda J, Craig E, Qualls C. (1993) Accuracy of Leopold maneuvers in screening for malpresentation: A prospective study. *Birth* 20(3), 132–135. doi: 10.1111/j.1523-536x.1993.tb00437.x
9. Watson WJ, Welter S, Day D. (2004) Antepartum identification of breech presentation. *The Journal of Reproductive Medicine* 49(4), 294–296.

10. Udompornthanakij P, Kongsomboon K, Hanprasertpong T. (2020) Accuracy and factors influencing Leopold's manoeuvres in determining vertex presentation during late third trimester of pregnancy. *Journal of Obstetrics and Gynaecology: The Journal of the Institute of Obstetrics and Gynaecology* 40(5), 639–643. doi: 10.1080/01443615.2019.1645102

11. Crichton D. (1974) A reliable method of establishing the level of the fetal head in obstetrics. *South African Medical Journal* 47(4), 784–787.

12. Tully G. (2010) *The Belly Mapping Workbook: How Kicks and Wiggles Reveal Your Baby's Position*. Minneapolis: Maternity House Publishing.

13. Sutton J, Scott P. (1996) *Understanding and Teaching Optimal Foetal Positioning*, 2nd revised edn. UK: Birth Concepts.

14. Tully G. (2021) *What Is Spinning Babies®?* Spinning Babies. https://www.spinningbabies.com/about/what-is-spinning-babies

15. Vitner D, Paltieli Y, Haberman S, Gonen R, Ville, Y Nizard J (2015) Prospective multicenter study of ultrasound-based measurements of fetal head station and position throughout labor. *Ultrasound in Obstetrics & Gynecology: The Official Journal of the International Society of Ultrasound in Obstetrics and Gynecology* 46(5), 611–615. doi: 10.1002/uog.14821

16. Fitzpatrick M, McQuillan K, O'Herlihy C. (2001) Influence of persistent occiput posterior position on delivery outcome. *Obstetrics and Gynecology* 98(6), 1027–1031. doi: 10.1016/s0029-7844(01)01600-3

17. Cheng YW, Shaffer BL, Caughey AB. (2006) Associated factors and outcomes of persistent occiput posterior position: A retrospective cohort study from 1976 to 2001. *The Journal of Maternal-Fetal & Neonatal Medicine: The Official Journal of the European Association of Perinatal Medicine, the Federation of Asia and Oceania Perinatal Societies, the International Society of Perinatal Obstetricians* 19(9), 563–568. doi: 10.1080/14767050600682487

18. Simpson CN, Chambers CN, Sharshiner R, Caughey AB. (2015) Effects of persistent occiput posterior position on mode of delivery. *Obstetrics & Gynecology* 125, 82S–83S.

19. Pilliod RA, Caughey AB. (2017) Fetal malpresentation and malposition: Diagnosis and Management. *Obstetrics and Gynecology Clinics of North America* 44(4), 631–643. doi: 10.1016/j.ogc.2017.08.003

20. Simkin P. (2010) The fetal occiput posterior position: State of the science and a new perspective. *Birth* 37(1), 61–71. doi: 10.1111/j.1523-536X.2009.00380.x

21. Martin JA, Hamilton BE, Osterman M, Driscoll AK. (2021) Births: Final data for 2019. *National Vital Statistics Reports: From the Centers for Disease Control and Prevention, National Center for Health Statistics, National Vital Statistics System* 70(2), 1–51.

22. Coates D, Makris A, Catling C, Henry A, Scarf V, Watts N, Fox D, Thirukumar P, Wong V, Russell H, Homer C. (2020) A systematic scoping review of clinical indications for induction of labour. *PloS One* 15(1), e0228196. doi: 10.1371/journal.pone.0228196

23. Madden JV, Flatley CJ, Kumar S. (2018) Term small-for-gestational-age infants from low-risk women are at significantly greater risk of adverse neonatal outcomes. *American Journal of Obstetrics and Gynecology* 218(5), 525.e1–525.e9. doi: 10.1016/j.ajog.2018.02.008

24. Al-Amin A, Hingston T, Mayall P, Araujo Júnior E, Fabrício Da Silva C, Friedman D. (2015) The utility of ultrasound in late pregnancy compared with clinical evaluation in detecting small and large for gestational age fetuses in low-risk pregnancies. *The Journal of Maternal-Fetal & Neonatal Medicine: The Official Journal of the European Association of Perinatal Medicine, the Federation of Asia and Oceania Perinatal Societies, the International Society of Perinatal Obstetricians* 28(13), 1495–1499. doi: 10.3109/14767058.2014.961007

25. Preyer O, Husslein H, Concin N, Ridder A, Musielak M, Pfeifer C, Oberaigner W, Husslein P. (2019) Fetal weight estimation at term - ultrasound versus clinical examination with Leopold's manoeuvres: A prospective blinded observational study. *BMC Pregnancy and Childbirth* 19(1), 122. doi: 10.1186/s12884-019-2251-5

26. Ray EM, Alhusen JL. (2016) The suspected macrosomic fetus at term: A clinical dilemma. *Journal of Midwifery & Women's Health* 61(2), 263–269. doi: 10.1111/jmwh.12414

27. Malin GL, Bugg GJ, Takwoingi Y, Thornton JG, Jones NW. (2016) Antenatal magnetic resonance imaging versus ultrasound for predicting neonatal macrosomia: A systematic review and meta-analysis. *BJOG: An International Journal of Obstetrics and Gynaecology* 123(1), 77–88. doi: 10.1111/1471-0528.13517

28. Matthews KC, Williamson J, Gupta S, Lam-Rachlin J, Saltzman DH, Rebarber A, Fox NS. (2017) The effect of a sonographic estimated fetal weight on the risk of cesarean delivery in macrosomic and small for gestational-age infants. *The Journal of Maternal-Fetal & Neonatal Medicine: The Official Journal of the European Association of Perinatal Medicine, the Federation of Asia and Oceania Perinatal Societies, the International Society of Perinatal Obstetricians* 30(10), 1172–1176. doi: 10.1080/14767058.2016.1208744

Assessing Progress in Labor

4

29. Buckley SJ. (2015) *Hormonal Physiology of Childbearing: Evidence and Implications for Women, Babies, and Maternity Care.* Washington, DC: Childbirth Connection Programs, National Partnership for Women & Families.

30. Yellon SM (2020) Immunobiology of cervix ripening. *Frontiers in Immunology* 10, 3156. doi: 10.3389/fimmu.2019.03156

31. Bishop EH. (1964) Pelvic scoring for elective induction. *Obstetrics and Gynecology* 24, 266–268.

32. Hughey MJ, McElin TW, Bird CC. (1976) An evaluation of preinduction scoring systems. *Obstetrics and Gynecology* 48(6), 635–641.

33. Laughon SK, Zhang J, Troendle J, Sun L, Reddy UM. (2011) Using a simplified Bishop score to predict vaginal delivery. *Obstetrics and Gynecology* 117(4), 805–811. doi: 10.1097/AOG.0b013e3182114ad2

34. Malapati R, Vuong YN, Nguyen TM. (2013) Reporting cervical effacement as a percentage: How accurate is it? *Open Journal of Obstetrics and Gynecology* 3(7), 569–572. doi: 10.4236/ojog.2013.37102

35. Meier K, Parrish J, D'Souza R. (2019) Prediction models for determining the success of labor induction: A systematic review. *Acta Obstetricia Et Gynecologica Scandinavica* 98(9), 1100–1112. doi: 10.1111/aogs.13589

36. Mishanina E, Rogozinska E, Thatthi T, Uddin-Khan R, Khan KS, Meads C. (2014) Use of labour induction and risk of cesarean delivery: A systematic review and meta-analysis. *CMAJ: Canadian Medical Association Journal = Journal de l'Association Medicale Canadienne* 186(9), 665–673. doi: 10.1503/cmaj.130925

37. Ezebialu IU, Eke AC, Eleje GU, Nwachukwu CE. (2015) Methods for assessing pre-induction cervical ripening. *The Cochrane Database of Systematic Reviews* 2015(6), CD010762. doi: 10.1002/14651858.CD010762.pub2

38. Caughey AB, Cahill AG, Guise JM, Rouse DJ American College of Obstetricians and Gynecologists. (2014) Safe prevention of the primary cesarean delivery. *American Journal of Obstetrics and Gynecology* 210(3), 179–193. doi: 10.1016/j.ajog.2014.01.026

39. Hanley GE, Munro S, Greyson D, Gross MM, Hundley V, Spiby H, Janssen PA. (2016) Diagnosing onset of labor: A systematic review of definitions in the research literature. *BMC Pregnancy and Childbirth* 16, 71. doi: 10.1186/s12884-016-0857-4

40. Zhang J, Landy HJ, Ware Branch D, et al. (2010) Contemporary patterns of spontaneous labor with normal neonatal outcomes. *Obstetrics & Gynecology* 116(6), 1281–1287.

41. Simkin P, Rohs K. (2018) *The Birth Partner: A Complete Guide to Childbirth for Dads, Partners, Doulas and Other Labor Companions*, 5th edn. Beverly, MA: The Harvard Common Press.

42. Sinclair C. (2004) *A Midwives' Handbook*. St Louis: Saunders.

43. Singata M, Tranmer J, Gyte GM. (2013) Restricting oral fluid and food intake during labour. *The Cochrane Database of Systematic Reviews* 2013(8), CD003930. doi: 10.1002/14651858.CD003930.pub3

44. Ciardulli A, Saccone G, Anastasio H, Berghella V. (2017) Less-restrictive food intake during labor in low-risk singleton pregnancies: A systematic review and meta-analysis. *Obstetrics and Gynecology* 129(3), 473–480. 10.1097/AOG.0000000000001898

45. Toohill J, Soong B, Flenady V. (2008) Interventions for ketosis during labour. *The Cochrane Database of Systematic Reviews* 2008(3), CD004230. doi: 10.1002/14651858.CD004230.pub2

46. Kobayashi S, Hanada N, Matsuzaki M, Takehara K, Ota E, Sasaki H, Nagata C, Mori R. (2017) Assessment and support during early labour for improving birth outcomes. *The Cochrane Database of Systematic Reviews* 4(4), CD011516. doi: 10.1002/14651858.CD011516.pub2

47. Zackler A, Flood P, Dajao R, Maramara L, Goetzl L. (2019) Suspected chorioamnionitis and myometrial contractility: Mechanisms for increased risk of cesarean delivery and postpartum hemorrhage. *Reproductive Sciences* 26(2), 178–183. doi: 10.1177/1933719118778819

48. Garite TJ, Weeks J, Peters-Phair K, Pattillo C, Brewster WR. (2000) A randomized controlled trial of the effect of increased intravenous hydration on the course of labor in nulliparous women. *American Journal of Obstetrics and Gynecology* 183(6), 1544–1548. doi: 10.1067/mob.2000.107884

49. Blankenship SA, Woolfolk CL, Raghuraman N, Stout MJ, Macones GA, Cahill AG. (2019) First stage of labor progression in women with large-for-gestational age infants. *American Journal of Obstetrics and Gynecology* 221(6), 640.e1–640.e11. doi: 10.1016/j.ajog.2019.06.042

50. Hobson SR, Abdelmalek MZ, Farine D. (2019) Update on uterine tachysystole. *Journal of Perinatal Medicine* 47(2), 152–160. doi: 10.1515/jpm-2018-0175

51. Osborne C, Ecker JL, Gauvreau K, Davidson KM., Lieberman E. (2011) Maternal temperature elevation and occiput posterior position at birth among low-risk women receiving epidural analgesia. *Journal of Midwifery & Women's Health* 56(5), 446–451. doi: 10.1111/j.1542-2011.2010.00064.x

52. Byrne D, Edmonds DK. (1990) Clinical method for evaluating progress in first stage of labour. *The Lancet* 335(8681), 122.

53. Nunes RD, Locatelli P, Traebert J. (2018) Use of the purple line to diagnose cervical dilatation and fetal head station during labor. *International Journal of Gynecology & Obstetrics* 141, 250–254.

54. Narchi NZ, da Costa Silveira de Camargo J, Salim NR, de Oliveira Menezes M, Bertolino MM. (2011) The use of the "purple line" as an auxiliary clinical method for evaluating the active phase of delivery. *Revista Brasileira de Saúde Materno Infantil* 11(3).

55. Kordi M, Irani M, Esmaily H, Tara F. (2013) Relationship between length of purple line and cervical dilation in active phase of labor. *The Iranian Journal of Obstetrics, Gynecology and Infertility* 15(37), 6–13.

56. Kordi M, Irani M, Tara F, Esmaily H. (2014) The diagnostic accuracy of purple line in prediction of labor progress in Omolbanin Hospital, Iran. *Iranian Red Crescent Medical Journal* 16(11).

57. Irani M, Kordi M, Esmaily H. (2018) Relationship between length and width of the purple line and foetal head descent in active phase of labour. *Journal of Obstetrics and Gynaecology* 38(1), 10–15.

58. Farrag RE, Eltohamy NAE. (2021) Accuracy of purple line to monitor labour progress: Longitudinal study. *Egyptian Journal of Health Care* 12(1), 30–44.

59. Housseine N, Punt MC, Browne JL, van 't Hooft J, Maaløe N, Meguid T, … Rijken MJ. (2019) Delphi consensus statement on intrapartum fetal monitoring in low-resource settings. *International Journal of Gynecology & Obstetrics* 146(1), 8–16.

60. Heazell A, Warland J, Stacey T, Coomarasamy C, Budd J, Mitchell EA, O'Brien LM. (2017) Stillbirth is associated with perceived alterations in fetal activity: Findings from an international case control study. *BMC Pregnancy and Childbirth* 17(1), 369. 10.1186/s12884-017-1555-6

61. American College of Obstetricians and Gynecologists. (2014) Practice bulletin no. 146: Management of late-term and postterm pregnancies. *Obstetrics and Gynecology* 124(2 Pt 1), 390–396. doi: 10.1097/01.AOG.0000452744.06088.48

62. Macones GA, Hankins GD, Spong CY, Hauth J, Moore T. (2008) The 2008 National Institute of Child Health and Human Development workshop report on electronic fetal monitoring: Update on definitions, interpretation, and research guidelines. *Journal of Obstetric, Gynecologic, and Neonatal Nursing: JOGNN* 37(5), 510–515. doi: 10.1111/j.1552-6909.2008.00284.x

63. American College of Obstetricians and Gynecologists. (2010) Practice bulletin no. 116: Management of intrapartum fetal heart rate tracings. *Obstetrics and Gynecology* 116(5), 1232–1240. doi: 10.1097/AOG.0b013e3182004fa9

64. Association of Women's Health, Obstetric and Neonatal Nurses. (2015) *Fetal Heart Monitoring Principles and Practices* (6th edn). Dubuque, IA: Kendall/Hunt.

65. American College of Nurse-Midwives (2015) Intermittent auscultation for intrapartum fetal heart rate surveillance. *Journal of Midwifery & Women's Health* 60(5), 626–632. doi: 10.1111/jmwh.12372

66. Dore S, Ehman W. (2020) No. 396: Fetal health surveillance: Intrapartum consensus guideline. *Journal of Obstetrics and Gynaecology of Canada: JOGC = Journal d'Obstetrique et Gynecologie du Canada: JOGC* 42(3), 316–348.e9. doi: 10.1016/j.jogc.2019.05.007

67. National Institute for Health and Care Excellence (NICE). (2014, updated 2017). Clinical guideline #190: Intrapartum care for healthy women and babies. London: NICE.

68. Ayres-de-campos D, Spong CY, Chandraharan E, & FIGO Intrapartum Fetal Monitoring Expert Consensus Panel. (2015) FIGO consensus guidelines on intrapartum fetal monitoring: Cardiotocography. *International Journal of Gynaecology and Obstetrics: The Official Journal of the International Federation of Gynaecology and Obstetrics* 131(1), 13–24. doi: 10.1016/j.ijgo.2015.06.020

69. Devane D, Lalor, JG, Daly, S, McGuire, W, Cuthbert, A, Smith, V (2017) Cardiotocography versus intermittent auscultation of fetal heart on admission to labour ward for assessment of fetal wellbeing. *The Cochrane Database of Systematic Reviews* 1(1), CD005122. doi: 10.1002/14651858.CD005122.pub5

70. Alfirevic Z, Devane D, Gyte GM, Cuthbert A. (2017) Continuous cardiotocography (CTG) as a form of electronic fetal monitoring (EFM) for fetal assessment during labour. *The Cochrane Database of Systematic Reviews* 2(2), CD006066. doi: 10.1002/14651858.CD006066.pub3

71. American College of Obstetricians and Gynecologists. (2009) Practice bulletin no. 106: Intrapartum fetal heart rate monitoring: Nomenclature, interpretation, and general management principles. *Obstetrics and Gynecology* 114(1), 192–202. doi: 10.1097/AOG.0b013e3181aef106

72. Liston R, Sawchuck D, Young D, Society of Obstetrics and Gynaecologists of Canada, & British Columbia Perinatal Health Program. (2007) Fetal health surveillance: Antepartum and intrapartum consensus guideline. *Journal of Obstetrics and Gynaecology of Canada: JOGC = Journal d'Obstetrique Et Gynecologie du Canada: JOGC* 29(9 Suppl 4), S3–S56.

73. Maude RM, Skinner JP, Foureur MJ. (2016) Putting intelligent structured intermittent auscultation (ISIA) into practice. *Women and Birth: Journal of the Australian College of Midwives* 29(3), 285–292. doi: 10.1016/j.wombi.2015.12.001

74. Hanson L. (2010) Risk management in intrapartum fetal monitoring: Accidental recording of the maternal heart rate. *The Journal of Perinatal & Neonatal Nursing* 24(1), 7–9. doi: 10.1097/JPN.0b013e3181cc4a95

75. Lawrence A, Lewis L, Hofmeyr GJ, Styles C. (2013) Maternal positions and mobility during first stage labour. *Cochrane Database of Systematic Reviews* 2013(8).

76. Cluett ER, Burns E, Cuthbert A. (2018) Immersion in water during labour and birth. *Cochrane Database of Systematic Reviews* 5(5).

77. Neumann Y. (2004). Doing a pelvic exam with a woman who has experienced sexual abuse. In: P Simkin, P Klaus (eds), *When Survivors Give Birth* (pp. 333–344). Seattle: Classic Day Publishing.

78. Goldberg J, Newman RB, Rust PF. (1997) Interobserver reliability of digital and endovaginal ultrasonographic cervical length measurements. *American Journal of Obstetrics and Gynecology* 177(4), 853–858. doi: 10.1016/s0002-9378(97)70282-5

79. Friedman E (1978). Normal labor. In: *Labor: Clinical Evaluation and Management*, 2nd edn. New York: Appleton-Century-Crofts, pp. 45–60.

80. Flint C. (1986) *Sensitive Midwifery*. Oxford: Butterworth-Heinemann Ltd.

81. Akmal S, Kametas N, Tsoi E, Hargreaves C, Nicolaides KH. (2003) Comparison of transvaginal digital examination with intrapartum sonography to determine fetal head position before instrumental delivery. *Ultrasound in Obstetrics & Gynecology: The Official Journal of the International Society of Ultrasound in Obstetrics and Gynecology* 21(5), 437–440. doi: 10.1002/uog.103

82. Hjartardóttir H, Lund SH, Benediktsdóttir S, Geirsson RT, Eggebø TM. (2021) When does fetal head rotation occur in spontaneous labor at term? Results of an ultrasound-based longitudinal study in nulliparous women. *American Journal of Obstetrics and Gynecology* 224(5), 514.e1–514.e9. doi: 10.1016/j.ajog.2020.10.054

83. Talaulikar VS, Arulkumaran S. (2015) Malpositions and malpresentations of the fetal head. *Obstetrics, Gynaecology & Reproductive Medicine* 25(6), 152–159.

84. Bamberg C, Sindhwani N, Teichgraeber U, Dudenhausen JW, Deprest J, Henrich W. (2014) Fetal head molding: Changes of fetal head diameters during active second stage of labour on open MRI scanner. *Ultrasound in Obstetrics & Gynecology* 44(S1), 318.

Chapter 5

Role of Physiologic and Pharmacologic Oxytocin in Labor Progress

Elise N. Erickson, PhD, CNM, FACNM and Nicole Carlson, PhD, CNM, FACNM, FAAN

Oxytocin is a hormone and neurotransmitter that stimulates uterine contraction during labor and after birth among other physiologic functions.[1] In its synthetic form, oxytocin is also an uterotonic medication (Pitocin/Syntocinon) that care providers may offer in situations where supportive care or physiologic interventions do not result in improvement in labor progress.[2] Synthetic oxytocin may also be used in conjunction with non-pharmacologic approaches to supporting labor progress (e.g. simultaneous oxytocin administration with ambulation or during water immersion). Oxytocin augmentation is typically offered in a hospital setting, as continuous fetal heart monitoring during administration is needed to ensure a healthy fetal response to enhanced uterine activity.[3–5]

The availability of pharmaceutical oxytocin has increased globally (which must be maintained in cold storage), and the drug is now utilized in a high percentage of births occurring in many high-resource countries, including the United States[6] and in a growing number of births in middle and lower resource countries.[7] Labor augmentation

Simkin's Labor Progress Handbook: Early Interventions to Prevent and Treat Dystocia, Fifth Edition. Edited by Lisa Hanson, Emily Malloy, and Penny Simkin.
© 2024 John Wiley & Sons Ltd. Published 2024 by John Wiley & Sons Ltd.

Uterine Tachysystole: more than 5 contractions in 10 minutes averaged over 30 minutes.

rates in the United States are not tracked systematically, however, over 30% of respondents from a national US survey said they were given oxytocin to speed labor.[6] A study in Norway documented labor augmentation with oxytocin between 30–40% for nulliparous labors and between 5–12% in multiparous labors.[8] Although oxytocin infusion can be a useful tool for helping prevent or treat labor dystocia, it is also true that oxytocin use can lead to excessive uterine activity (uterine tachysystole),[3,4] which can lead to fetal intolerance to labor and urgent need for delivery and also increase the likelihood of uterine atony or postpartum hemorrhage through receptor down regulation. Therefore, when offering oxytocin augmentation of labor, a balance between immediate clinical needs, alternative strategies for advancing labor progress, and potential for future risks must be considered. This chapter will review the function of endogenous oxytocin in physiologic labor and clinical use of synthetic oxytocin in the setting of spontaneous labor onset as a method to help promote labor progress. Considerations for individualizing the use of oxytocin augmentation by maternal characteristics, including obesity and maternal age, will also be discussed. Oxytocin use in labor induction is addressed in terms of dosing and care to various special populations of laboring people. Breastfeeding considerations and risks for postpartum hemorrhage are also addressed.

HISTORY OF OXYTOCIN DISCOVERY AND USE IN HUMAN LABOR

In 1906, a British physiologist, Sir Henry Dale, first identified oxytocin as an important biological substance.[9] He demonstrated in experiments with a pregnant cat that the substance excreted from the pituitary also caused the uterus to contract. From this point onward, oxytocin has been inextricably linked to the processes of childbirth. During the early part of the 20th century, the "substance" also known as "pitressin," was used in humans for isolated cases of prolonged labor or to expel a demised fetus.[10] Importantly, the limited record detailing the use of this pure pituitary extract is linked to devastating outcomes (uterine rupture)[11] as it likely also contained arginine vasopressin (AVP) which shares a very similar structure to oxytocin and was administered in an uncontrolled fashion. It was not until nearly 50 years later that the pharmaceutical form of oxytocin was synthesized, by American biochemist, Vincent du Vigneaud, a discovery for which he was awarded the Nobel Prize.[10] The development of stable and standardized quantities of oxytocin has since led to the widespread use of the medication in childbirth, whether it is for promotion of labor contractions or to prevent or manage postpartum uterine bleeding.

STRUCTURE AND FUNCTION OF OXYTOCIN

Oxytocin is a small peptide made up of only nine amino acids.[12] The peptide is formed primarily by the hypothalamus in mammals and is transported into the posterior pituitary and then released into circulation to function as a hormone by binding to *oxytocin receptors* throughout the body.[13] It is noted that oxytocin is released by the pituitary in a pulsatile pattern and usually in response to some external or internal stimulus.[14,15] During lactation, nipple stimulation is able to cause oxytocin release from the maternal hypothalamus and pituitary that leads to milk ejection (let-down).[16] Oxytocin also plays a role within the brain, as it binds to oxytocin receptors on adjacent neurons acting as a neurotransmitter in many important regions.[17,18] From these actions, endogenously produced oxytocin has gained a reputation for influencing certain behaviors including care of offspring and social behaviors as well as homeostatic regulation of glucose, engaging parasympathetic nervous system (lowering heart rate and blood pressure), modulating the hypothalamic-pituitary-adrenal axis (tempering cortisol/glucocorticoid secretion), and enhancing serotonin and dopamine function.[19–21]

OXYTOCIN RECEPTORS

Oxytocin must exert its effect (brain and/or body) upon available oxytocin receptors.[1] The oxytocin receptor is classified as a G-protein coupled receptor. The effect of binding oxytocin on the receptor produces two main intracellular actions, the first is a rise in intracellular calcium, which triggers smooth muscle contraction when the receptor is located on a muscle cell (or depolarization in the case of neurons). In addition, receptor binding leads to second messenger cascades, which are important for vasodilation, ion channel regulation, prostaglandin synthesis among other processes.[1] The fetal hypothalamus also makes oxytocin and prepares before birth by increasing oxytocin receptor levels as well.[22,23] Some neuroscience researchers have proposed that endogenous oxytocin helps protect the fetal brain from cell death that may occur during temporary low oxygen levels experienced during labor and birth by inhibiting neuronal activation (depolarization) which may occur in response to periods of transient hypoxemia.[24–26] Using rat pup models, endogenous oxytocin has also been shown to exert an analgesic effect on newborn pups after birth.[27]

Oxytocin receptors, when bound by oxytocin, will be temporarily unavailable for biding again (called receptor saturation). If receptors become widely bound, the body will respond to this saturation by instructing the cell to remove the receptor from the cell membrane, through a process known as internalization.[28,29] These receptors are then often degraded by the cell's lysosomes. In the presence of high concentrations of oxytocin, the nucleus of the cell further regulates receptors by decreasing the messenger RNA (the code transcribed from DNA) responsible for making more oxytocin receptors.[30] These processes are clearly complex in nature, but nonetheless important considerations as they represent one of the body's self-regulatory mechanisms. Clinicians using oxytocin during labor should appreciate these principles as the implications of receptor saturation or downregulation are important for titrating oxytocin, during prolonged labor and for postpartum uterine tone/hemorrhage.[28,31] This is particularly important because in the course of labor, passage of time is often a key consideration, and restoring downregulated or desensitized receptors can take several hours. An "oxytocin holiday" or "rest" has been studied, McAdow (2020) and colleagues found that among individuals having a labor induction and a prolonged latent phase (at least eight hours of oxytocin without cervical change), stopping oxytocin for at least eight hours was related to a 67% reduction in cesarean birth compared those who were not given a rest.[32] Further studies by Balki et al. (2016) showed that uterine tissue samples obtained during cesarean births had decreased uterine activity after initial exposure to oxytocin which persisted for 6 hours.[33] Recent research from large clinical databases supports this finding as it was shown that during low-risk labor and vaginal birth, higher rates of postpartum hemorrhage are seen after only 4 hours of labor augmentation.[34]

OXYTOCIN AND SPONTANEOUS LABOR ONSET AND PROGRESSION

Oxytocin is often discussed as being important for the normal physiologic labor process.[35] However, this belief has been challenged by several reports. Researchers have shown that genetically modified mice (that lack the oxytocin receptors) are able to achieve pregnancy and give birth as expected, however, they lacked both the ability to produce milk or to provide appropriate maternal care, resulting in pup death.[36] Interestingly, these studies also found genetically altered mice, lacking oxytocin receptors, went on to develop obesity, which had led to interesting work on the connection between oxytocin and metabolism.[37,38] In humans, a case series of four pregnant individuals with dysfunctional pituitary glands also found that labor initiation took place in the absence of what would be normal oxytocin secretion from the maternal hypothalamus.[39] On the other hand, prostaglandin receptor deficient mice (genetically modified) do not start labor spontaneously.[40] Notably, the placenta can also synthesize oxytocin thus, it may play a localized role in the progression of labor, particularly in prostaglandin production from within the uterine lining tissue formed during early gestation (decidua) or by causing uterine muscle contraction.[41] This evidence underscores that oxytocin likely plays a supporting role in the physiology of labor *onset*. While oxytocin *can* cause uterine contractions, other fetal/placental hormonal signals precede the upregulation of oxytocin receptors, for example, higher estradiol, prostaglandin formation, and corticotrophin releasing hormone. Researchers have shown that the maternal hypothalamus produces oxytocin in higher quantities when labor is more established, that is, during the late first stage, second, and third stages in particular,[35] Classic experiments with pregnant cow, sheep, and goat models demonstrated that vaginal distension (not cervical dilation) with a balloon catheter causes oxytocin to release into circulation from the maternal brain (i.e. Ferguson reflex).[42] In human birth, vaginal distension typically occurs in the final minutes/hours of labor, therefore it seems that this reflex may be important for helping accomplish the second stage and to help expel the placenta. The most compelling role for oxytocin in perinatal physiology is actually after the birth, for the onset of lactation as well for typical maternal behaviors and stress modulation,[43] at least in experimental models.

PROMOTING ENDOGENOUS OXYTOCIN FUNCTION IN SPONTANEOUS LABOR

Many studies link oxytocin secretion to warm and positive social interactions.[44,45] However, oxytocin is also released from the hypothalamus during periods of stress. This oxytocin (in the hypothalamus) helps to counter future stress-linked hormone release (i.e. cortisol).[46] However, during periods of excessive stress, fear or panic the stress hormones like epinephrine (B-adrenergic receptor agonists) may potentially counteract the effect of available oxytocin by causing uterine relaxation.[47,48] This link between stress and oxytocin is the topic of many research studies in psychology and neurobiology, particularly in the context of childbearing and postpartum care.[49–51] It is important to note that much of what is understood regarding oxytocin function has been generated from rodent or other animal research, and it is hypothesized to apply to human experience, but many experiments of this nature would be unethical in pregnant humans. Stress does appear to inhibit parturition progress in some mammals[52,53] (and can inhibit milk ejection as well).[54] Regardless, in the context of childbirth, from this neurobiological perspective, supporting the laboring person's oxytocin secretion may serve to counterbalance the stress of labor but also serve to promote some labor progress.[55,56]

Researchers have linked social support in labor to more effective labor progress and less need for pain relief.[57–59] Some speculate that dedicated support may influence oxytocin function and stress responses as well as promoting the right counter-balance to the stress of labor and uterine contractility.[56] Conversely, severe stress, abuse, anxiety or isolation may be associated with abnormal labor progress or perception of greater severity of pain.[60] A lack of supportive care may also connect oxytocin dysregulation or excessive adrenergic stimulation with abnormal labor progress.[56]

Suggestions for promoting effective oxytocin function include activities that either directly help release oxytocin or those that limit anxiety or fear may include:

- Continuous social support
- Feeling of safety, addressing safety concerns
- Slow controlled inhalation and exhalation
- Limiting fear-inducing stimuli: loud noises, harsh lights
- Light touch on arms/legs (depending on if a person likes this kind of touch)
- Foot massage
- Nipple stimulation
- Pleasant smells (essential oils)

However, each person's neuro-hormonal response for any of these suggestions may be based on their prior experiences with certain stimuli.[45,61] For example, if light touch or nipple stimulation is associated with a prior trauma, a laboring individual may in fact find these methods fear-inducing (triggering) rather than helping limit fear/anxiety. There is some evidence that individuals with post-traumatic stress have different oxytocin function than those without past trauma.[62–68]

ETHICAL CONSIDERATIONS IN OXYTOCIN ADMINISTRATION

Synthetic oxytocin has been an important piece of the obstetric toolkit for nearly 70 years.[2] However, this medication also represents an example of the "too much too soon, too little too late" shortcomings of obstetric care from the global view.[69]

Long delays in the initiation of indicated labor augmentation may pose risks to maternal or fetal health including:

- intra-amniotic infection (chorioamnionitis), sepsis
- newborn NICU admission
- more difficult cesarean births
- obstetric fistula (more common in areas where cesarean is not readily available)
- postpartum hemorrhage (particularly in the setting of infection or cesarean after long labor)

5

However, the ubiquitous use of oxytocin for labor management can also lead to:

- labor that is faster or more painful than necessary (and possible need for more pharmacologic pain management)
- more restrictions on the laboring person's movement
- iatrogenic fetal intolerance to labor due to hyperstimulation of the uterus (and possible need for urgent delivery)
- increased likelihood of postpartum hemorrhage or need for additional postpartum uterotonic medications.

For these reasons, some laboring people (and some care providers) may be reluctant to use oxytocin, particularly when other non-pharmacologic options have not been tried, or the rationale for use of oxytocin has not been explained. It is therefore important that when oxytocin use is clinically indicated, a process of shared decision making be initiated with the laboring person and their support team to discuss the rationale for use, alternatives, risks, and benefits.[70] Following shared decision making, if a person declines oxytocin, the right of the laboring person to nonpharmacologic augmentation should be honored. Another opportunity to individualize oxytocin dosing, or minimize duration (and possibly the risks associated with it) would be to trial discontinuing oxytocin after active phase labor is reached. Although more research is needed, researchers have demonstrated that this strategy may help minimize fetal intolerance to oxytocin-stimulated uterine contractions and uterine tachysystole; though the length of active labor may be longer on average, neonatal outcomes do not appear to differ in terms of cord blood acidosis.[71]

OXYTOCIN USE

Considerations for starting oxytocin during labor may include many of the items listed below. Depending on the answers to these questions, oxytocin administration may or may not be the optimal solution to the labor progress issue. Table 5.1 provides an overview of the considerations with oxytocin use that will be presented in this section:

- What phase of labor is the person in? Oxytocin augmentation should be reserved for active phase labor. If initiated in latent phase, oxytocin is used as part of a labor induction.
- For how long has progress of cervical dilation, effacement or station been unchanged?
- What is the fetal health status?
- Are there concerns about intraamniotic infection (chorioamnionitis)?
- What is the status of the bag of water?
- Is an epidural in use?

Table 5.1. Key considerations and opportunities to individualize oxytocin administration.

Indications	Considerations	Alternatives	Actions
Fatigue Fever Prolonged or prelabor rupture of membranes Prolonged labor Maternal request	What definition of prolonged labor is being used to assess normal progress? Has the definition of abnormal labor been met or highly likely to occur? Is the cervix ripened? If NOT, reconsider oxytocin in favor of ripening methods. Is there any evidence of fetal compromise? If YES: reconsider risks of augmentation and move to delivery via Cesarean or assisted vaginal birth if appropriate	Endogenous oxytocin function • nipple stimulation • massage • promotion of safety Hydration, energy (food) Ambulation Position changes Amniotomy (if appropriate)	Shared decision making, consent given prior to augmentation of labor Individualize dosing strategy Consider higher doses as appropriate (BMI) Consider discontinuation after having sufficient progress in labor Watch for abnormal fetal heart tracing Anticipate post-birth uterine atony

- Are there concerns about maternal exhaustion or dehydration with ongoing labor?
- Are there any characteristics of the laboring person which might lead to slower labor, including above-normal range BMI? If so, consider watchful waiting as part of an individualized labor approach.

An important consideration when offering oxytocin is whether or not the bag of waters is intact or ruptured. If intact, depending on parity, the phase of labor, contraction pattern and station of the fetal head, amniotomy may be a reasonable alternative to oxytocin to release prostaglandins and stimulate more endogenously driven contractility for labor augmentation. Breast or nipple massage/stimulation may also be a source for helping a labor progress as well via endogenous oxytocin production, though, may not be effective in all circumstances.

OXYTOCIN USE DURING LATENT PHASE LABOR

In latent labor, the cervix may dilate slowly as effacement and softening are often required prior to advanced dilation in spontaneous labor. Because latent phase (onset of labor to 5–6 centimeters) may take up to 18 hours in non-obese and 20–25 hours or more in obese laboring individuals people,[72] use of oxytocin may be indicated based on factors unrelated to a specific length of time. Use of oxytocin during latent phase labor (or following rupture of membranes/prodromal labor) might be better characterized as a labor induction rather than augmentation. It is important to consider cervical status before starting oxytocin in this setting; ripening of the cervix (with prostaglandins or other mechanical methods) to a Bishop score of 6 (multiparous) or 8 (nulliparous) is advised before oxytocin is initiated in latent phase.[73]

Indications for labor induction during latent labor include:

- Up to 18 hours of latent labor (20–25 hours or more in person with obesity) without achieving active phase labor
- Maternal exhaustion (in this situation, therapeutic rest may also be reasonable)
- Fever, signs of intra-amniotic infection
- Prelabor rupture of membranes (PROM):
  ◦ Note that PROM does not necessitate labor interventions, but should be part of a process of shared decision making.[74] A period of expectant management and watchful waiting is often appropriate and may lead to less use of other interventions (i.e. oxytocin, epidural etc.)[75]

OXYTOCIN USE DURING ACTIVE PHASE LABOR

Indications for labor augmentation with oxytocin in active phase labor (6 cm or more) may include:

- Inadequate uterine contractions following epidural placement (after 2 hours)
- Following no cervical change in active phase for 2–4 hours when the condition of the laboring person and fetus are reassuring.
- For multiparous (history of prior labor), consider that dilation typically advances more rapidly in the active phase. Therefore, no change in 2 hours in a multiparous active phase labor may be considered slow/protracted.[76]

Importantly, a provider should consider progress in further effacement or fetal station in addition to a dilation. One should also consider variability in cervical assessment between different examiners before deeming that progress is adequate or inadequate.

- Fever, signs of intra-amniotic infection
- Physiologic labor typically accelerates after 6 cm, therefore augmentation for lack of cervical change should be considered after a shorter interval of time than in latent first stage
- A partograph-based approach may be useful in determining the appropriate waiting time relative to the phase of labor.[77]

OXYTOCIN USE DURING SECOND STAGE LABOR

At times, a labor may reach full dilation and then a period of rest or spacing of uterine contractions may occur in those without epidural. In this setting, assuming fetal status is reassuring, a period of watchful waiting, offering time to rest or position changes will lead to a resumption of labor and an urge to push. Rotation of a mal-positioned fetus may help resume labor progress in the 2nd stage, ensuring adequate hydration or need for glucose (energy) may also help resolve the problem without need for oxytocin administration. Once active pushing begins:

- Labor progress is assessed hourly in the expulsive second stage.
- Assessment may be made by visualization (presence of perineal/rectal bulging, visualization of fetal scalp), and thus does not always require internal examination.
- Oxytocin may be indicated if uterine contractions become spaced out (>5min apart), maternal exhaustion or weak expulsive efforts are noted.
- If no progress is noted in 1 hour of pushing, offering oxytocin augmentation of the second stage may help avoid cesarean birth, prolonged pushing, onset of infection (particularly when labor had already been prolonged) and/or maternal exhaustion.
- Physiologic doses of oxytocin (<12mU/min) in the second stage tend to work well for laboring persons who have not yet received oxytocin augmentation.
- Laboring persons who receive more than 4 hours of oxytocin augmentation in first stage labor will likely require higher doses of oxytocin in the second stage.

CHANGES IN CONTEMPORARY POPULATIONS AND LABOR PROGRESS

One critically important consideration in the decision to recommend oxytocin to a particular person is whether or not their labor pattern is truly slower than normal, unless another rationale exists for labor augmentation (i.e. prolonged ruptured membranes or maternal exhaustion). Definitions of prolonged labor have been reassessed with recent research in modern populations.[76] Given that oxytocin is labeled a "high-alert medication," and inappropriate use is a primary cause of preventable perinatal harm,[78,79] providers should avoid ordering oxytocin according to outdated definitions of abnormal labor progress to prevent iatrogenic harm whenever possible.

Compared to historic studies of labor duration, investigators of modern labor studies demonstrate that progress through labor is slower and active phase labor initiates at more advanced cervical dilatation. The reasons for this are multifold, including increased use of labor interventions including early labor hospital admission and epidurals in contemporary populations. Epidural use is highly linked to oxytocin administration, with more than 75% of labors involving epidural were also having labor induced or augmented with oxytocin in a United States population study from 2003.[80]

However, the most profound factor associated with slower progression in contemporary laboring individuals is higher maternal weight at the time of labor. Research has demonstrated that labor lengthens with higher body mass index (BMI) (Table 5.2). For example, nulliparous individuals who have a BMI of >35 kg/m^2 can take up to 7 hours longer than people with a BMI of <30 kg/m^2 to dilate from 4–10 cm, while people with a BMI (25–30) labor will likely only be up to 0.6 hours longer.[72] As a result of their naturally slower labors, laboring people with high BMIs are more often augmented with oxytocin than people in lower weight ranges.[81,82] The greatest difference in dilation speed among larger-bodied laboring people compared to those who are smaller-bodied occurs during latent and early first stage labor (4–7 cm), while transition and 2nd stage labor tend to proceed similarly, regardless of BMI. Thus, most larger-bodied people will not initiate active phase labor until at least 6 cm dilation.

Slow labor progress for people with a BMI over 30 is theorized to be the result of less forceful and less coordinated uterine muscle cell function. Multiple physiologic alterations occurring in pregnant people of size appear to cause less forceful and coordinated myometrial contractions (myometrial dysfunction), including decreased uterine muscle mass,[83] leptin resistance,[84] hypercholesterolemia,[84] and changes in fatty acid activation.[85,86] Individuals of size may also have altered levels of endogenous oxytocin production or may have genetic differences in oxytocin function (oxytocin receptor genotype).[87–90]

Table 5.2.   Adjusted median duration of labor in hours by body mass index (kg/m^2).

	BMI at Labor Onset					*p* value for trend
	< 25.0	**25.0–29.9**	**30.0–34.9**	**35.0–39.9**	**≥ 40**	
Nulliparous	5.4 (18.2)	5.7 (18.8)	6.0 (19.9)	6.7 (22.2)	7.7 (25.6)	< .0001
Multiparous	4.6 (17.5)	4.5 (17.4)	4.7 (17.9)	5.0 (19.0)	5.4 (20.6)	< .0001

Note: Adjusted for age, height, race, gestational age, diabetes, induction, augmentation, epidural (first stage), operative vaginal delivery, and birthweight. Adapted from "Contemporary Labor Patterns: The Impact of Maternal Body Mass Index," by M. A. Kominiarek et al., 2011, *American Journal of Obstetrics and Gynecology, 205*, p. 244.e.1–244.e8.

OXYTOCIN DOSING

When given intravenously during labor, oxytocin is dosed in milliUnits/minute (mU/min), typically administered via pump or by visually counting infused drops per minute if an electronic IV pump is not available (Table 5.3). One unit (1000 mU) is equal to 1.67 micrograms of synthetic oxytocin.[35] The "physiologic" level of oxytocin produced endogenously during spontaneous labor is equivalent to a synthetic oxytocin infusion rate of 5–10 mU/min and a rate of 11–13 mU/min is identified as where most people with achieve adequate contractions and birth[35,91]; however, as mentioned previously, endogenous oxytocin levels (and density of receptors) during the labor process demonstrate wide variations according to the person's age, Bishop score, gestational age, BMI, genetic factors, and parity.[92] Therefore, it is important that providers closely observe the response of the laboring person and their fetus during oxytocin infusion.

High dose/low dose

Dosing protocols for oxytocin to augment labor fall into two general categories: high dose or low dose. In a high-dose regimen, the oxytocin infusion rate is initiated at 6 mU/min, then increased by 1–6 mU/min every 15–40 minutes with a maximum dose of 40 mU/min. In a low-dose regimen (Table 5.2), oxytocin is initiated at a rate of 0.5–1 mU/min, then increased by 1–2 mU/min every 15–40 minutes to a maximum dose of 20–40 mU/min. Although supported by obstetrics professional organizations,[93,94] these dosing protocols are not based on the pharmacokinetics of synthetic oxytocin, and the high-dose protocol violates the principle of using the lowest dose possible of a drug which achieves a desired effect. In a Cochrane meta-analysis of high- vs. low-dose oxytocin regimens, investigators found that high-dose regimens were associated with uterine hyperstimulation, but were not different for cesarean birth or maternal/neonatal morbidity/mortality compared to low-dose regimens.[95] Given that oxytocin has a half-life of 10–12 minutes and it takes 30–60 minutes to achieve a steady state of this medication after any titration change,[2,35] the high-dose oxytocin regimen may increase maternal and fetal risks, especially if they are maintained over long periods of time. Table 5.3 contains a comparison of low-dose guidelines for the use of synthetic oxytocin.

VARIATION IN OXYTOCIN DOSING AMONG SPECIAL POPULATIONS

Higher body mass index

There is evidence that laboring people with obesity require higher doses of oxytocin, infused for longer periods of time, to achieve vaginal birth.[82,97] For example, in a retrospective analysis of oxytocin doses in 118 laboring people in spontaneous labor with arrest of dilation,[98] those who with morbid obesity (BMI ≥ 35 kg/m2) required significantly more oxytocin than groups with lower BMI ranges during the first 3 hours of infusion (800 mU vs. 500–600 mU, *P* = .003), yet nevertheless had the highest rates of unplanned cesarean birth following oxytocin augmentation (69.6% vs. 11.4%–34.3% among groups of people with lower BMI ranges). In a recent study,[99] the mean

Table 5.3. Clinical guidance for use of synthetic oxytocin.

Low-Dose Oxytocin Protocols				Clinical Guidance
	AWHONN	ACOG	SOGC[96]	The "physiologic" level of oxytocin produced endogenously during spontaneous labor is equivalent to a synthetic oxytocin infusion rate of 5–10 mU/min[35,91]
Starting dose (mU/min)	1	0.5–2	1–2	Infusion rates of 8–13 mU/min cause most laboring people to experience adequate contractions and cervical change.
Increment dose (mU/min)	1–2	1–2	1–2	After active phase labor acceleration, consider an oxytocin holiday by reducing or discontinuing the infusion rate to possibly decrease risk of adverse side effects.
Frequency of dose increase (minutes)	30–60	15–40	30	**Potential Adverse Side Effects** • Uterine tachysystole • Fetal heart rate changes • Meconium staining of amniotic fluid • Placental abruption
Maximum dose (mU/min)	20	None	30	• Amniotic fluid embolism • Water intoxication and hyponatremia (provide electrolyte solution IV or orally)

Abbreviations: ACOG, American College of Obstetricians and Gynecologists; AWHONN, Association of Women's Health, Obstetric and Neonatal Nurses; SOGC, The Society of Obstetricians and Gynaecologists of Canada; IOL, induction of labor; SOL, spontaneous onset of labor; mU, milliunits; min, minutes.

cumulative oxytocin dose increased with BMI group (2278 U normal weight BMI, 3108 mU overweight, 4082 mU obese, $P < .001$), and these differences were predicted by higher fetal birth weights, more frequent use of epidural analgesia, and the less advanced cervical dilation when oxytocin was initiated. Thus, delaying the use of epidural and using physiologic labor interventions may assist laboring people with obesity to avoid exposure to excess oxytocin. For example, in otherwise healthy nulliparous people with obesity, hydrotherapy use in the latent-to-active phase transition (4–6 cm dilation) by midwifery care providers decreased rates of oxytocin augmentation compared to similar people laboring with physician providers who used less hydrotherapy.[100]

Although intrauterine pressure catheters are recommended to ascertain if contractions are "adequate" during labor augmentation for labor dystocia,[101] there is evidence that laboring people with obesity have a longer labor course than people with non-obese BMIs, despite having contractions with similar strength. Thus, the best approach to a long labor course in an otherwise healthy laboring person with obesity is to provide supportive care, reassurance, and patience as suggested in a "watchful waiting"[102] model of care while delaying oxytocin initiation using physiologic interventions for as long as possible, then infusing oxytocin over longer periods of time to achieve vaginal birth safely.

Nullipara

It is well known that labor proceeds more slowly for individuals having their first birth (including first vaginal birth after cesarean) compared to others who are multiparous. It is therefore important that oxytocin augmentation be individualized based on parity. When augmentation is used, there is some evidence from a large US cohort that higher-dose compared to low-dose oxytocin protocols decreased the duration of first stage labor in nulliparous people (compared to regimen starting at 1 mU/min, regimen starting at 2 mU/min was 0.8 hours faster (95% confidence interval 0.5–1.1) and regimen starting at 4 mU/min was 1.3 hours faster [1.0–1.7]).[103] However, providers should remember that oxytocin is far more likely to be successful (owing to adequate oxytocin receptors) when there is a Bishop score of ≥ 8 for nulliparous individuals.[73]

Maternal age

Increasing maternal age is significantly related to higher likelihood of having Cesarean birth. However, higher age is not necessarily linked to longer labor. One study of individuals who achieved full dilation found that advancing age was associated with shorter duration of labor, or faster progress (this study considered induced and spontaneous labors together). In that study, investigators found that nulliparous individuals who are less than 20 years of age labored for more than 2 hours longer than those who are 30–40 years old (17.2 hours in ≤20 year group vs. 15.1 hours in 30–40 year group at 95% median traverse times for dilation from 4–10 cm).[104] A limitation of that study is that people who were undergoing Cesarean before full dilation were not included, thus we cannot say if all labors progress more quickly with age. In fact, another interpretation of the study is that care providers were willing to be more patient with younger individuals in labor and more likely to move to cesarean with older aged people. However, other studies of human tissue and rodent models show that response to oxytocin does appear to decrease with advancing age.[105–108] Researchers think this may have to do with higher cholesterol or lipids in the tissue, which may reduce the uterine muscle's effectiveness. Given that individuals of advanced age are often recommended to have labor induction for obstetric or medical reasons or to minimize risk for unexplained stillbirth (associated with advanced maternal age), a high dosing strategy (increases by 2 or 4mU/min) thus might be worth considering in parturient individuals over 35 or 40.

EPIDURAL

Use of epidural in latent phase is often followed by oxytocin augmentation, as contractions may weaken or space out after epidural placement.[109–111] This phenomenon occurs commonly and may be due to a number of variables including:

- Decreased blood flow to the uterus as epidural blocks sympathetic nerves (T10-L1) and lowers catecholamine release, which can result in a decreased blood pressure or cause fetal bradycardia[112]
- Lower levels of oxytocin in circulation[113] (if labor is not being augmented)
- Lower levels of cortisol, which may be a stimulus for oxytocin release[114,115]
- Fluid boluses given intravenously during epidural placement
- Inability to ambulate or with a recumbent posture

Some practitioners will opt to actively manage labor once epidural is placed, regardless of any objective findings (lack of cervical change). However, more recent research indicates that patient-controlled epidural pumps may have less inhibition on uterine activity.[116] Thus, providers should use patient-controlled epidural pumps when available, and consider delaying oxytocin augmentation for several hours after epidural placement to allow fluid and oxytocin levels to normalize. If oxytocin augmentation is initiated post-epidural, providers should carefully titrate dosing to avoid uterine overstimulation.

PROBLEMS ASSOCIATED WITH HIGHER DOSES OR LONGER OXYTOCIN INFUSION

Postpartum hemorrhage

Due to receptor saturation or downregulation that occurs during both longer labor and with more than a few hours of oxytocin during labor, higher doses of oxytocin are often necessary to achieve an effective uterine contraction after the birth during the third/fourth stages. This pharmacologic issue is one of the more concerning recent trends in oxytocin use.[34,117] With longer intrapartum exposure or higher dosage, the uterus is more likely to become atonic after delivery and result in postpartum hemorrhage (PPH) and be less responsive to postpartum oxytocin treatment.[118] Indeed, recent research showed that oxytocin labor augmentation for as little as 4 hours was associated with a 2.4 times increased odds for postpartum hemorrhage among low-risk labors resulting in vaginal birth.[34] Thus, providers need to be aware that using oxytocin for prevention/treatment of postpartum bleeding may be less effective and to include this kind of information in the risk/benefit discussion when recommending oxytocin augmentation.

Fetal Intolerance to labor

Another adverse event commonly linked to labor augmentation with oxytocin is fetal heart rate abnormalities or "fetal intolerance to labor." With every contraction, the blood flow to the spaces between the maternal surface of the placenta is greatly decreased when pressure reaches 35 mmHg and is absent above 60 mmHg.[119] Therefore, it follows logically that increasing the frequency with which contractions occur with labor augmentation will result in progressively less oxygenated blood flow and the potential for buildup of fetal carbon dioxide and lactate.[120] When this occurs, the fetal heart tracing may begin is show signs suggesting acidemia (i.e. minimal variability or recurrent decelerations). Indeterminate (Category II) fetal tracings make up a large percentage of the indications for cesarean birth,[121,122] however, Category II tracings have low sensitivity to predict a poor outcome or impending acidemia, that is, most cesareans for category II tracings result in the birth of an uncompromised newborn.[123] It is probable that a fetus who is not tolerating oxytocin-stimulated labor may not have tolerated a spontaneous "non-stimulated" labor. However, the likelihood for over stimulation of the uterus much higher with oxytocin use. Unfortunately, evidence is limited on how to appropriately treat tachysystole.[124] Recently emphasis has been placed on titrating oxytocin for adequate contractions patterns but also for ensuring adequate rest between contractions (at least 60 seconds between the completion of one contraction to the beginning of the next).

If oxytocin administration has been helpful in advancing labor, but fetal heart rate tracing or hypertonus of the uterus are concerns, titrating the medication down (half the current dose[2]) is appropriate to ensure adequate rest. Other strategies for helping support a fetus through stronger uterine contractions include:

- Position changes (particularly lateral side-lying or hands and knees)
- Fluid bolus (500 mL lactated ringers or normal saline)
- Encourage taking slow breaths to help keep well-oxygenated, avoid panic or breath-holding due to fear or pain (however, use of exogenous oxygen has not been found to be helpful according to new research).[125]
- In some circumstances (fetal bradycardia or worsening repetitive decelerations) oxytocin should be discontinued until the fetal heart patterns stabilize.

Oxytocin holiday

During the acceleration of active phase labor when uterine oxytocin receptors are activated, oxytocin infusions can be discontinued or decreased to help minimize possible risks. While this strategy has been studied in the setting of labor induction,[71,126,127] it may also be helpful in the setting of labor augmentation to decrease rates of cesarean birth particularly in the setting of fetal intolerance of labor related to uterine activity or tachysystole.

Breastfeeding and beyond

Despite the knowledge of receptor desensitization in uterine tissues during labor stimulation with oxytocin, little is known about oxytocin receptor responses within other tissues of the body.[43] Concerns have been raised in the experimental literature as well as in popular media about longer-term concerns about oxytocin use during labor. Despite these discussions, very little can be concluded from the existing research data. Among most studies that have considered the relationship between oxytocin use and breastfeeding, it is notable that no studies have demonstrated that breastfeeding performance or longevity has been improved when oxytocin is given during labor.[128] However, this does not mean that oxytocin administration necessarily harms the onset or duration of lactation. There are many intertwined variables involved when considering why labor augmentation is needed or used and also why breastfeeding is successful or not.

A few studies have noted that newborn feeding reflexes appear diminished after oxytocin use leading to being less likely to achieve an early post-birth latch.[129–131] Some of these have noted that this effect may also be related epidural analgesia administration. Whether this has a lasting impact on lactation overall is still being investigated, though some studies have not found an association with early cessation after controlling for other factors like BMI or cesarean birth without labor.[132,133]

Some studies have been conducted examining the role for oxytocin function in maternal mood or development of postnatal depression.[134] Indeed oxytocin function/dysfunction has been linked in animal work as well as in human samples to depressed mood or maternal behavior.[135–137] Oxytocin given during the labor has been linked to postpartum depression[138,139] but one should consider that differences in oxytocin function before pregnancy might influence one's tendency to develop a mood disorder or to require more oxytocin in labor as well. More research in this domain is needed before firm conclusions can be made. What birth care providers and companions can take way from this ongoing area of research is that people with more complex labors may need additional support for achieving a successful transition to milk production and mood stability and anticipatory guidance for resources and support should be offered.

NEW AREAS OF OXYTOCIN RESEARCH

Emerging research in how oxytocin is regulated in the body may one day influence how labor is managed. For example, oxytocin receptor genotype research[140,141,142] has found that some individuals may be more likely to require higher doses of oxytocin during labor because of genetic differences in their receptor gene compared to those who do not require high doses. Pharmaceutical researchers have also been studying a more potent oxytocin form (with a much longer half-life) for the prevention or treatment of postpartum hemorrhage (carbetocin).[143] Furthermore, blocking the oxytocin receptor has been an area of interest in helping avoid preterm birth by using an oxytocin antagonist (atosiban). Though this research has not proved that atosiban is highly effective in all cases of preterm birth, it may be given in certain countries in an attempt to slow preterm labor.[144]

CONCLUSION

Oxytocin, both in endogenous and exogenous forms, plays an important role in the birth tool kit for helping promote physiologic labor progress or treat labor dystocia or prolonged labor. An appreciation of the regulation of oxytocin function is important to both physiologic and pharmacologically stimulated labor. Understanding when oxytocin use is indicated as well as the contraindications and alternatives to oxytocin infusion will help maximize the likelihood of safe use of this medication and healthy vaginal birth. Labor augmentation with oxytocin should occur in the setting of informed consent, access to continuous fetal heart rate monitoring and access to surgical services. Providers should aim to individualize their use of oxytocin including using the most suitable dose for the appropriate length of time. Finally, providers should anticipate and respond appropriately to complications including uterine tachysystole, abnormal fetal heart tracings or postpartum hemorrhage.

REFERENCES

1. Arrowsmith S, Wray S. (2014) Oxytocin: Its mechanism of action and receptor signalling in the myometrium. *Journal of Neuroendocrinology* 26(6), 356–369. doi: 10.1111/jne.12154
2. Page K, McCool WF, Guidera M. (2017) *Examination of the Pharmacology of Oxytocin and Clinical Guidelines for Use in Labor.* Vol. 200. American College of Nurse-Midwives. 9. doi: 10.1111/jmwh.12610
3. Clark SL, Meyers JA, Frye DK, Garthwaite T, Lee AJ, Perlin JB. (2015) Recognition and response to electronic fetal heart rate patterns: Impact on newborn outcomes and primary cesarean delivery rate in women undergoing induction of labor. *American Journal of Obstetrics and Gynecology* 212(4), 494.e1–6. doi: 10.1016/j.ajog.2014.11.019
4. Sundin C, Mazac L, Ellis K, Garbo C. (2018) Implementation of an oxytocin checklist to improve clinical outcomes. *MCN American Journal of Maternal/Child Nursing* 43(3), 133–138. doi: 10.1097/NMC.0000000000000428
5. World Health Organization, (ed) (2014) *WHO Recommendations for Augmentation of Labour.* World Health Organization.
6. Declercq ER, Sakala, C, Corry, MP, Applebaum, S, Herrlich, A. (2014) Major survey findings of listening to mothers(SM) III: New mothers speak out: Report of national surveys of women's childbearing experiences conducted October-December 2012 and January-April 2013. *Journal of Perinatal Education* 23(1), 17–24.

7. Litorp H, Sunny AK, Kc, A. (2021) Augmentation of labor with oxytocin and its association with delivery outcomes: A large-scale cohort study in 12 public hospitals in Nepal. *Acta Obstetricia Et Gynecologica Scandinavica* 100(4), 684–693. doi: 10.1111/aogs.13919

8. Rossen J, Østborg TB, Lindtjørn E, Schulz J, Eggebø TM. (2016) Judicious use of oxytocin augmentation for the management of prolonged labor. *Acta Obstetricia Et Gynecologica Scandinavica* Published online. doi: 10.1111/aogs.12821

9. Ottenhausen M, Bodhinayake I, Banu MA, Stieg PE, Schwartz TH. (2015) Vincent du Vigneaud: Following the sulfur trail to the discovery of the hormones of the posterior pituitary gland at Cornell Medical College. *Journal of Neurosurgery* Published online October. 124, 1–5.

10. Douglas RG, Bonsnes RW. (1955) Natural and synthetic oxytocin: Preliminary report on the use of both for the induction and stimulation of labor. *obstetrics* Published online January. http://journals.lww.com/greenjournal/Abstract/1955/09000/Natural_and_Synthetic_Oxytocin__Preliminary_report.2.aspx

11. Holmes JM. (1954) The use of continuous intravenous oxytocin in obstetrics. *The Lancet* 264(6850), 1191–1193. doi: 10.1016/S0140-6736(54)92258-8

12. Insel T. (1992) Oxytocin–a neuropeptide for affiliation: Evidence from behavioral, receptor autoradiographic, and comparative studies. *Psychoneuroendocrinology* 17(1), 3–35.

13. Swaab D, Pool C, Nijveldt F. (1975) Immunofluorescence of vasopressin and oxytocin in the rat hypothalamo-neurohypophypopseal system. *Journal of Neural Transmission* 36(3–4), 195–215.

14. Neumann ID, Wigger A, Torner L, Holsboer F, Landgraf R. (2000) Brain oxytocin inhibits basal and stress-induced activity of the hypothalamo-pituitary-adrenal axis in male and female rats: Partial action within the paraventricular nucleus. *Journal of Neuroendocrinology* Published online. doi: 10.1046/j.1365-2826.2000.00442.x

15. Jonas W, Johansson LM, Nissen E, Ejdebäck M, Ransjö-Arvidson AB, Uvnäs-Moberg K. (2009) Effects of intrapartum oxytocin administration and epidural analgesia on the concentration of plasma oxytocin and prolactin, in response to suckling during the second day postpartum. *Breastfeeding Medicine* 4(2), 71–82. doi: 10.1089/bfm.2008.0002

16. Bruckmaier RM. (2005) Normal and disturbed milk ejection in dairy cows. *Domestic Animal Endocrinology* 29(2), 268–273.

17. Feldman R, Monakhov M, Pratt M, Ebstein RP. (2016) Oxytocin pathway genes: Evolutionary ancient system impacting on human affiliation, sociality, and psychopathology. *Biological Psychiatry* 79(3), 174–184. doi: 10.1016/j.biopsych.2015.08.008

18. Ludwig M. (2014) Dendritic release of the neuropeptides vasopressin and oxytocin. In: WE Armstrong, JG Tasker (eds.), *Neurophysiology of Neuroendocrine Neurons.* John Wiley & Sons, Ltd, 207–223. http://doi.wiley.com/10.1002/9781118606803.ch9

19. Quintana DS, Guastella AJ. (2020) An allostatic theory of oxytocin. *Trends in Cognitive Sciences* Published online. doi: 10.1016/j.tics.2020.03.008

20. Carter CS. (2018) Oxytocin and human evolution. *Current Topics in Behavioral Neurosciences* 35, 291–319. doi: 10.1007/7854_2017_18

21. Ding C, Leow MKS, Magkos F. (2019) Oxytocin in metabolic homeostasis: Implications for obesity and diabetes management. *Obesity Reviews* 20(1), 22–40. doi: 10.1111/obr.12757

22. Schubert F, George JM, Rao MB. (1981) Vasopressin and oxytocin content of human fetal brain at different stages of gestation. *Brain Research* 213(1), 111–117.

23. Endoh H, Fujioka T, Endo H, Inazuka Y, Furukawa S, Nakamura S. (2008) Stimulation of fetal hypothalamus induces uterine contractions in pregnant rats at term. *Biology of Reproduction* 79(4), 633–637.

24 Tyzio R, Cossart R, Khalilov I, et al. (2006) Maternal oxytocin triggers a transient inhibitory switch in GABA signaling in the fetal brain during delivery. *Science* Published online. doi: 10.1126/science.1133212

25. Kenkel WM, Perkeybile AM, Yee JR, et al. (2019) Behavioral and epigenetic consequences of oxytocin treatment at birth. *Science Advances* 5(5), 1–11. doi: 10.1126/sciadv.aav2244

26. Rokicki J, Kaufmann T, Glasø de Lange AM, et al. (2021). Oxytocin receptor expression patterns in the human brain across development. Published online. doi: 10.31219/osf.io/j3b5d

27. Mazzuca M, Minlebaev M, Shakirzyanova A, et al. (2011) Newborn analgesia mediated by oxytocin during delivery. *Frontiers in Cell Neurosciences* 5, 3–3.

28. Robinson C, Schumann R, Zhang P, Young R. (2003) Oxytocin-induced desensitization of the oxytocin receptor. *American Journal of Obstetrics and Gynecology* 188(2), 497–502.

29. Phaneuf S, Asboth G, Carrasco M et al. (1998) Desensitization of oxytocin receptors in human myometrium. *Human Reproduction Update* 4(5), 625–633.

30. Phaneuf S, Europe-Finner GN, Carrasco MP, Hamilton CH, Lopez Bernal A. (1995) Oxytocin signalling in human myometrium. *Advances in Experimental Medicine and Biology* 395, 453–467.

31. Erickson EN, Lee CS, Emeis CL. (2017) Role of prophylactic oxytocin in the third stage of labor: Physiologic versus pharmacologically influenced labor and birth. *Journal of Midwifery & Women's Health* 62(4), 418–424. doi: 10.1111/jmwh.12620

32. McAdow M, Xu X, Lipkind H, Reddy UM, Illuzzi JL. (2020) Association of oxytocin rest during labor induction of nulliparous women with mode of delivery. *Obstetrics & Gynecology* 135(3), 569–575. doi: 10.1097/AOG.0000000000003709

33. Balki M, Ramachandran N, Lee S, Talati C. (2016) The recovery time of myometrial responsiveness after oxytocin-induced desensitization in human myometrium in vitro. *Anesthesia and Analgesia* 122(5), 1508–1515. doi: 10.1213/ANE.0000000000001268

34. Erickson EN, Carlson NS. Predicting postpartum hemorrhage after low-risk vaginal birth by labor characteristics and oxytocin administration. *Journal of Obstetric Gynecologic and Neonatal Nursing* Published online September 2020 doi: 10.1016/j.jogn.2020.08.005

35. Uvnäs-Moberg K, Ekström-Bergström A, Berg M, et al. (2019) Maternal plasma levels of oxytocin during physiological childbirth - A systematic review with implications for uterine contractions and central actions of oxytocin. *BMC Pregnancy Childbirth* 19(1). doi: 10.1186/s12884-019-2365-9

36. Takayanagi Y, Yoshida M, Bielsky IF, et al. (2005) Pervasive social deficits, but normal parturition, in oxytocin receptor-deficient mice. *Proceedings of the National Academy Sciences* 102(44), 16096–16101. doi: 10.1073/pnas.0505312102

37. Takayanagi Y, Kasahara Y, Onaka T, Takahashi N, Kawada T, Nishimori K. (2008) Oxytocin receptor-deficient mice developed late-onset obesity. *Neuroreport* 19(9), 951–955.

38. Blevins JE, Baskin DG. (2015) Translational and therapeutic potential of oxytocin as an anti-obesity strategy: Insights from rodents, nonhuman primates and humans. *Physiology and Behavior* 152, 438–449. doi: 10.1016/j.physbeh.2015.05.023

39. Shinar S, Many A, Maslovitz S. (2016) Questioning the role of pituitary oxytocin in parturition: Spontaneous onset of labor in women with panhypopituitarism – A case series. *European Journal of Obstetrics & Gynecology and Reproductive Biology* 197, 83–85. doi: 10.1016/j.ejogrb.2015.11.028

40. Yoshida M, Takayanagi Y, Ichino-yamashita A, et al. (2019) Functional hierarchy of uterotonics required for successful parturition in mice. *Endocrinology* Published online doi: 10.1210/en.2019-00499

41. Pasca AM, Penn AA. (2010) The placenta: The lost neuroendocrine organ. *NeoReviews* 11(2), e64–e77. doi: 10.1542/neo.11-2-e64

42. Peeters G, De Vos N, Houvenaghel A, States U, Code US, Act C. (1971) Elimination of the Ferguson reflex by section of the pelvic nerves in the lactating goat. *Journal of Endocrinology* 265(12), 1529–1529. doi: 10.1677/joe.0.0490125

43. Bell AF, Erickson EN, Carter CS. (2014) Beyond labor: The role of natural and synthetic oxytocin in the transition to motherhood. *Journal of Midwifery & Women's Health* 59(1), 35–42. doi: 10.1111/jmwh.12101

44. Guastella AJ, Mitchell PB, Mathews F. (2008) Oxytocin enhances the encoding of positive social memories in humans. *Biological Psychiatry* Published online. doi: 10.1016/j.biopsych.2008.02.008

45. Portnova GV, Proskurnina EV, Sokolova SV, Skorokhodov IV, Varlamov AA. (2020) Perceived pleasantness of gentle touch in healthy individuals is related to salivary oxytocin response and EEG markers of arousal. *Experimental Brain Research* 238(10), 2257–2268. doi: 10.1007/s00221-020-05891-y

46. Cox EQ, Stuebe A, Pearson B, Grewen K, Rubinow D, Meltzer-Brody S. (2015) Oxytocin and HPA stress axis reactivity in postpartum women. *Psychoneuroendocrinology* 55, 164–172. doi: 10.1016/j.psyneuen.2015.02.009

47. Shnider M, Wright RG, Levinson G, et al. (1979) Uterine blood flow and plasma norepinephrine changes during maternal stress in the pregnant Ewe. *Anesthesiology* 50(6), 524–527. doi: 10.1097/00000542-197906000-00010

48. Saxton A, Fahy K, Hastie C. (2014) Effects of skin-to-skin contact and breastfeeding at birth on the incidence of PPH: A physiologically based theory. *Women Birth* 27(4), 250–253. doi: 10.1016/j.wombi.2014.06.004

49. Slattery DA, Neumann ID. (2008) No stress please! Mechanisms of stress hyporesponsiveness of the maternal brain. *Journal of Physiology* 586, 377–385. doi: 10.1113/jphysiol.2007.145896

50. Barba-Müller E, Craddock S, Carmona S, Hoekzema E. (2019) Brain plasticity in pregnancy and the postpartum period: Links to maternal caregiving and mental health. *Archives of Women's Mental Health* 22(2), 289–299. doi: 10.1007/s00737-018-0889-z

51. Babb JA, Carini LM, Spears SL, Nephew BC. (2014) Transgenerational effects of social stress on social behavior, corticosterone, oxytocin, and prolactin in rats. *Hormones and Behavior* 65(4), 386–393. doi:10.1016/j.yhbeh.2014.03.005

52. Martínez-Burnes J, Muns R, Barrios-García H, Villanueva-García D, Domínguez-Oliva A, Mota-Rojas D. (2021) Parturition in mammals: Animal models, pain and distress. *Animal Open Access Journal MDPI* 11(10), 2960. doi: 10.3390/ani11102960

53. Nagel C, Aurich C, Aurich J. (2019) Stress effects on the regulation of parturition in different domestic animal species. *Animal Reproduction Science* 207, 153–161. doi: 10.1016/j.anireprosci.2019.04.011

54. Nagel EM, Howland MA, Pando C, et al. (2021) Maternal psychological distress and lactation and breastfeeding outcomes: A narrative review. *Clinical Therapeutics* S0149-2918(21)00461-6. Published online December 19. doi: 10.1016/j.clinthera.2021.11.007

55. Sakala C, Romano AM, Buckley SJ. (2016) Hormonal physiology of childbearing, an essential framework for maternal-newborn nursing. *Journal of Obstetric Gynecologic and Neonatal Nursing JOGNN NAACOG* 45(2), 264–275.

56. Olza I, Uvnas-Moberg K, Ekström-Bergström A, et al. (2020) Birth as a neuro-psycho-social event: An integrative model of maternal experiences and their relation to neurohormonal events during childbirth. *PLoS ONE* 15(7). doi: 10.1371/journal.pone.0230992

57. Bohren MA, Hofmeyr GJ, Sakala C, Fukuzawa RK, Cuthbert A. (2017) Continuous support for women during childbirth. *Cochrane Database of Systematic Reviews* (7). Art. No.: CD003766. doi: 10.1002/14651858.CD003766.pub6

58. Garfield L, Holditch-Davis D, Carter CS, et al. (2019) Pilot study of oxytocin in low income women with a low birth weight infant: Is oxytocin related to posttraumatic stress? *Advance Neonatal Care Official Journal of National Association Neonatal Nurses* 19(4), E12–E21. doi: 10.1097/ANC.0000000000000601

59. Seng JS. (2010) Posttraumatic oxytocin dysregulation: Is it a link among posttraumatic self disorders, posttraumatic stress disorder, and pelvic visceral dysregulation conditions in women? *Journal of Trauma Dissociation Official Journal International Society Study Dissociation ISSD* 11(4), 387–406. doi: 10.1080/15299732.2010.496075

60. Grant EN, Tao W, Craig M, McIntire D, Leveno K. (2015) Neuraxial analgesia effects on labor progression: Facts, fallacies, uncertainties, and the future. *BJOG International Journal of Obstetrics and Gynaecology* 122(3), 288–293. doi: 10.1111/1471-0528.12966

61. Shamay-Tsoory SG, Abu-Akel A. (2016) *The Social Salience Hypothesis of Oxytocin.* Vol. 79. 202. doi: 10.1016/j.biopsych.2015.07.020

62. Fragkaki I, Verhagen M, van Herwaarden AE, Cima M. (2019) Daily oxytocin patterns in relation to psychopathy and childhood trauma in residential youth. *Psychoneuroendocrinology* 102, 105–113. doi: 10.1016/j.psyneuen.2018.11.040

63. Smearman EL, Almli LM, Conneely KN, et al. (2016) Oxytocin receptor genetic and epigenetic variations: Association with child abuse and adult psychiatric symptoms. *Child Development* 87(1), 122–134. doi: 10.1111/cdev.12493

64. Heim C, Young LJ, Newport DJ, Mletzko T, Miller AH, Nemeroff CB. (2008). Lower CSF oxytocin concentrations in women with a history of childhood abuse. Published online. doi:10.1038/mp.2008.112

65. Yirmiya K, Motsan S, Zagoory-Sharon O, Feldman R. (2020). Human attachment triggers different social buffering mechanisms under high and low early life stress rearing. Published online. doi:10.1016/j.ijpsycho.2020.04.001

66. Lara-Cinisomo S, Zhu K, Fei K, Bu Y, Weston AP, Ravat U. (2018) Traumatic events: Exploring associations with maternal depression, infant bonding, and oxytocin in Latina mothers. *BMC Womens Health* 18(1). doi: 10.1186/s12905-018-0520-5

67. Krause S, Boeck C, Gumpp AM, et al. (2018) Child maltreatment is associated with a reduction of the oxytocin receptor in peripheral blood mononuclear cells. *Frontiers in Psychology* 9, 173–173. doi: 10.3389/fpsyg.2018.00173

68. Simons RL, Lei MK, Beach SRH, Cutrona CE, Philibert RA. (2017) Methylation of the oxytocin receptor gene mediates the effect of adversity on negative schemas and depression. *Development and Psychopathology* Published online. doi: 10.1017/S0954579416000420

69. Miller S, Abalos E, Chamillard M, et al. (2016) Beyond too little, too late and too much, too soon: A pathway towards evidence-based, respectful maternity care worldwide. *Lancet Lond Engl* 388(10056), 2176–2192. doi: 10.1016/S0140-6736(16)31472-6

70. Megregian M, Emeis CL, Nieuwenhuijze M. (2020) The impact of shared decision making in perinatal care: A scoping review. *Journal of Midwifery Women's Health.* Nov; 65(6), 777–788. doi: 10.1111/jmwh.13128

71. Boie S, Glavind J, Velu AV, et al. (2018) Discontinuation of intravenous oxytocin in the active phase of induced labour. *Cochrane Database of Systematic Reviews* 8, CD012274. doi: 10.1002/14651858.CD012274.pub2

72. Kominiarek MA, Zhang J, Vanveldhuisen P, Troendle J, Beaver J, Hibbard JU. (2011) Contemporary labor patterns: The impact of maternal body mass index. *American Journal of Obstetrics and Gynecology* 205(3), 244.e1–8. doi: 10.1016/j.ajog.2011.06.014

73. Smith H, Peterson N, Lagrew D, Main E. (2016) Toolkit to support vaginal birth and reduce primary cesareans: A quality improvement toolkit. Appendix R: Induction of labor algorithm. Stanford, CA: California Maternal Quality Care Collaborative.

74. Practice C on O. (2017) ACOG Committee Opinion No. 687: Approaches to limit intervention during labor and birth. *Obstetrics & Gynecology* 129(2), e20–e28.

75. American College of Nurse-Midwives. (2012) Supporting healthy and normal physiologic childbirth: A consensus statement by the American college of nurse-midwives, midwives alliance of North America, and the national association of certified professional midwives. *Journal of Midwifery & Women's Health* 57(5), 529–532. doi: 10.1111/j.1542-2011.2012.00218.x

76. Zhang J, Landy HJ, Ware Branch D, et al. (2010) Contemporary patterns of spontaneous labor with normal neonatal outcomes. *Obstetrics & Gynecology* 116(6), 1281–1287. doi: 10.1097/AOG.0b013e3181fdef6e

77. Tolba SM, Ali SS, Mohammed AM, et al. (2018) Management of spontaneous labor in primigravidae: Labor scale versus WHO partograph (SLiP Trial) Randomized controlled trial. *American Journal of Perinatology* Published online. doi: 10.1055/s-0037-1605575

78. Clark SL, Simpson KR, Knox GE, Garite TJ. (2009) Oxytocin: New perspectives on an old drug. *American Journal of Obstetrics and Gynecology* 200(1), 35.e1–6. doi: 10.1016/j.ajog.2008.06.010

79. Hayes E, Weinstein L. (2008) Improving patient safety and uniformity of care by a standardized regimen for the use of oxytocin. *American Journal of Obstetrics and Gynecology* 198(6).

80. Osterman MJK, Martin, JA (2008). *Epidural and Spinal Anesthesia Use During Labor: 27-State Reporting Area, 2008.*

81. Frolova AI, Wang JJ, Conner SN, et al. (2018) Spontaneous labor onset and outcomes in obese women at term. *American Journal of Perinatology* 35(1), 59–64. doi: 10.1055/s-0037-1605574

82. Carlson NS, Corwin EJ, Lowe NK. (2017) Oxytocin augmentation in spontaneously laboring, nulliparous women: Multilevel assessment of maternal BMI and oxytocin dose. *Biological Research for Nursing* 19(4), 382–392. doi: 10.1177/1099800417701831

83. Gam CMBF, Larsen LH, Mortensen OH, et al. (2017) Unchanged mitochondrial phenotype, but accumulation of lipids in the myometrium in obese pregnant women. *Journal of Physiology* 595(23), 7109–7122. doi: 10.1113/JP274838

84. Padol AR, Sukumaran SV, Sadam A, et al. (2017) Hypercholesterolemia impairs oxytocin-induced uterine contractility in late pregnant mouse. *Reproduction Camb Engl* 153(5), 565–576. doi: 10.1530/REP-16-0446

85. Muir R, Liu G, Khan R, et al. (2018) Maternal obesity-induced decreases in plasma, hepatic and uterine polyunsaturated fatty acids during labour is reversed through improved nutrition at conception. *Scientific Reports* 8(1), 3389. doi: 10.1038/s41598-018-21809-9

86. Carlson NS, Frediani JK, Corwin EJ, Dunlop A, Jones D. (2020) Metabolic pathways associated with term labor induction course in African American women. *Biological Research for Nursing* 22(2), 157–168. doi: 10.1177/1099800419899730

87. Maestrini S, Mele C, Mai S, et al. (2018) Plasma Oxytocin concentration in Pre- and Postmenopausal Women: Its relationship with obesity, body composition and metabolic variables. *Obesity Facts* 11(5), 429–439. doi: 10.1159/000492001

88. Fu-Man D, Hong-Yu K, Bin-Hong D, Da-Na L, Xin-Yang Y. (2019) Associations of oxytocin with metabolic parameters in obese women of childbearing age. *Endokrynologia Polska* 70(5), 417-422. doi: 10.5603/EP.a2019.0028. Epub 2019 May 28. PMID: 31135057.

89. Çatli G, Acar S, Cingöz G, et al. (2021) Oxytocin receptor gene polymorphism and low serum oxytocin level are associated with hyperphagia and obesity in adolescents. *International Journal of Obesity 2005* 45(9), 2064–2073. doi: 10.1038/s41366-021-00876-5

90. Bush NR, Allison AL, Miller AL, Deardorff J, Adler NE, Boyce WT. (2017) Socioeconomic disparities in childhood obesity risk: Association with an oxytocin receptor polymorphism. *JAMA Pediatrics* 171(1), 61–67. doi: 10.1001/jamapediatrics.2016.2332

91. Simpson KR. (2011) Clinicians' guide to the use of oxytocin for labor induction and augmentation. *Journal of Midwifery & Women's Health* 56(3), 214–221. doi: 10.1111/j.1542-2011.2011.00052.x

92. Blanks AM, Thornton S. (2003) The role of oxytocin in parturition. *BJOG: An International Journal of Obstetrics and Gynaecology* 110, 46–51. doi: 10.1016/S1470-0328(03)00024-7

93. Simpson KR. (2020) Cervical ripening and labor induction and augmentation, 5th Edition. *Nursing for Women's Health* 24(4), S1–S41. doi: 10.1016/j.nwh.2020.04.005

94. American College of Obstetrics and Gynecology. (2009) ACOG Practice Bulletin No. 107: Induction of labor. *Obstetrics & Gynecology* 114(2 Pt 1), 386–397. doi: 10.1097/AOG.0b013e3181b48ef5

95. Budden A, Chen LJY, Henry A. (2014) High-dose versus low-dose oxytocin infusion regimens for induction of labour at term. *Cochrane Database of Systematic Reviews* Published online. doi: 10.1002/14651858.CD009701.pub2

96. Leduc D, Biringer A, Lee L, Dy J. (2013) Clinical practice obstetrics committee, special contributors. Induction of labour. *Journal of Obstetrics and Gynaecology Can JOGC Journal of Obstetrics and Gynaecology Can JOGC* 35(9), 840–857. doi: 10.1016/S1701-2163(15)30842-2

97. Roloff K, Peng S, Sanchez-Ramos L, Valenzuela GJ. (2015) Cumulative oxytocin dose during induction of labor according to maternal body mass index. *International Journal of Gynecology and Obstetrics Official Organ International Federation of Gynecology and Obstetrics* 131(1), 54–58. doi: 10.1016/j.ijgo.2015.04.038

98. Soni S, Chivan N, Cohen WR. (2013) Effect of maternal body mass index on oxytocin treatment for arrest of dilatation. *Journal of Perinatal Medicine* 41(5), 517–521. doi: 10.1515/jpm-2013-0024

99. Ramö Isgren A, Kjölhede P, Carlhäll S, Blomberg M. (2021) Maternal body mass index and oxytocin in augmentation of labour in nulliparous women: A prospective observational study. *BMJ Open* 11(3), e044754. doi: 10.1136/bmjopen-2020-044754

100. Carlson NS, Corwin EJ, Lowe NK. (2017) Labor intervention and outcomes in women who are nulliparous and obese: Comparison of nurse-midwife to obstetrician intrapartum care. *Journal of Midwifery & Women's Health* 62(1), 29–39. doi: 10.1111/jmwh.12579

101. Spong CY, Berghella V, Wenstrom KD, Mercer BM, Saade GR. (2012) Preventing the first cesarean delivery: Summary of a joint eunice kennedy shriver national institute of child health and human development, society for maternal-fetal medicine, and American College of Obstetricians and Gynecologists Workshop. *Obstetrics and Gynecology* 120(5), 1181–1193. doi: 10.1097/AOG.0b013e3182704880y

102. Carlson NS, Lowe NK. (2014) A concept analysis of watchful waiting among providers caring for women in labour. *Journal of Advanced Nursing* 70(3), 511–522. doi: 10.1111/jan.12209

103. Zhang J, Branch DW, Ramirez MM, et al. (2011) Oxytocin regimen for labor augmentation, labor progression, and perinatal outcomes. *Obstetrics & Gynecology* Published online doi: 10.1097/AOG.0b013e3182220192

104. Zaki MN, Hibbard JU, Kominiarek, MA. (2013) Contemporary Labor Patterns and Maternal Age. *Obstetrics & Gynecology* 122(5), 1018–1024. doi: 10.1097/AOG.0b013e3182a9c92c

105. Crankshaw DJ, O'Brien YM, Crosby DA, Morrison JJ. (2015) Maternal age and contractility of human myometrium in pregnancy. *Reproductive Sciences* 22(10), 1229–1235. doi: 10.1177/1933719115572483

106. Patel R, Moffatt JD, Mourmoura E, et al. (2017) Effect of reproductive ageing on pregnant mouse uterus and cervix. *Journal of Physiology* 595(6), 2065–2084. doi: 10.1113/JP273350

107. Elmes M, Szyszka A, Pauliat C, et al. (2015) Maternal age effects on myometrial expression of contractile proteins, uterine gene expression, and contractile activity during labor in the rat. *Physiology Reports* 3(4). doi: 10.14814/phy2.12305

108. Arrowsmith S, Robinson H, Noble K, Wray S. (2012) What do we know about what happens to myometrial function as women age? *Journal of Muscle Research and Cell Motility* 33(3–4), 209–217. doi: 10.1007/s10974-012-9300-2

109. Lowensohn R, Paul R, Fales S, Yeh S, Hon E. (1974) Intrapartum epidural anesthesia. An evaluation of effects on uterine activity. *Obstetrics & Gynecology* 44(3), 388–393.

110. Schellenberg J. (1977) Uterine activity during lumbar epidural analgesia with bupivacaine. *American Journal of Obstetrics and Gynecology* 127(1), 26–31.

111. Arici G, Karsli B, Kayacan N, Akar M. (2004) The effects of bupivacaine, ropivacaine and mepivacaine on the contractility of rat myometrium. *International Journal of Obstetric Anesthesia* 13(2), 95–98. doi: 10.1016/j.ijoa.2003.10.007

112. Hawkins JL. (2010) Epidural analgesia for labor and delivery. *New England Journal of Medicine* 362(16), 1503–1513.

113. Rahm V, Hallgren A, Hogberg H, Hurtig I, Odlind V. (2002) Plasma oxytocin levels in women during labor with or without epidural analgesia: A prospective study. *Acta Obstetricia Et Gynecologica Scandinavica* 81(11), 1033–1039.

114. Miller NM, Fisk NM, Modi N, Glover V. (2005) Stress responses at birth: Determinants of cord arterial cortisol and links with cortisol response in infancy. *BJOG International Journal of Obstetrics and Gynaecology* Published online. doi: 10.1111/j.1471-0528.2005.00620.x

115. Bell A, McFarlin BL. (2006) Maternal and fetal stress responses during birth: Adaptive or Maladaptive? *Journal of Midwifery & Women's Health* Published online. doi: 10.1016/j.jmwh.2006.06.005

116. Qian X, Li P, Shi SQ, Garfield RE, Liu H. (2017) Uterine and abdominal muscle electromyographic activities in control and PCEA-treated nulliparous women during the second stage of labor. *Reproductive Sciences Thousand Oaks Calif* 24(8), 1214–1220. doi: 10.1177/1933719116682875

5

117. Graugaard HL, Maimburg RD. Is the increase in postpartum hemorrhage after vaginal birth because of altered clinical practice?: A register-based cohort study. *Birth* Published online March 2021:birt.12543-birt.12543. doi: 10.1111/birt.12543

118. Grotegut CA, Paglia MJ, Johnson LNC, Thames B, James AH. (2011) Oxytocin exposure during labor among women with postpartum hemorrhage secondary to uterine atony. *American Journal of Obstetrics and Gynecology* 204(1), 56.e1–56.e6. doi: 10.1016/j.ajog.2010.08.023

119. Li H, Gudmundsson S, Olofsson P. (2003) Uterine artery blood flow velocity waveforms during uterine contractions. *Ultrasound in Obstetrics and Gynecology* 22(6), 578–585. doi: 10.1002/uog.921

120. Wiberg-Itzel E, Pembe AB, Järnbert-Pettersson H, Norman M, Wihlbäck AC, Hoesli I, Todesco Bernasconi M, Azria E, Åkerud H, Darj E. (2016) Lactate in amniotic fluid: predictor of labor outcome in oxytocin-augmented primiparas' deliveries. *PLoS One.* Oct 26; 11(10), e0161546. doi: 10.1371/journal.pone.0161546. PMID: 27783611; PMCID: PMC5082650.

121. Barber EL, Lundsberg LS, Belanger K, Pettker CM, Funai EF, Illuzzi JL. (2011) Indications contributing to the increasing cesarean delivery rate. *Obstetrics & Gynecology* 118(1), 29–38. doi: 10.1097/AOG.0b013e31821e5f65

122. Zhang J, Troendle J, Reddy UM, et al. (2010) Contemporary cesarean delivery practice in the United States. *American Journal of Obstetrics and Gynecology* 203(4), 326.e1–326.e10. doi: 10.1016/j.ajog.2010.06.058

123. Shilkrut AG, Hsu RC, Fuks AM. (2021) Fetal heart rate tracing category II: A broad category in need of stratification. *NeoReviews* 22(2), e88–e94. doi: 10.1542/neo.22-2-e88

124. Leathersich SJ, Vogel JP, Tran TS, Hofmeyr GJ. (2018) Acute tocolysis for uterine tachysystole or suspected fetal distress. *Cochrane Database of Systematic Reviews* 7, CD009770. doi: 10.1002/14651858.CD009770.pub2

125. Raghuraman N, López JD, Carter EB, et al. (2020) The effect of intrapartum oxygen supplementation on category II fetal monitoring. *American Journal of Obstetrics and Gynecology* 223(6), 905.e1–905.e7. doi: 10.1016/j.ajog.2020.06.037

126. Bor P, Ledertoug S, Boie S, Knoblauch NO, Stornes I. (2016) Continuation versus discontinuation of oxytocin infusion during the active phase of labour: A randomised controlled trial. *BJOG International Journal of Obstetrics and Gynaecology* Published online. doi: 10.1111/1471-0528.13589

127. Saccone G, Ciardulli A, Baxter JK, et al. (2017) Discontinuing oxytocin infusion in the active phase of labor: A systematic review and Meta-analysis. *Obstetrics & Gynecology* 130(5), 1090–1096. doi: 10.1097/AOG.0000000000002325

128. Erickson EN, Emeis CL. (2017) Breastfeeding outcomes after oxytocin use during childbirth: An integrative review. *Journal of Midwifery & Women's Health* 62(4), 397–417. doi: 10.1111/jmwh.12601

129. Bell AF, White-Traut R, Rankin K. (2013) Fetal exposure to synthetic oxytocin and the relationship with prefeeding cues within one hour postbirth. *Early Human Development.* Mar; 89(3), 137–143. doi: 10.1016/j.earlhumdev.2012.09.017. Epub 2012 Oct 16. PMID: 23084698.

130. Marín Gabriel MA, Olza Fernández I, Malalana Martínez AM, et al. (2015) Intrapartum synthetic oxytocin reduce the expression of primitive reflexes associated with breastfeeding. *Breastfeed Medicine Official Journal of Academic Breastfeed Medicine* 10(4), 209–213. doi: 10.1089/bfm.2014.0156

131. Brimdyr K, Cadwell K, Widström AM, et al. (2015) The association between common labor drugs and suckling when skin-to-skin during the first hour after birth. *Birth Berkeley Calif* 42(4), 319–328. doi: 10.1111/birt.12186

132. Gomes M, Trocado V, Carlos-Alves M, Arteiro D, Pinheiro P. (2018) Intrapartum synthetic oxytocin and breastfeeding: A retrospective cohort study. *Journal of Obstetrics and Gynaecology* 38(6), 745–749. doi: 10.1080/01443615.2017.1405924

133. Fernández-Cañadas Morillo A, Durán Duque M, Hernández López AB, et al. (2018). Cessation of breastfeeding in association with oxytocin administration and type of birth. A prospective cohort study. Published online. doi:10.1016/j.wombi.2018.04.017

134. Stuebe AM, Grewen K, Pedersen CA, Propper C, Meltzer-Brody S. (2012) Failed lactation and perinatal depression: Common problems with shared neuroendocrine mechanisms? *Journal of Womens Health* 21(3), 264–272. doi: 10.1089/jwh.2011.3083

135. Kim S, Soeken TA, Cromer SJ, Martinez SR, Hardy LR, Strathearn L. (2014) Oxytocin and postpartum depression: Delivering on what's known and what's not. *Brain Research* 1580, 219–232. doi: 10.1016/j.brainres.2013.11.009

136. Kimmel M, Clive M, Gispen F, et al. (2016) Oxytocin receptor DNA methylation in postpartum depression. *Psychoneuroendocrinology* 69, 150–160. doi: 10.1016/j.psyneuen.2016.04.008

137. Thul TA, Corwin EJ, Carlson NS, Brennan PA, Young LJ. (2020) Oxytocin and postpartum depression: A systematic review. *Psychoneuroendocrinology* 120, 104793. doi: 10.1016/j.psyneuen.2020.104793

5

138. Kroll-Desrosiers AR, Nephew BC, Babb JA, Guilarte-Walker Y, Moore Simas TA, Deligiannidis KM. (2017) Association of peripartum synthetic oxytocin administration and depressive and anxiety disorders within the first postpartum year. *Depress Anxiety* 34(2), 137–146. doi: 10.1002/da.22599

139. Gu V, Feeley N, Gold I, et al. (2016) Intrapartum synthetic oxytocin and its effects on maternal well-being at 2 months postpartum. *Birth* 43(1), 28–35. doi: 10.1111/birt.12198

140. Erickson EN, Krol KM, Perkeybile AM, Connelly JJ, Myatt L. (2022) Oxytocin receptor single nucleotide polymorphism predicts atony-related postpartum hemorrhage. *BMC Pregnancy and Childbirth* 22(1), 884. doi: 10.1186/s12884-022-05205-w

141. Grotegut CA, Ngan E, Garrett ME, Miranda ML, Ashley-Koch AE, Swamy GK. (2017) The association of single-nucleotide polymorphisms in the oxytocin receptor and G protein–coupled receptor kinase 6 (GRK6) genes with oxytocin dosing requirements and labor outcomes. *American Journal of Obstetrics and Gynecology* 217(3), 367.e1–367.e9. doi: 10.1016/j.ajog.2017.05.023

142. Reinl EL, Goodwin ZA, Raghuraman N, et al. (2017) Novel oxytocin receptor variants in laboring women requiring high doses of oxytocin. *American Journal of Obstetrics and Gynecology* Published online doi: 10.1016/j.ajog.2017.04.036

143. Jin B, Du Y, Zhang F, Zhang K, Wang L, Cui L. (2016) Carbetocin for the prevention of postpartum hemorrhage: A systematic review and meta-analysis of randomized controlled trials. *Journal of Maternal-Fetal and Neonatal Medicine* 29(3), 400–407. doi: 10.3109/14767058.2014.1002394

144. Romero R, Sibai B, Sanchez-Ramos L, et al. (2000) An oxytocin receptor antagonist (atosiban) in the treatment of preterm labor: A randomized, double-blind, placebo-controlled trial with tocolytic rescue. *American Journal of Obstetrics and Gynecology* 182(5), 1173–1183.

Chapter 6

Prolonged Prelabor and Latent First Stage

Ellen L. Tilden, PhD, RN, CNM, FACNM, FAAN, Jesse Remer, BS, CD(DONA), BDT(DONA), LCCE, FACCE, and Joyce K. Edmonds, PhD, MPH, RN

Simkin's Labor Progress Handbook: Early Interventions to Prevent and Treat Dystocia, Fifth Edition. Edited by Lisa Hanson, Emily Malloy, and Penny Simkin.
© 2024 John Wiley & Sons Ltd. Published 2024 by John Wiley & Sons Ltd.

THE ONSET OF LABOR: KEY ELEMENTS OF RECOGNITION AND RESPONSE

The onset of labor marks a transformational shift from pregnancy to active labor to birth. This time of transition can affect the overall emotional and physical tenor of the journey toward birth. While the processes of prelabor, labor onset, and the latent phase of labor generally do not receive the same scientific or clinical attention as active labor and delivery, birth attendants with expertise in physiologic labor understand the critical importance of these processes. If childbearing were a race, prelabor, labor onset, and the latent phase of labor are the critically important stretching and warm up activities that make for success during the sprint of active labor. Birthing people who have the capacity and support to conserve their physical and emotional energies during prelabor, labor onset, and the latent phase of labor are often better prepared and more resilient during active labor and birthing. Well-managed and well-tolerated prelabor, labor onset, and latent phase of labor also help low-risk birthing people remain out of the hospital until active labor—a factor that is important for avoiding unnecessary cesarean birth. Learning to identify and effectively support people during prelabor, labor onset, and the latent phase of labor are key skills to support physiologic birth. The focus of this chapter is to share common symptoms of labor onset and subsequent events of the latent phase of labor as well as relevant science and clinical pearls for helping to manage or support these processes.

One of the greatest challenges for pregnant people, their families, and their caregivers is identification of labor onset. Birth attendants and support people find that the subtle and often unique constellation of each person's onset of labor signs and symptoms makes it difficult to give concise preparation guidance on what to expect. From a provider's perspective, the diagnosis of labor onset is like painting a picture or doing a puzzle—each sign adding something to the greater understanding of progress and, ultimately, a definitive confirmation of labor onset. For example, a pregnant person may report to their doula a distinct feeling of being "done" with their pregnancy, an intense urge to clean and cook, and cramping "down low," while a visit to the midwife might confirm a loss of their mucus plug and softening or thinning of the cervix. It's not uncommon for the midwife, physician, or doula to receive a photo from a pregnant person with the question: "Is this my mucus plug?" Pregnant people, their families, and their caregivers are tasked with attending to and connecting these various "puzzle pieces" to help identify the prelabor, labor onset, and the latent phase of labor transitions. If labor onset is defined as contractions that cause dilation of the cervix, the precise moment when this process begins can be challenging to detect. Despite extensive research, the exact mechanisms causing labor onset are not well understood. The most recent evidence about identifying labor's onset is revealed through a collaborative perspective between the pregnant person reporting physical and emotional changes and their care provider noting changes in the cervix.

The uterus contracts off and on throughout pregnancy, with contractions generally becoming more noticeable and more frequent late in pregnancy until the individual is in labor and gives birth. The onset and progression of labor contractions are driven by complex and dynamic biological, neurohormonal, and physiologic processes driving the transition from pregnancy to late pregnancy to labor. Thus, the pregnant person's body evolves into labor. While it is nearly impossible to identify the precise moment in time that the cervix begins dilating, the laboring person's symptom experience is essential to recognizing the onset of labor and is of central importance in people's experience of their labor and in subsequent clinical decision making.[1] The challenge of identifying the exact onset of labor and identifying when to transition to the birth setting can be daunting and often creates emotional uncertainty.[2] For example, it can bring up feelings of excitement and anxiousness similar to the first trimester confirmation of pregnancy. Questions like "Is this labor? Will I stay in labor? Will it progress?" are common. Birth attendants and workers spend time supporting pregnant people through this assessment stage. Many birthing people feel torn between the worry of arriving at the birth setting "too late" and the worry of premature hospital admission leading to a cascade of unnecessary intervention.[2]

Defining labor onset

The latent phase of the first stage of labor begins with regular contractions that lead to progressive cervical change as they become stronger, longer, and closer together. Criteria commonly used to diagnose labor onset have only recently been scientifically evaluated for their reliability. One prospective study sought to evaluate the reliability of commonly used criteria in identifying labor.[3] The researchers evaluated usual criteria that do not require a medical exam. These criteria were: regular intervals between contractions; decreasing intervals between contractions;

increasing abdominal pain; backache; pain relief from walking; vomiting; changes in intestinal habits over the previous 24 hours; and changes in breathing pattern and body position during contractions. The findings showed that the only criteria consistently associated with hospital admission for active labor were decreasing intervals between contractions and increasing contraction intensity. In addition to tracking symptoms, the authors also evaluated signs: premature rupture of the membranes; loss of the mucus plug (not associated with exam); cervical dilation; and effacement. Of those criteria, only cervical effacement and dilation were positively associated with labor onset.

Signs of impending labor

Common behaviors and physical changes may characterize imminent labor onset, although there is lack of agreement about the specific indicators of approaching labor and wide variability in experiences. Commonly reported signs of imminent labor include lower back pain, an increase in watery or blood-stained vaginal discharge ("bloody show,") diarrhea, passage of the mucus plug, feeling nervous and/or excited, and altered sleep patterns.[4] Some people also report bursts of energy and feelings of excitement, apprehension, and anxiety that can accompany a desire to "nest."[5] Nesting is considered an instinct that helps pregnant people prepare their environment for the upcoming birth and can be accompanied by a sense of urgency to organize and make plans for the new baby's arrival. In their studies of pregnant and non-pregnant women in Canada, Anderson and Rutherford found that women in late pregnancy had a preference for being in familiar places, close to home, and a strong preference for kin and close friends during impending labor.[6]

Prelabor

Prelabor, which is sometimes called prodromal, false, or early labor, refers to contractions that are not associated with cervical dilation. Prelabor contractions are often characterized as being unpredictable in intensity, duration, and frequency. Prelabor is unpredictable in duration and may be hours or days. It is also common for prelabor to repeatedly begin and stop. People with prelabor symptoms may believe that their labor has begun; however, caregivers generally await signs and symptoms other than contractions, such as cervical dilation or changes in the nature of the contractions (e.g., duration, strength, and frequency), before diagnosing labor onset. Once the cervix begins to progressively dilate with contractions (beyond the first few centimeters that commonly occur in late pregnancy), the latent phase of labor has begun.

Prelabor vs labor: the dilemma

The most reliable symptom distinguishing prelabor from labor is regular contractions and the most reliable indicator of labor onset is progressive cervical dilation. While the experience of regular contractions is often accompanied by the sign of progressive cervical dilation, it is also quite common that the laboring person's perception of regular contractions is not paired with cervical dilation. Respectfully and kindly navigating this common discrepancy between the laboring person's understanding of labor onset versus the clinician's understanding of labor onset is important. People who believe that their prelabor symptoms signal true labor onset can feel disrespected, shamed, discouraged, or uncertain when their provider disagrees.[2] These feelings can lead to isolation, exhaustion, and/or anxiety, can damage the patient/provider relationship, or decrease the laboring person's satisfaction with their overall birth experience. To help prevent these negative experiences and feelings, it is recommended during prenatal care to provide anticipatory guidance about the varying symptoms and processes that occur during prelabor, labor onset, and the latent phase of labor. Normalizing the uncertainty that often characterizes these transitions and emphasizing how common it is to present to the hospital thinking one is in labor only to be sent home with the news that one is in prelabor or latent labor can help pregnant people navigate prelabor.

Delaying latent labor hospital admissions

Home birth parents must decide when to call their midwife—not too early and not too late—and the midwife bases their decision about when to join the family on the information conveyed during the phone call. The overall dilemma about prelabor versus labor becomes more complex related to the timing of hospital or birth center admission. Once a laboring individual suspects that they are in labor, they often call their health care provider for advice regarding when to arrive at their place for birth and/or how to cope with early labor at home. The goal is to arrive at one's chosen place of birth in a timely manner relative to labor onset and progression. Parents frequently find the decision about arrival at their intended place of birth stressful.[2] This decision can be influenced by factors such as how a pregnant person is coping with latent labor discomforts, the perceptions and desires of those who are with the laboring person, and concerns about travel time to the hospital.

Many laboring people present to the hospital or birth center only to be sent home because labor is not sufficiently advanced to warrant admission.[7,8] In normal labors with good outcomes, prelabor and the latent phase of labor may continue for much longer than previously understood, until as much as 5–6 cm of dilation, before the active phase begins.[9] Therefore, arriving at the optimal time can reduce unnecessary interventions in childbirth, while arriving "too soon" might lead to a cascade of unnecessary interventions and negative experiences.[10,11] Further, caregivers in busy labor units can find it inefficient to spend limited staff time and resources triaging people who are not in active labor. Most challenging of all, for both caregivers and parents, prelabor may continue for a very long time. In such cases inappropriate interventions are sometimes used to accelerate what is normal latent labor. Clinical experience strongly suggests that a frank, pregnancy-timed conversation about prelabor versus labor that emphasizes the *protective value* of coping with latent labor at home and reserving hospital admission for when active labor is well-established can go a long way in helping laboring people understand that being sent home in latent labor is a mark of high-quality maternity care, not a critique of the individual.

ANTICIPATORY GUIDANCE

The key elements of prelabor, labor onset, and the latent phase of labor anticipatory guidance will be described (Box 6.1).[12] While this guidance can be shared during any time during labor, a recent review of evidence-based labor management prior to labor onset recommends offering anticipatory guidance and education during pregnancy.[13] It is helpful to begin anticipatory guidance by communicating the immense value of prelabor, labor onset, and the latent phase of labor. Pregnant and laboring people need to understand that these elements are essential for birth. And framing the uncertainty that people often experience prior to active labor onset as *expected and normal* can help to decrease uncertainty-related distress prior to active labor. Anticipatory guidance can also include information about Simkin's six ways to progress in labor, identifying and using appropriate coping strategies, and the Sommer's New Year's Eve technique, explained below.

Box 6.1.   Necessary information for expectant parents to improve their chances of timely admission to hospital/ birth center or timely arrival of the midwife for a home birth

Laboring people and their families need to know:

1. How to recognize uterine contractions (periodic wave-like tightenings of the entire abdomen that are accompanied by pain, generally in the lower abdomen or back and rarely in the thighs).
2. How to time and record contractions correctly—using pencil, paper, and clock with a second hand, or one of the many contraction apps for computers or smart phones (obtainable by searching the Internet):
    a. number of minutes from the beginning of one contraction to the beginning of the next;
    b. noting the duration (in seconds) of the contractions;
    c. recognition by the pregnant person of whether their contractions are increasing in intensity over time.
3. To time and record five or six contractions in a row to identify a pattern, then wait until the pattern seems to have changed (longer, more intense, more frequent contractions), and time five or six more to detect changes.
4. To continue timing off and on until a pattern emerges, in which the contractions are clearly progressing—that is, over time, they consistently exhibit at least two of the following:
    a. continually becoming more intense (according to the laboring person's perception);
    b. continuing to become longer in duration;
    c. continuing to become closer together (fewer minutes between beginning of one to the beginning of the next). These contractions are progressing and are a sign that the cervix is likely beginning to dilate.

5. Specific comfort and calming measures for early progressing labor at home (please also see, "Anticipatory Guidance for Coping Prior to Active Labor," below).
6. Whom to call (caregiver or hospital maternity department) and when, in terms of contraction pattern and the correct phone numbers.
7. What information to give when calling: contraction pattern and how it has changed over time, any leaking of fluid or blood.

Simkin's six ways to progress in prelabor, labor onset, and the latent phase of labor

Contractions without dilation are frustrating and discouraging to a laboring person and their caregivers, who may believe that a lack of dilation means no progress. Penny Simkin developed these six strategies for re-envisioning progress prior to active labor. These six ways of understanding progress prior to active labor can be shared with pregnant people and their families as part of anticipatory guidance:

Six Ways to Progress:

1. The cervix moves from a posterior (pointing toward the laboring person's back) to an anterior (pointing toward the laboring person's front) position.
2. The cervix ripens or softens.
3. The cervix effaces.
4. The cervix dilates.
5. The fetal head prepares for descent (rotates, flexes, and molds).
6. The fetus descends, rotates further, and is born.

The first three steps in Simpkin's Six Ways to Progress are preparing the cervix to dilate. If the cervix is not yet dilating, even with continuing contractions, the pregnant person is in prelabor, and will need reassurance and suggestions from their caregiver that these contractions are accomplishing the necessary task of preparing the cervix to dilate. One of the first suggestions is to remind the pregnant person of the physiological steps, starting with pregnancy weeks they have already completed. Ask the person to put their hands on their belly and imagine when they were in their first trimester. Could they imagine their belly being this big? Encourage them to notice how small incremental changes, like the way fetal development occurs in each trimester, make a significant impact on the health of the overall journey and create capacity in their bodies to nurture a baby to term. And now—just the same—incremental changes in prelabor effacement of the cervix make the body ready for bigger dilation later in labor and create capacity to birth. Invite them to trust the process with each small change.

In pragmatic terms, until contractions progress and dilation begins, support measures should focus on educating the pregnant person about the six ways to progress, encouraging them to engage in distracting activities, helping them to be patient and accept the slow progress of early labor as a normal variation, preventing exhaustion, meeting nutritional needs, and keeping them comfortable. The first four elements of the Bishop Score are the same as the first four of the Six Ways to Progress. Understanding these elements provides valuable information for the pregnant person who is having contractions. If the cervix has ripened or moved forward (even if there are no other changes), the pregnant person can be encouraged that changes are beginning. Steps 5—rotation/flexion—and 6—molding and descent of the fetal head—take place in active labor and second stage.

Anticipatory guidance for coping prior in prelabor

Identifying physical, emotional, informational, and distraction strategies to help cope with the time before active labor can be very helpful. These strategies may be most effective when they reflect the pregnant person's own "love language" (time, touch, service, words or gifts). *Physical strategies* include walking, resting, massage, comfort positions, bathing, singing, dancing, cooking, and any number of enjoyable physical activities as defined by the laboring person. Special attention can be spent on forward leaning and hip opening positions to encourage optimal fetal positioning as the labor progresses. For some, intimacy with a partner including cuddling and nipple stimulation can also encourage oxytocin and, if combined with intercourse with a partner with a penis (as long as the bag of waters is intact), can potentially offer cervical softening due to the prostaglandins in semen. The focus of any physical contact should be what feels pleasurable to the laboring person, not on the potential benefit of sperm near the cervix. One clinical pearl is to avoid excessive walking during prelabor. Some pregnancy sources recommend walking as a means to speed labor, and some people interpret this to mean that they should walk a great deal before active labor. This can lead to exhaustion during active labor. *Emotional strategies* can include social connections like playing games, spending time with loved ones, art projects, or preparing baby items. *Informational strategies* can come in the form of connecting with their support team or provider, to have a touch stone on how things have changed, understand where they are in the process, or receive new ideas for distracting activities. *Distraction strategies* could include a longer cooking or baking project, watching a movie, and/or engaging with an involved project such as a complex puzzle. A distraction that the laboring person finds very funny or engaging can be particularly helpful for distinguishing prelabor from labor because most people in active labor are no longer interested in such activities. So, for example, if contractions are mild enough to make the laboring person briefly pause during a distraction activity but they quickly resume interest in the activity when the contraction is completed, this could be a sign of prelabor. However, if the laboring person loses all interest in the distraction activity, this could be a sign of labor onset.

Sommer's New Year's Eve technique

While many pregnant people are focused on preparing for pain during childbearing, fewer may be as well prepared for coping with fatigue during childbearing. Anticipatory guidance related to increasing opportunities to rest and conserving energy during prelabor, labor onset, and the latent phase of labor can be helpful, especially for those who ultimately experience longer labors. Mary Sommers, Certified Professional Midwife (CPM), created the New Year's Eve technique to help make this aspect of anticipatory guidance easy for most people to understand and remember.[14] The point of this technique is to help pregnant people who are just beginning to notice prelabor symptoms to conserve their physical and emotional energy by imagining that they are planning to be up all night for a New Year's Eve party. Here is an example script for offering this anticipatory guidance:

"When you start to feel mild cramping, I want you to pretend that it's New Year's Eve and you will be up all night long. The first thing you should do is go to sleep, or if you can't fall asleep at least rest in a dark, quiet space. If your cramping is interrupting your sleep, try a warm bath or shower and then get into bed. Stay in bed sleeping or resting for as long as you can. If it is possible, invite your partner or support people to rest as well. Everyone who will be at this 'New Year's Eve party' should rest as much as they can! When you can't stay in bed any longer, I want you to get up and eat something nutritious. In many hospitals food is restricted during active labor and also many people in active labor are not very hungry. So, use this time to eat well. After you have eaten, find something interesting or distracting to do. Don't use this time to: 1) write down the time of each contraction, 2) call friends or family and announce that you are 'in labor', 3) post on social media that you are 'in labor', or 4) use any of the resources you plan to use during active labor—these plans and resources should exclusively be saved for use in active labor. This time is for quietly and calmly preparing for a burst of energy later. If your symptoms stop entirely, just go back to your normal day and know that your body has made some important progress in getting ready for labor. If your prelabor symptoms persist, continue rotating through sleeping or resting, eating, and distraction. When your symptoms change and become more consistent with an active labor pattern, contact your care provider. Think of this special time as cocooning or gathering what you need in preparation for the burst of energy and activity that happens during active labor."

PROLONGED PRELABOR AND THE LATENT PHASE OF LABOR

How long is too long for prelabor or the latent phase of labor? This question perplexes researchers, clinicians, and laboring people. There are not definitive answers. The challenges of pinpointing the onset of labor and distinguishing it from prelabor make using hours, or range of hours, as the diagnostic criterion imprecise. A 2016 systematic review of the international literature noted variation in the definition of labor onset.[15] These authors recommended that future labor onset research use laboring people's self-reported latent labor symptoms to identify labor onset. Informed by this recommendation, Tilden and colleagues[16] described latent phase duration among 1281 low-risk women in spontaneous labor. The researchers found that the median duration of the latent phase of labor was 9.0 hours among nulliparous women, the median duration of the latent phase of labor was 6.8 hours among multiparous women, and that there was wide variation in latent labor duration regardless of parity.

Recent estimates suggest that the 95th percentile of latent labor duration was 30.0 hour among nulliparas and 24.5 hours among multiparas.[16,17] Subsequently, Tilden et al analyzed a larger, Swedish sample of 67,267 people in spontaneous labor. This research suggested that among nulliparous people the median duration of the latent phase of labor was 16.0 hours and the 95th percentile of latent labor duration was 57.0 hours while among multiparous people the median duration of the latent phase of labor was 9.4 hours and the 95th percentile of latent labor duration was 33.0 hours. Wider replication studies are needed before these findings are used to shape clinical care. While the science on these topics is too early to recommend specific clinical strategies, clinical expertise recommends focusing on the person's immediate physical and emotional needs during prolonged prelabor and the latent phase while considering factors that might be contributing to longer than usual prelabor processes. For example, some may not receive adequate hydration or nutrition during prolonged prelabor. A reminder to eat and stay hydrated (by oral or intravenous fluids) can be helpful. Acknowledging the uncertainty that the laboring person is likely experiencing is also critical. It takes unique and personalized care for each pregnant person to understand what is most emotionally supportive. Doulas may also play a crucial part in closing the gap in this early phase of labor as emotional caregivers and providing physical comfort. As doula programs around the country grow, advocacy and continuous care for the entire labor process are emphasized.

Therapeutic rest is one longstanding clinical option to support prolonged prelabor, and recent research affirms the effectiveness, safety, and satisfaction of this approach. The caregiver might also explore factors that could contribute to prolonged labor. The associations between longer duration of the latent phase of labor and chorioamnionitis and fetal malposition require vigilance and, if possible, correction of fetal malposition during labor.[16,17] Another clinical pearl is to pay attention to the possibility that there is someone with the laboring person who is making them uncomfortable. Anecdotally, labor progress can slow or even stop if the laboring person does not feel trust and ease with everyone in their space.

Fetal factors that may prolong early labor

In some cases, it is possible before labor to identify conditions that increase the likelihood of prolonged early labor. For example, the occiput posterior (OP) or occiput transverse (OT) position of the fetus, or a brow, face, or compound presentation, a large unengaged or unflexed fetal head often cause a "poor fit" of the fetus in the pelvis.[18] OP and OT fetal position has been associated with significantly longer durations of the latent phase of labor. It is unclear if the fetal malposition leads to longer latent phase or if longer latent phase leads to fetal malposition.[16,17] Though most OP or OT fetal positions resolve spontaneously before birth, labor with OP or OT fetal positions frequently require more time and more contractions.

Optimal fetal positioning: prenatal features

The concept of "optimal fetal positioning" (OFP), as described by Sutton and Scott[19] and Scott,[20] applies to both late pregnancy and intrapartum positions and movements that are recommended to increase the likelihood of the fetus being in the left occiput anterior (LOA) or left occiput transverse (LOT) position at the onset of labor and throughout. The concept of OFP was developed based on a theoretical understanding of anatomy and physiology relating to childbirth and their clinical experience as midwives. OFP principles recommend that pregnant people spend very little time during late pregnancy in supine or semi-reclining positions. They suggest that these positions actually encourage the fetus into an OP (occiput posterior) position. Rather, in late pregnancy the pregnant person is encouraged to spend most of their time in forward-leaning, vertical, and lateral positions, such as those seen in Fig. 6.1. These postures propose to use gravity to increase the space at the pelvic brim, within the pelvis, and at the outlet. OFP advocates exercise during pregnancy, such as walking, swimming in a prone position, and yoga, while discouraging prenatal squatting and long car trips sitting in a bucket seat.

While this approach to optimizing the fetal position is commonly practiced in many midwifery communities, may be helpful in individual circumstances, and is unlikely to be harmful, it should be noted that evidence in support of this approach is limited. Only two studies have examined any aspect of the lifestyle practices recommended by OFP.[21,22] Among their limitations, these studies did not investigate the sweeping postural and lifestyle

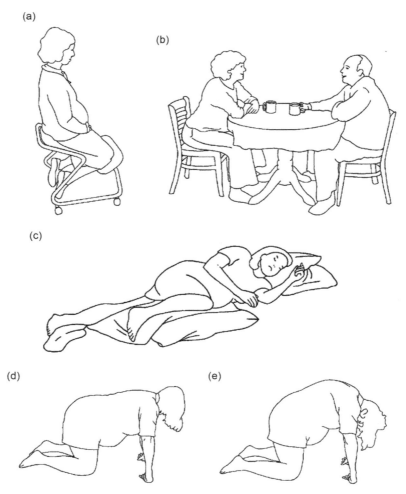

Fig. 6.1. Helpful positions for later pregnancy: (**a**) sitting upright; (**b**) sitting leaning forward; (**c**) semiprone on left side; (**d**), (**e**) doing the pelvic rocking exercise ("cat-cow" in yoga).

teachings of Sutton and Scott. Neither found any long-lasting benefit (i.e., lasting OA positions in labor) from using the hands and knees positions for brief periods, whether with pelvic rocking or abdominal stroking on a daily basis in late pregnancy. The lack of evidence of benefit has led the Royal College of Midwives to withhold support of Sutton and Scott's recommendations for pregnancy positions and movements.[23] The earlier analyses of both Gardberg[24] and Simkin[18] found that fetal position at the onset of labor does not predict fetal position at birth. Studies of side-lying positions have yielded mixed results. LeRay studied the effect of having the birthing person side-lie for one hour on the side opposite the fetal spine, with the bottom leg extended straight and the top leg flexed at 90 degrees and elevated by a peanut ball, leg rest, or pillows.[25] This intervention did not result in a change in fetal position either in labor or for birth. However, Bueno-Lopez studied the effectiveness of having the birthing person side lie on the same side as the fetal back for 40 minutes, and found that half of fetuses rotated to OA, compared to only 22% in the control group.[26] This study used only patients with epidurals and may not be generalizable to those without epidurals.

A recent systematic review and meta-analysis on this topic affirmed these earlier studies, finding that antenatal OFP interventions did not lead to optimal fetal position at birth.[27] For these reasons, those who wish to recommend OFP are advised to have a "light touch" on this topic with the people they are counseling. Some pregnant people will be quite diligent in doing everything recommended by their care providers and may be vulnerable to taking OFP activities quite seriously. This can set pregnant people up for feeling that they failed in OFP if their fetus remains OP or OT. It is important for those considering these steps to appreciate the lack of evidence in support of OFP so that if they choose this approach, they can engage with this practice understanding that it will not hurt and it might help but that results are not guaranteed.

Miles circuit (Fig 6.2)

Another option that has been proposed to help with optimizing fetal positioning is the Miles Circuit (Fig. 6.2). The Miles Circuit can be applied during prelabor or the latent phase of labor. Miles Circuit is a series of three positions done over 90 minutes (30 minutes each) for use when contractions space out or stall in order to rotate the fetus into an optimal position.[28] First the pregnant person spends 30 minutes in knee–chest position with the knees widely spread. The next 30 minutes are spent in an exaggerated far left side-lying position with the knees on pillows. Finally, 30 minutes of asymmetric pelvic opening movements such as side-step lunges up the stairs are done to open the pelvis. Available at https://www.milescircuit.com. The use of the Miles Circuit has not been scientifically studied.

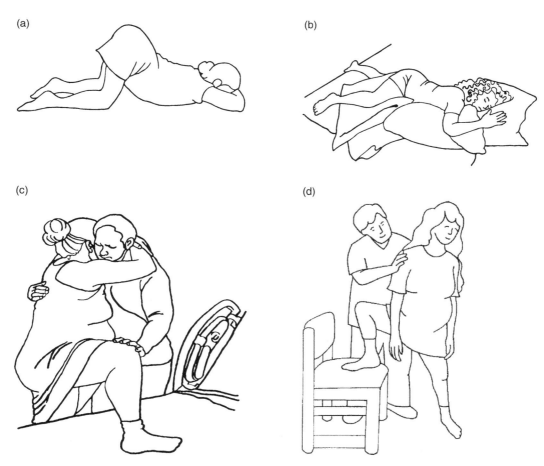

(a)

(b)

(c)

(d)

Fig. 6.2.   Miles circuit. (**a**) Exaggerated open knee chest. (**b**) Exaggerated side-lying. (**c**) Standing lunge on bed. (**d**) Standing lunge.

SUPPORT MEASURES FOR PREGNANT PEOPLE WHO ARE AT HOME IN PRELABOR AND THE LATENT PHASE (CHART 6.1)

In the absence of medical contraindications, these suggestions can help laboring people maintain normal progress and confidence while conserving the emotional and physical energy they will need in active labor:

- Continue normal restful activities (even if they cannot sleep) for as long as possible, while avoiding overexertion.
- Receive physical, emotional, and informational encouragement from their primary support people (partner, friend, relative, or doula) who may remain in close contact with them.
- Rest as much as possible through the night, including on the bed, couch, on a yoga mat, in the bathtub, or in familiar surroundings with the comforts of home. (Please note: Immersion in water in early labor may temporarily stop contractions and give the laboring person some rest.[29–31] This is an advantage if they need rest but may be a disadvantage if conditions exist that make it important that the labor progresses, for example, prolonged pregnancy or prolonged rupture of membranes).
- Allow for the pregnant person's spontaneous relaxation techniques, rhythms, and rituals to develop.
- Educate on Six Ways to Progress.
- Nurture self: eat, drink.
- Optimal Fetal Positioning and/or the Miles Circuit to encourage comfort, rest and potentially fetal rotation.
- Labor-stimulating measures such as intimacy, nipple stimulation, intercourse (if waters are intact), orgasm.
- Mental distractions such as games, media, singing, reading aloud, dancing, cooking, art projects, shopping, visiting with friends/family, going for a short drive, sitting in peaceful areas, and forest bathing in nature.
- Physical supports including massage and movement. There are many parks and walking trails that are famous for "getting into labor." Walking a local labyrinth, outdoor "art walk," or healing garden can be grounding to pass the time. Walking around the house or leaning over the back of a chair or sitting on a birth ball are also supportive movements. Very eager laboring people should be reminded that walking during prelabor should be balanced with rest; (please see "Anticipatory Guidance.") Receiving comforting touch like anchoring touch, acupressure points, gentle effleurage stroking, "waterfall" stroking down the back, or progressive relaxation "wiping" away tension can be helpful. Hair braiding, brushing, or other hygiene activities like a manicure/hand massage or pedicure/foot massage can be soothing.
- Emotional support to release fears and build confidence such as verbal affirmations, humor, hypnotherapy scripts, meditations or visualizations, close contact with partners, helpers, or pets.
- Regular check-points with their provider ("Let's talk in the morning unless you notice new symptoms or a change in your contractions") and a plan for possible progress checks.
- Remind the pregnant person of the providers' guidelines for when to come to the birthing place. If consistent with these guidelines, consider a cervical exam and assessment if this information would be useful for decision making and/or reassuring to the laboring person.
- More advanced focused labor coping techniques may begin when distraction is no longer possible and walking and talking through contractions without pausing at the peaks is no longer easy for the laboring person. Relaxation and self-calming techniques, breath awareness, and attention-focusing are appropriate at this time. Examples include: counting breaths, breathing in a color, breathing to a body part, focusing on the exhale, focal point objects, "finding the edge" of the pain, hot and cold therapy on the back, massage tools, aromatherapy, mantras, hypnotherapy scripts, counter pressure on the hips by a support person, slow dancing, leaning over a ball, all-fours, supported squats, and numerous other labor positions become essential to "pacing" the labor.
- As labor sensations become more distinct, periodically time consecutive contractions for duration, frequency, and interval to determine if they are "stronger, longer and closer together" and are signs of labor progress. Contraction-timing apps are available online; they allow those present with the laboring person to focus on things besides the mathematical calculations required to detect a contraction pattern. And the original noticing of "Start of One to the Start of the Next" is an easy formula to monitor. A clinical pearl is to emphasize to those laboring that monitoring contraction duration, frequency, and intervals only needs to be accomplished periodically and only when their symptoms intensify. Diligent and continuous monitoring of contractions can distract some from the self-care; "cocooning" activities strongly recommended during prelabor and latent labor.

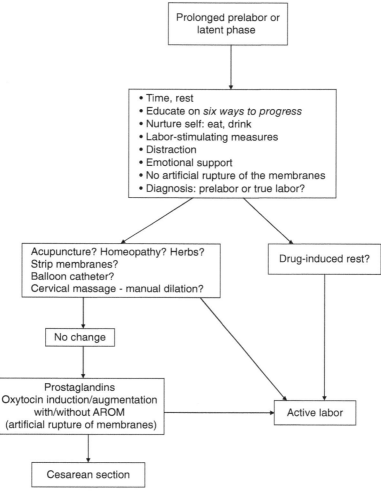

Chart 6.1.   Prolonged prelabor or latent phase.

Chart 6.1 contains an overview of prolonged pre-labor or latent phase labor. In the following sections factors that can present challenges to latent labor progress will be discussed.

SOME REASONS FOR EXCESSIVE PAIN AND DURATION OF PRELABOR OR THE LATENT PHASE

For some pregnant people, prelabor or latent phase is extremely painful and prolonged for a variety of reasons including iatrogenic, cervical, and other soft tissue factors. Those having excessively painful non-progressing pre-labor or early labor often appear to be much further along in labor than they truly are. The contractions may be so intense that the laboring person must rely on coping strategies that others might not use until late in the first stage. Of course, they can also become exhausted, discouraged, and hopeless as it becomes clear that they are not progressing as they had believed. The caregiving team's choices in language and tone are critical at these moments. It is important that caregivers express compassion and patience for those experiencing excessive pain and duration of prelabor or latent labor. It is important that caregivers avoid labeling the laboring person's ability to cope, either as a 'low pain tolerance', 'frail', 'poor coping', or in any other way discount the person's pain. Judgments do not help the laboring person and will only result in their feeling inadequate or unsupported.

Iatrogenic factors

There is evidence that walking and upright positions can reduce the duration of the first stage of labor.[32,33] Occasionally, outdated policies, labor management protocols, and practices can prevent freedom of mobility in labor and restrict laboring people to bed during prelabor or latent labor. Common reasons may include maternal and fetal monitoring (e.g., continuous fetal monitoring), maternal obstetric complications (e.g., gestation hypertension), and hospital customs or institutional routines (e.g., intravenous hydration). However, in most cases, restriction to bed is inappropriate or detrimental, particularly for low-risk pregnant people in spontaneous labor.[32]

Cervical factors

An unripe cervix at term may indicate insufficient connective tissue remodeling, which causes cervical resistance, even as intrauterine pressures increase with contractions.[34–38] Alternatively, it may indicate the presence of muscle fibers in the cervix, which cause cervical contractions during uterine contractions.[39] Throughout most of the pregnancy, the cervix typically contracts when the uterus contracts. These contractions keep the cervix firm, closed, and long, and protect against preterm labor. Cervical contractions usually decline in late pregnancy as the muscle cells in the cervix undergo the remodeling process. Remodeling, a hormonally driven transformation of cervical tissue, results in cervical ripening, effacement, and dilation. If contractions begin before the transformation has occurred, the cervix is not yet ready or ripe. So, while the cervix undergoes those early changes that prepare it to dilate, pre- or early labor can be prolonged. Cervical status may explain why some people have noticeable uterine contractions without going into premature labor (i.e., their cervix still contains muscle cells). In contrast, others have a preterm delivery with relatively few prior noticeable uterine contractions (because their cervix has undergone the remodeling process earlier than is optimal).

Management of cervical stenosis or the "zipper" cervix

Another cervix-related factor that may prolong pre- and early labor is scar tissue in the cervix, possibly from previous surgery (e.g., cauterization, cryosurgery, cone biopsy, loop electrosurgical excision procedure [LEEP], or other procedures). Cervical scars sometimes increase the resistance of the cervix to effacement and the first few centimeters of dilation.[40] Contractions of great intensity for many hours or days may result. Laboring people, doulas, and caregivers sometimes misinterpret these contractions as advanced labor, only to discover with a cervical exam that the cervix has hardly changed! If change does not occur with support, time, patience, and/or prelabor appropriate intervention, (e.g., therapeutic rest) then cervical massage to gently soften scar tissue or prostaglandins may be required to overcome this resistance. After these interventions, dilation often proceeds normally.

Cervical massage in the case of stenosis: When the cervix is completely effaced, the caregiver can gently massage the cervix in a circular motion to release adhesions from scaring. This will cause less discomfort for the laboring person if it is done between contractions. Another approach is to insert one or two fingers into the cervical os in order to gently stretch it open. As the adhesions release, the cervical os opens like a zipper, sometimes dilating several centimeters during a single contraction.

Other soft tissue (ligaments, muscles, fascia) factors

The degree of balance and symmetry of support (i.e., flexibility, tension, and torque) provided by pairs of ligaments, muscles, and fascial structures in and around the pelvis and uterus, may play a crucial role in fetal positioning and mobility within the uterus and pelvis. Though these factors have been subjected to little scientific experimentation, some practitioners (i.e., midwives, physical therapists, chiropractors, massage therapists, and other body workers) have devised numerous ways to assess and correct soft tissue factors that may impede labor progress.[41–44] These approaches are based on a detailed understanding of anatomy and kinesiology as well as how fetal position may be influenced by and may influence maternal soft tissue structures. Manual techniques and maternal movements are used to release tension, relieve musculoskeletal pain, increase flexibility or improve the balance and function of these structures within the laboring person's body. The goal is to create conditions within the body that will provide the fetus with the room and soft tissue resiliency necessary to negotiate the twisting, turning path through the birth canal.

Emotional dystocia

Extreme fear, anxiety, loneliness, stress, or anger before or during labor may lead to a buildup of catecholamines and slow labor progress.[45,46] Fear of pain and pain-related anxiety has been associated with labor pain catastrophization.[47] Pregnant people who are not supported emotionally or who have experienced previous difficult childbirths; traumatic experiences such as emotional, physical, or sexual abuse; substance abuse; multiple hospitalizations; or other adverse life experiences may find early labor unexpectedly painful or traumatic.[48–54] Exhaustion, discouragement, and feelings of hopelessness may result from a long prelabor or latent phase. The laboring person's optimism and coping ability can diminish and pain can worsen as time goes on without apparent labor progress. It is helpful to ask the laboring person about their emotional state during latent labor. Their answer may assist the caregiver in diagnosing emotional distress.[55] Between contractions, questions such as "What was going through your mind during that contraction?" or "How are you feeling right now?" or "Why do you think this labor is going slowly right now?" may reveal that the pregnant person is frightened or worried over specific concerns. Knowing these concerns can reveal opportunities for the caregiver to offer the laboring person more effective reassurance and/or emotional support.

The next section offers suggestions to improve labor progress or reduce discomfort in early labor. Of course, if fetal distress, macrosomia, malpresentation, inadequate contractions, or other complications are diagnosed, supportive measures should be tailored to account for these factors.

TROUBLESHOOTING MEASURES FOR PAINFUL PROLONGED PRELABOR OR LATENT PHASE

- For the pain and discouragement that may accompany some longer early labors, labor inductions or an unripe or scarred cervix, reassure the pregnant person that under these circumstances early labor is more challenging, but that it does not necessarily mean that active labor will be abnormal.[55] Those experiencing such labor patterns also need validation, intense emotional support, and physical comfort. Care providers should try not to contribute to self-doubt or worries by suggesting that something is wrong or that they are at fault and that their behavior is making it worse.
- If they are discouraged over slow dilation or non-progressing contractions, remind the laboring person that before their cervix can dilate, it must move forward, ripen, and efface—each of which is a positive sign of progress. Be sure to disclose any progress in these areas to the laboring person whenever you check their cervix. Use the "The Six Ways to progress in labor—prelabor to birth" earlier in this chapter.
- Avoid the term "false labor" because it implies that the laboring person's contractions are somehow "not real" and that because their cervix is not dilating, the contractions are not accomplishing anything significant. Such implications are most discouraging to the person who is experiencing prelabor or prolonged latent labor symptoms. In fact, if the cervix is changing at all, these prelabor contractions are preparing the cervix for dilation.
- Encourage the laboring person to seek and use positions or movements that they find more comfortable.
- Offer a bath, shower, or massage as a temporary relaxer and pain reliever.
- Transcutaneous electrical nerve stimulation (TENS) may be especially useful to relieve back pain during early labor. TENS is more useful for back pain than for other labor pain and is more beneficial when introduced early in labor.
- If at all possible, do not restrict movement to the bed. There is no evidence that reclining positions during labor will prevent cord prolapse, so this is not an appropriate reason to encourage lying down even after membranes are ruptured. If there is provider or patient anxiety about walking or standing after membranes are ruptured, the caregiver might auscultate the fetal heart and assess fetal movement with the laboring person in an upright position. An upright position may actually protect against a prolapsed cord, as gravity may help keep the head applied to the cervix, thus preventing the cord from slipping through.

- Assess the laboring person's emotional state during early labor; if they are distressed, try to address their concerns and/or offer appropriate measures to help improve their emotional state.
- For exhaustion, discouragement, and hopelessness, you can suggest a change of activity or environment: suggest a change of positions every twenty minutes, bathing, comb hair, brush teeth, take a walk, play some upbeat music. These measures are especially effective as the sun comes up after a long night with little progress. The new day can renew spirits.
- Offering an attentive conversation with the laboring person and their birth companions, encouraging them to express their feelings. Acknowledge and validate their feelings of frustration, discouragement, fatigue, or even anger at the staff for not "doing something" to correct the problem. They may benefit from a good cry, followed by a pep talk and perhaps a visit from a friend or family member who is rested and optimistic.
- If the above measures are unsuccessful, therapeutic rest with a sleep medication or pain reliever may be an appropriate choice.

MEASURES TO ALLEVIATE PAINFUL, NON-PROGRESSING, NON-DILATING CONTRACTIONS IN PRELABOR OR LATENT PHASE

If early contractions are painful and irregular with little or no progress in dilation, it makes sense to consider persistent asynclitism, a deflexed fetal head, or another unfavorable fetal position, such as OP (Fig. 6.3).

Synclitism and asynclitism

Labor normally begins with the fetal head in asynclitism (i.e., the head is angled so that one of the parietal bones, rather than the vertex, presents at the pelvic inlet, as shown in Fig. 6.4). This facilitates passage of the fetal head through the pelvic inlet, and then the head usually shifts into synclitism (Fig. 6.5) so that the vertex presents as the head descends further. However, sometimes the asynclitism persists and, if so, it can keep the fetus from rotating

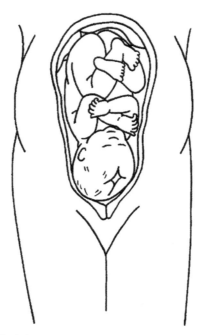

Fig. 6.3.   Right occiput posterior, abdominal view.

(a)   (b)

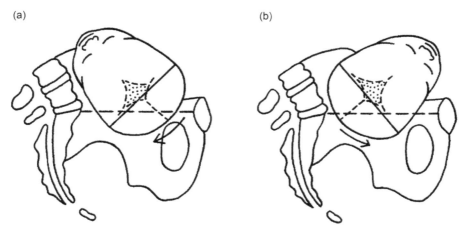

Fig. 6.4. (**a**) Posterior asynclitism. (**b**) Anterior asynclitism.

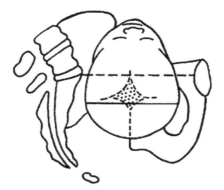

Fig. 6.5. Synclitism.

and descending.[56] Without descent, the head may not be well applied to the cervix and contractions often become irregular and ineffective. At this stage of labor, it is difficult or impossible (and not considered very clinically important) to assess the angle and position of the fetal head. However, if contractions are irregular and ineffective for a long time, position changes and movements may correct the problem and improve the contraction pattern.

If the laboring person is having their first labor or has good abdominal muscle tone, suggesting forward leaning positions can help move the fetus's center of gravity forward, encouraging the head to pivot into a more favorable position (Figs 6.6–6.9). This may evenly disperse or increase the head-to-cervix force, leading to more regular, more effective contractions.

If the pregnant person's abdomen is presenting as pendulous, the fetus's center of gravity may fall so far forward that the fetus is not well aligned with the pelvic inlet. There may be benefit from assuming a semi-reclining position (Fig. 6.9). Having them "lean back" in this way may move the fetus's center of gravity toward their back, thus aligning the fetus with the pelvis and allowing the head to put more pressure on the cervix during contractions. This repositioning in itself may lead to more regular, more effective contractions.

King suggests abdominal lifting (Fig. 6.10) with a pelvic tilt during contractions at any time in labor if there is back pain in association with pendulous abdominal muscles, a short waist, a previous back injury, or a

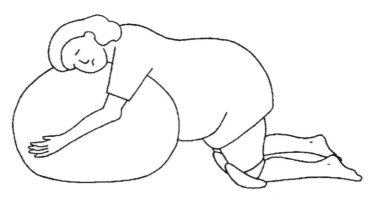

Fig. 6.6. Kneeling with a ball and knee pads to correct possible posterior asynclitism.

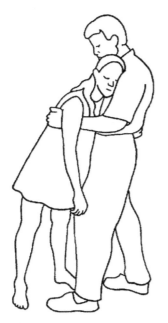

Fig. 6.7. Standing, leaning forward on partner.

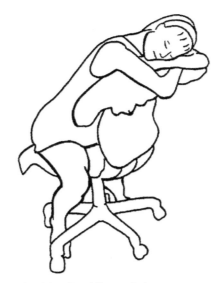

Fig. 6.8. Straddling a chair.

malpositioned baby.[57] Abdominal lifting should only be performed by a skilled maternity care attendant. When it works well, abdominal lifting helps to realign the fetus's torso in relation to the angle of the pelvic inlet.[58] The contractions then become more efficient in pressing the baby's head onto the cervix. We suggest that fetal heart tones be checked periodically by the nurse or midwife during a contraction with abdominal lifting. In the remote possibility that the heart rate decelerates, it might be due to anterior placement of the umbilical cord. The fetus might become markedly more active if this is the case, or the heart rate may slow. If so, the pressure on the low abdomen from the abdominal lift could compress the cord; therefore, abdominal lifting should be discontinued.

(a) (b)

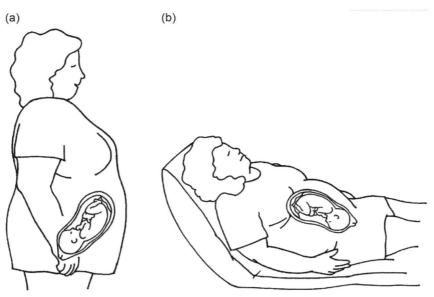

Fig. 6.9. **(a)** Pregnant person with poor abdominal muscle tone and pendulous abdomen, standing. Fetal center of gravity falls away from pelvic inlet. **(b)** Pregnant person with poor abdominal muscle tone and pendulous abdomen, semi-reclining. Fetal center of gravity aligns with pelvic inlet.

(a) (b)

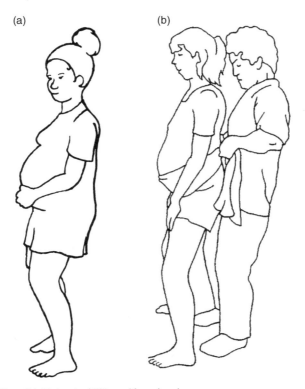

Fig. 6.10. **(a)** Abdominal lifting. **(b)** Abdominal lifting with a shawl.

OPEN KNEE–CHEST POSITION

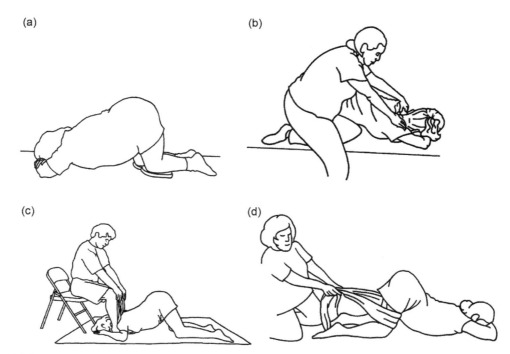

(a)

(b)

(c)

(d)

Fig. 6.11. (**a**) Open knee–chest position. (**b**) Partner's hands-on aid to maintaining the position. (**c**) Open knee–chest position, shoulders resting on partner's shins. (**d**) Open knee–chest with sheet or shawl around thighs and partner pulling back.

El Halta[59] suggested the open knee–chest position for specific symptoms in prelabor or the latent phase, when there is a long period of frequent, irregular, and brief uterine contractions, usually accompanied by severe persistent backache but resulting in little or no dilation. This contraction pattern seems to be associated with a fetal malposition. The position takes advantage of gravity to allow the fetus to "back out" of the laboring person's pelvis, rotate, and descend again in a more favorable position.

When the laboring person's stomach is empty (to avoid reflux), they spend 30–45 minutes in an open knee–chest position: their hips are flexed to an angle greater than 90 degrees (Fig. 6.11a). This position has been associated with rapid reduction of the back pain. Because the position is difficult to maintain for 30 or more minutes, the laboring person will find it easier if is assisted in any of these ways:

1. The birth companion, partner, or doula stands beside the bed with the laboring person in the open knee-chest position. The partner places their hands on the top of the laboring person's shoulders, and leans back, letting their upper body weight pull back on the laboring person's shoulders to support their weight and reduce effort to maintain the position (Fig. 6.11b).
2. The partner or doula sits on a straight chair, feet flat on the floor about 10 inches apart. The laboring person gets onto hands and knees and leans forward, placing their head between their partner's ankles with their shoulders supported by the support person's shins (padded with small towels), so that they can support much of the weight of the laboring person's upper body (Fig. 6.11c). The laboring person can place hands around the support person's ankles and rest their head on their hands.

3. The laboring person lies on the bed, in the open knee–chest position. Their support partner or doula wraps a shawl, fabric tie or sheet around their upper thighs close to the hips but below the belly and gently pulls back to help support the open knee–chest position.

Caution: Do not fold the scarf into a narrow band and place it beneath their belly and across their groin. The pressure it will cause in this area could impair the circulation through their groin area, especially if the position is held for a half hour or more. Widening the scarf over the thighs disperses the pressure evenly and safely.

The open knee–chest position tilts the pelvis forward with the inlet lower than the outlet. This allows gravity to encourage the unengaged OP fetal head out of the pelvis and may allow the head to reposition more favorably toward OA before re-entering the pelvis.

CLOSED KNEE–CHEST POSITION

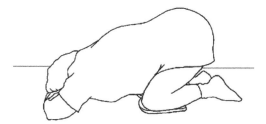

Fig. 6.12. Closed knee–chest position with knee pads. Pressure of the thighs on the abdomen may interfere with fetal rotation.

By contrast, a "closed knee–chest position" (Fig. 6.12) causes the laboring person's hips and knees to be flexed so that their thighs are beneath their abdomen and the pelvic inlet is higher than the outlet. This does not encourage the fetus to move out of the pelvis and removes the gravity effect.

SIDE-LYING RELEASE

Gail Tully devised the side-lying release (Fig 6.13) for many purposes in her Spinning Babies® approach including for hip and back pain in pregnancy, fetal malpresentations or malposition, labor contractions without progress, and others. The technique utilizes a side-lying position on a firm surface, with the top leg dangling unsupported over the side, which allows for passive stretching and tension release in deep structures (muscles, ligaments, fascia) in the hip and low back. It should be done on both sides. The technique requires two people and is quite detailed.[41]

Prolonged prelabor and the latent phase of labor by themselves rarely indicate a complication, although they are discouraging and exhausting for the laboring person. Suggestions are given for coping with the discouragement and early measures are described that may correct possible fetal malposition. Most of the measures suggested here

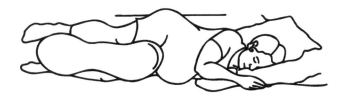

Fig. 6.13. Side-lying Release.

are well tolerated in labor but if they are distressing or uncomfortable, the laboring person should be encouraged to do what they find most helpful.

WHEN PROGRESS IN PRELABOR OR LATENT PHASE REMAINS INADEQUATE

If progress seems particularly slow when a pregnant person is in the prelabor or latent phase, there are several strategies that can be used if the situation warrants. The latent phase of labor is now recognized to be longer than previously thought, and pregnant people may become discouraged and fatigued.[16,17] The strategies that will be described are therapeutic rest, nipple stimulation, and membrane sweeping and avoidance of the artificial rupture of membranes (AROM).

Therapeutic rest

The pregnant person may be exhausted, discouraged, and frustrated if progress has not improved after a variety of measures are tried. Assuming all else is normal and latent labor is not progressing, the caregiver may use medications that broadly fit under the term "therapeutic rest" to promote comfort while enhancing labor progress. While "therapeutic rest" is not clearly defined, generally, the term is used to describe the use of medication to alleviate painful contractions, promote rest, or relieve the pain, anxiety, or insomnia in the latent phase of labor.[60] The goal of this therapy is sleep rather than analgesia. A variety of medications may be used and the choice of medications will vary by clinical setting.[60] Medication must be carefully selected to enhance benefits and minimize risks as there is no clear indication for use, and currently there is insufficient knowledge on the maternal and neonatal side-effects associated with "therapeutic rest."[60] However, a prospective cohort study of 66 individuals receiving intramuscular morphine sulfate and promethazine as outpatients in early labor suggested that therapeutic rest is a well-tolerated and effective option for outpatient pain control in early labor.[61]

Nipple stimulation

Nipple stimulation can be used to augment labor when contractions are inadequate. A Cochrane review included five trials with a total of 719 pregnant people in whom breast stimulation was compared with no intervention, and two trials where breast stimulation was compared to oxytocin.[62] When the cervix was favorable and breast stimulation was compared to no intervention, the number of pregnant people not in labor by 72 hours was significantly reduced by the use of nipple stimulation. There was also a significantly lower rate of postpartum hemorrhage. There were no significant differences in the rates of cesarean birth, meconium-stained amniotic fluid, or hyperstimulation of the uterus. When breast stimulation was compared with oxytocin, no significant differences were found on the outcomes of labor initiation by 72 hours, cesarean rate, or meconium-stained fluid. Since the publication of the Cochrane review, Demirel and Guler[63] conducted a randomized control trial of 390 pregnant people in Turkey, who were randomized to either nipple stimulation, uterine stimulation, or neither.[63] Those in both the nipple stimulation group and the uterine stimulation group had shorter labors, were less likely to need augmentation with oxytocin, and had fewer cesarean sections than those in the control group.[63] Therefore, nipple stimulation is a viable option to attempt before considering oxytocin augmentation of labor. Because several fetal deaths were reported in a study that included high-risk laboring people, the authors of the Cochrane review concluded that breast stimulation should not be used in that subgroup until further research verifies the safety of the intervention. There is a potential risk of uterine hyperstimulation and tachysystole when using nipple stimulation because the amount of oxytocin released cannot be controlled. Existing protocols are focused on diminishing this risk through the use of rest periods and ceasing stimulation when a contraction starts and resuming when the contraction subsides.

While nipple stimulation appears to be beneficial in initiating labor, protocols vary between sources and a standardized definition is lacking.[64] Several specific protocols have been described as a part of research studies. One approach uses an electric breast pump unilaterally for 15 minutes on each breast.[65] Alternatively, either manual stimulation or an electric breast pump unilaterally (on the lowest setting) for 10 minutes followed by 5 minutes of rest can be used.[66] This pattern is repeated up to four times or until contractions are less than 3 minutes apart. Manual stimulation can be done by the pregnant person or by the partner either by gently stroking the nipple directly or indirectly through clothing.

Other protocols described by practitioners include instructions for the pregnant person to stop the nipple stimulation if a contraction occurs or to stimulate the nipples only between contractions.[64] There is no evidence for the efficacy of one protocol over another, and research in this area is needed.[64]

Membrane sweeping

Membrane "sweeping" or "stripping" is a mechanical way to induce or augment labor in which the care provider inserts one or two fingers into the cervix and "sweeps" the fingers in a circular motion around the cervix to separate the membrane, or bag of water, from the cervix. The goal of membrane sweeps is to cause the release of prostaglandins or a small amount of "bloody show" to stimulate cervical ripening or contractions without medications. A 2020 Cochrane review by Finucane and colleagues concluded that while there is limited evidence, membrane sweeping may be helpful in causing spontaneous contractions.[67] Candidates for consideration of membrane sweeping should be full term, with no evidence of placenta previa and no active infection such as HIV or Herpes. Prior cesarean and planned vaginal birth after cesarean and/or, Group B Streptococcus colonization are not contraindications to membrane sweeping, although individual assessment of candidates is recommended. Membrane sweeping may be preferred by pregnant people who hope to avoid induction of labor using medication. It is unclear how many membrane sweeps are needed or at what frequency they should be offered. Some care providers offer membrane sweeping at term in the office prior to labor as a means of encouraging labor to start. Membrane sweeping or cervical massage may also be used during early latent labor to cause stronger contractions. Prior to membrane sweeping, the caregiver must explain the procedure, risks and benefits, and obtain informed consent. The caregiver must assure the pregnant person that the procedure can be stopped at any time. Some pregnant people find membrane sweeping invasive and uncomfortable, while others tolerate it well.

Artificial rupture of membranes in latent labor

Amniotomy is a procedure used to purposely break the amniotic sac or bag of water using a small hook that nicks the membrane to release fluid and is done to speed up labor. Amniotomy is also known as artificial rupture of membranes (AROM) or by the description "breaking the water" and should not be routinely used for laboring people in normally progressing spontaneous labor or when labor has become prolonged.[68] While the primary goal of AROM is to speed up contractions and shorten the length of labor, the World Health Organization does not recommend routine amniotomy for prevention or delay of labor because of the lack of sufficient evidence.[69] In latent labor, AROM can disturb or interfere with the physiologic process of labor and start a cascade of intrapartum interventions.[70,71] Laboring people may need pain relief to help cope with stronger and more painful contractions that can follow AROM. Laboring people become closely monitored once the procedure is performed, and their labors are placed on time limits. Laboring people also can have unpredictable responses to the procedure, and it is associated with potential risks, including fetal heart deceleration, increased cesarean delivery rates for fetal distress, increases in ascending infections, an increased chance of cord prolapse, and increased discomfort and pain.[72] Laboring people should not feel pressured to commit to having AROM and a laboring person's verbal consent must be obtained before AROM is performed. If the maternal and fetal status is reassuring, the preferred course of events is letting the labor process unfold without AROM.

CAN PRENATAL ACTIONS PREVENT SOME POSTDATES PREGNANCIES, PROLONGED PRELABORS, OR EARLY LABORS?

Prenatal preparation of the cervix for dilation

The prospect of remaining pregnant beyond the due date or having a prolonged prelabor or early labor worries expectant parents and their caregivers. Rather than patiently awaiting labor, parents may feel impatient and/or receive pressure and advice on ways they can hasten ripening of the cervix or start labor themselves. Recent research suggests that induction of labor at 39 weeks gestation or 40 weeks gestation may increase chances of vaginal birth.[73,74] These findings might increase interest in prenatal interventions to encourage cervical ripening. As well, induction of labor is recommended in some pregnancies, based on medical recommendations and/or personal wishes of the pregnant person. It is also important to remember that despite a scheduled or recommended induction of labor, some pregnant people may still hope to avoid induction of labor and strive for a less interventive birth. We will focus here on those circumstances when an induction is indicated and planned.

Pregnant people may try complementary alternative medicine (CAM) techniques to hasten the ripening and effacement of the cervix, or to start labor. Most of these non-pharmacologic measures have not received sufficient scientific study to establish their efficacy in priming the cervix or improving the course of prelabor and early labor. Many of these are self-administered remedies while others require the guidance and expertise of a professional. Table 6.1 contains descriptions of some of these non-pharmacologic techniques, along with each technique's suspected mechanism of action, potential risks, and effectiveness as reported in the scientific literature. Some of the techniques have not been subjected to any scientific scrutiny, and fall into the category of "folk remedies" or traditional knowledge.

Table 6.1. Self-administered techniques to ripen the cervix and induce labor.

Self-administered method and how it is done	How it is thought to work	Effectiveness	References
Acupressure Intermittent finger pressure on meridians. A frequently used labor point for labor induction or augmentation is Spleen 6 (SP6), located on the medial aspect of the lower leg, three to four fingerbreadths above the ankle. Protocols vary, but firm pressure is held on the SP6 point during contractions, by the midwife or care provider. *Caution*: It is advised that women avoid this stimulation unless they are at term and there is a plan to do a medical induction. It is theoretically possible to start labor prematurely if done too early.	Acupressure stimulates meridians as defined within Chinese medicine. Spleen 6 is understood to increase contraction strength and decreased anxiety. Acupressure is believed to have originated in Japan in the early 1900s.[75] *There is more on this procedure in Chapter 11.*	A 2017 Cochrane review on acupuncture and acupressure did not find that these approaches were associated with decreases in rates of labor intervention, including cesarean.[76] A 2020 Cochrane review on acupuncture and acupressure indicates that either technique may slightly reduce labor pain.[77] Overall, more studies are needed but acupressure is a low-risk, readily available option to try to increase contractions or help with labor pain during a long latent phase.	Smith et al.[76] Smith et al.[77]
Breast/nipple stimulation Light manual stroking or breast pumping of one or both breasts; pause when contractions begin, resume after contractions end	Increases oxytocin production to causecontractions	A 2005 Cochrane review of breast Stimulation, compared to placebo or no intervention, suggests that breast stimulation significantly reduced number of women not in labor 72 hours later if cervix was favorable when started. Also there was less postpartum hemorrhage.[62] Safe for low-risk women. May be unsafe for women with high-risk pregnancies. A small study (n = 42) showed that breast simulation was associated with an increase in salivary oxytocin[78]	Kavanagh et al.[62] Takahata et al.[78]
Sexual activity (intercourse, fellatio, clitoral) Ejaculation of semen into vagina or mouth; manual stimulation of the clitoris leading to orgasm. Intercourse is risky if membranes have ruptured	Semen contains prostaglandins, which ripen the cervix. Clitoral stimulation and orgasm increases oxytocin release	Though contractions often result from sexual activity, a recent systematic review and meta-analysis of randomized controlled trials did not show that sexual activity increased spontaneous labor onset.[79]	Carbone et al.[79]

Table 6.1. Alternative and complementary approaches* to ripen cervix or induce labor.

Method	How it is thought to work	Effectiveness	References
	Method How it is thought to work		
Acupuncture			
Requires a skilled, certified acupuncturist who painlessly inserts fine needles into many points on the body. Sometimes needles are heated with a smoldering herbal paste (also painless) or with electrical current (causing tingling sensations). Treatments at full-term are daily or every other day for a few treatments	By stimulating points on certain meridians, energy (qi or chi) is released. A staple of Eastern medicine, acupuncture is used for a variety of conditions, including induction of labor, believed to be caused by alterations of energy flow along the meridians. Western health specialists try to explain acupuncture's success in Western medical terms, including an increase of endorphin production, or a reduction in inflammation, or other explanations	A 2017 Cochrane review on acupuncture and acupressure did not find that these approaches were associated with decreases in rates of labor intervention, including cesarean.[73] A 2020 Cochrane review on acupuncture and acupressure indicates that either technique may slightly reduce labor pain.[74] Overall, more studies are needed but acupuncture is unlikely to cause harm and may be helpful.	Smith et al.[76] Smith et al.[77]
Homeopathy			
Based on the idea that "like cures like." Giving very dilute doses of a substance that would cause adverse reactions in undiluted doses enhances the body's regulation/regulatory processes. Use of caulophyllum and pulsatilla are commonly used to ripen the cervix. Caulophyllum is thought to convert prelabor contractions to dilating contractions. Cimicifuga has been recommended for when the cervix is rigid or tightly closed and/or does not dilate. Cimicifuga has also been used to decrease labor fear among those with a history of traumatic childbirth, miscarriage, or abortion.[78] Homeopathics are generally given in pill or liquid form	To prevent non-productive irregular contractions at term, these substances may be given to "tone" the uterus and help produce productive contractions	"There is insufficient evidence to recommend the use of homoeopathy as a method of induction."[80] Trials were not of high quality and clinically meaningful outcomes were not measured. No harm was reported	Smith CA[80] Mallory DJ[81]
Castor oil (sometimes with verbena oil added): "induction cocktail"			
Castor oil is mixed with fruit juice (sometimes with baking soda added to reduce oiliness) or into a smoothie. It may be given two or three times before effects occur. When combined with verbena oil, the mix may be as follows: 2T. 3 castor oil, 5 drops lemon-verbena oil, 11/4 4 cups water, 3/ cup apricot juice and 2T. almond butter Importantly, castor oil should not be used until after the due date is passed and labor induction is chosen or indicated	For centuries castor oil has been used as a cathartic to cause contractions, possibly by increasing prostaglandin production from strongly contracting intestines. It causes nausea, cramps, and diarrhea and sometimes leads to labor. An active ingredient, ricinoleic acid, was recently discovered in castor oil. It stimulates smooth muscle cells to contract (as are found in the intestines and in the uterus)[79]	A small observational study (n = 293) showed that 90% of those who consumed castor oil to induce labor delivered vaginally.[82] And a small RCT (n = 81) found that castor oil consumption significantly increased the odds of entering spontaneous active labor among multips but not among nulips.[83] While no maternal fetal harms were noted in castor oil studies, sample sizes were underpowered to identify risk patterns. Oil of verbena has not been studied for its safety and efficacy	Tunaru et al.[84] DeMaria et al.[82] Gilad et al.[83]

(Continued)

Table 6.1. *(Continued)*

Method	How it is thought to work	Effectiveness	References
	Method How it is thought to work		
Evening primrose oil			
Evening primrose oil (EPO) is taken as capsules inserted into the vagina so that the oil bathes the cervix in the last week of pregnancy. Often used with other methods in this table	Widely used by midwives for cervical ripening. May reduce inflammation, helps ripen and efface the cervix. Contains gamma-linoleic acid, which is a precursor of prostaglandins. Recommended not be taken orally; otherwise considered safe when given vaginally	The efficacy and safety of evening primrose oil is unclear. One small (n = 40) RCT did not show that EPO was associated with higher Bishop scores[85] while a second small (n = 86) RCT including nulliparous women showed that vaginal EPO use was significantly associated with higher Bishop scores.[86] More research is needed to draw conclusions.	Kalati et al.[85] Najafi et al.[86]
Herbal teas and tinctures or foods			
Numerous herbs are used as tinctures and teas. Some prenatal mixtures of teas may ripen and efface the cervix if taken over a 5- or 6-week period until labor begins (i.e., squaw vine, blessed thistle, black cohosh, pennyroyal herb, false unicorn root, red raspberry leaf, and lobelia). Others are used to start labor. These and many others are used too induce contractions. Emerging research suggests that date consumption may encourage labor onset[89]	Mechanisms of action seem to be poorly understood, with trial-and-error and empirical observations of associated effects seemingly the main rationales for acceptance	Method based on a long tradition of use without scientific scrutiny Mostly categorized as traditional knowledge or folk remedies. Few scientific studies of effectiveness and mechanism of action exist. Raspberry leaf tea use did not show harm nor benefit in trials that include pregnant people (Bowman et al.),[87] however, a 2019 systematic review suggests that raspberry leaf tea is associated with increased risk for cesarean and that use of the herbal medicine Mwanaphepo was associated with maternal illness and neonatal death (Munoz Balbontin et al.)[88] If herbs will be used, a professional herbalist or caregiver with added training in use of these herbs should be involved, as undesired effects may occur if selection, timing, and dosage of the product are inappropriate. A 2019 systematic review and meta-analysis indicates that date fruit consumptions significantly increased cervical dilation at hospital admission, rates of spontaneous labor onset, and decreased the length of second stage[86]	Bowman et al.[87] Munoz Balbontin et al.[88] Nasiri et al.[89]

*Note: These techniques require provider knowledge and/or intervention.

If complementary or alternative methods do not succeed in ripening the cervix sufficiently, or in initiating labor, then the following techniques can be considered:

- Mechanical cervical stimulation, such as balloon catheter cervical dilators or laminaria.
- Sweeping or stripping the membranes.
- Artificial rupture of the membranes.
- Oral or intravaginal prostaglandins
- Synthetic oxytocin intravenous drips.

It is beyond the scope of this book to provide an in-depth discussion of these methods.

REFERENCES

1. Hundley V, Downe S, Buckley SJ. (2020) The initiation of labour at term gestation: Physiology and practice implications. *Best Practice & Research. Clinical Obstetrics & Gynaecology* 67, 4–18. doi: 10.1016/j.bpobgyn.2020.02.006
2. Eri TS, Bondas T, Gross MM, Janssen P, Green JM. (2015) A balancing act in an unknown territory: A metasynthesis of first-time mothers' experiences in early labour. *Midwifery* 31(3), e58–e67. doi: 10.1016/j.midw.2014.11.007
3. Ragusa A, Mansur M, Zanini A, Musicco M, Maccario L, Borsellino G. (2005) Diagnosis of labor: A prospective study. *MedGenMed: Medscape General Medicine* 7(3), 61.
4. Edmonds JK, Zabbo G. (2017) Women's descriptions of labor onset and progression before hospital admission. *Nursing for Women's Health* 21(4), 250–258. doi: 10.1016/j.nwh.2017.06.003
5. Gross MM, Haunschild T, Stoexen T, Methner V, Guenter HH. (2003) Women's recognition of the spontaneous onset of labor. *Birth (Berkeley, Calif.)* 30(4), 267–271. doi: 10.1046/j.1523-536x.2003.00257.x
6. Anderson MV, Rutherford MD. (2011) Recognition of novel faces after single exposure is enhanced during pregnancy. *Evolutionary Psychology: An International Journal of Evolutionary Approaches to Psychology and Behavior* 9(1), 47–60.
7. Beebe KR, Humphreys J. (2006) Expectations, perceptions, and management of labor in nulliparas prior to hospitalization. *Journal of Midwifery & Women's Health* 51(5), 347–353. doi: 10.1016/j.jmwh.2006.02.013
8. Nyman V, Downe S, Berg M. (2011) Waiting for permission to enter the labour ward world: First time parents' experiences of the first encounter on a labour ward. *Sexual & Reproductive Healthcare: Official Journal of the Swedish Association of Midwives* 2(3), 129–134. doi: 10.1016/j.srhc.2011.05.004
9. Zhang J, Landy HJ, Ware Branch D, Burkman R, Haberman S, Gregory KD, Hatjis CG, Ramirez MM, Bailit JL, Gonzalez-Quintero VH, Hibbard JU, Hoffman MK, Kominiarek M, Learman LA, Van Veldhuisen P, Troendle J, Reddy UM, Consortium on Safe Labor. (2010) Contemporary patterns of spontaneous labor with normal neonatal outcomes. *Obstetrics and Gynecology* 116(6), 1281–1287. doi: 10.1097/AOG.0b013e3181fdef6e
10. Bailit JL, Dierker L, Blanchard MH, Mercer BM. (2005) Outcomes of women presenting in active versus latent phase of spontaneous labor. *Obstetrics and Gynecology* 105(1), 77–79. doi: 10.1097/01.AOG.0000147843.12196.00
11. Miller YD, Armanasco AA, McCosker L, Thompson R. (2020) Variations in outcomes for women admitted to hospital in early versus active labour: An observational study. *BMC Pregnancy and Childbirth* 20(1), 469. doi: 10.1186/s12884-020-03149-7
12. Berghella V, Di Mascio D. (2020) Evidence-based labor management: Before labor (Part 1). *American Journal of Obstetrics & Gynecology MFM* 2(1), 100080. doi: 10.1016/j.ajogmf.2019.100080
13. Beake, R, Chang, BYS, Cheyne, RM, Spiby, H, Sandall, H, Bick, D. (2018) Experiences of early labour management from perspectives of women, labour companions and health professionals: A systematic review of qualitative evidence. *Midwifery* 57, 69–84. https://0-doi-org.libus.csd.mu.edu/10.1016/j.midw.2017.11.002
14. Sommers M. Personal communication Mary Sommers 10/12/2021.
15. Hanley GE, Munro S, Greyson D, Gross MM, Hundley V, Spiby H, Janssen PA. (2016) Diagnosing onset of labor: A systematic review of definitions in the research literature. *BMC Pregnancy and Childbirth* 16, 71. doi: 10.1186/s12884-016-0857-4
16. Tilden EL, Phillippi JC, Ahlberg M, King TL, Dissanayake M, Lee CS, Snowden JM, Caughey AB. (2019) Describing latent phase duration and associated characteristics among 1281 low-risk women in spontaneous labor. *Birth (Berkeley, Calif.)* 46(4), 592–601. doi: 10.1111/birt.12428

17. Tilden EL, Caughey AB, Ahlberg M, Lundborg L, Wikström AK, Liu X, Ng K, Lapidus J, Sandström A. (2023) Latent phase duration and associated outcomes: a contemporary, population-based observational study. *American Journal of Obstetrics and Gynecology*, 228(5S), S1025–S1036.e9. doi: 10.1016/j.ajog.2022.10.003

18. Simkin P. (2010) The fetal occiput posterior position: State of the science and a new perspective. *Birth (Berkeley, Calif.)* 37(1), 61–71. doi: 10.1111/j.1523-536X.2009.00380.x

19. Sutton J, Scott P. (1996) *Understanding and Teaching Optimal Foetal Positioning*. Birth Concepts.

20. Scott P. (2003) *Sit up and Take Notice!: Positioning Yourself for a Better Birth*. Great Scott Publications.

21. Andrews CM, Andrews EC. (1983) Nursing, maternal postures, and fetal position. *Nursing Research* 32(6), 336–341.

22. Kariminia A, Chamberlain ME, Keogh J, Shea A. (2004) Randomised controlled trial of effect of hands and knees posturing on incidence of occiput posterior position at birth. *BMJ (Clinical Research Ed.)* 328(7438), 490. doi: 10.1136/bmj.37942.594456.44

23. Munro J, Jokinen M. (2012) Persistent lateral and posterior fetal positions at the onset of labour. In: *Evidence Based Guidelines for Midwifery-led Care in Labour*. Royal College of Midwives Trust.

24. Gardberg M, Laakkonen E, Sälevaara M. (1998) Intrapartum sonography and persistent occiput posterior position: A study of 408 deliveries. *Obstetrics and Gynecology* 91(5 Pt 1), 746–749. doi: 10.1016/s0029-7844(98)00074-x

25. Le Ray C, Lepleux F, De La Calle A, Guerin J, Sellam N, Dreyfus M, Chantry AA. (2016) Lateral asymmetric decubitus position for the rotation of occipito-posterior positions: Multicenter randomized controlled trial EVADELA. *American Journal of Obstetrics and Gynecology* 215(4), 511.e1–511.e5117. doi: 10.1016/j.ajog.2016.05.033

26. Bueno-Lopez V, Fuentelsaz-Gallego C, Casellas-Caro M, Falgueras-Serrano AM, Crespo-Berros S, Silvano-Cocinero AM, Alcaine-Guisado C, Zamoro Fuentes M, Carreras E, Terré-Rull C. (2018) Efficiency of the modified Sims maternal position in the rotation of persistent occiput posterior position during labor: A randomized clinical trial. *Birth (Berkeley, Calif.)* 45(4), 385–392. doi: 10.1111/birt.12347

27. Levy AT, Weingarten S, Ali A, Quist-Nelson J, Berghella V. (2021) Hands-and-knees posturing and fetal occiput anterior position: A systematic review and meta-analysis. *American Journal of Obstetrics & Gynecology MFM* 3(4), 100346. doi: 10.1016/j.ajogmf.2021.100346

28. Miles MH, Muza S, Dewey K. (n.d.) *The Miles Circuit*. https://www.milescircuit.com

29. Kelly AJ, Kavanagh J, Thomas J. (2013) Castor oil, bath and/or enema for cervical priming and induction of labour. *The Cochrane Database of Systematic Reviews* 2013(7), CD003099. doi: 10.1002/14651858.CD003099.pub2

30. Cluett ER, Burns E. (2009) Immersion in water in labour and birth. *The Cochrane Database of Systematic Reviews* (2), CD000111. doi: 10.1002/14651858.CD000111.pub3

31. Odent M. (1997) Can water immersion stop labor? *Journal of Nurse-Midwifery* 42(5), 414–416. doi: 10.1016/s0091-2182(97)00051-7

32. Lawrence A, Lewis L, Hofmeyr GJ, Styles C. (2013) Maternal positions and mobility during first stage labour. *The Cochrane Database of Systematic Reviews* (10), CD003934. doi: 10.1002/14651858.CD003934.pub4

33. Ondeck M. (2019) Healthy birth practice #2: Walk, move around, and change positions throughout labor. *The Journal of Perinatal Education* 28(2), 81–87. doi: 10.1891/1058-1243.28.2.81

34. Oláh K. (1991) Measurement of the cervical response to uterine activity in labour and observations on the mechanism of cervical effacement. *Journal of Perinatal Medicine* 19(Suppl. 2), 245.

35. Oláh KS, Gee H, Brown JS. (1993) Cervical contractions: The response of the cervix to oxytocic stimulation in the latent phase of labour. *British Journal of Obstetrics and Gynaecology* 100(7), 635–640. doi: 10.1111/j.1471-0528.1993.tb14229.x

36. Ulmsten U. (1994) The forces of labor, resistance of the cervix and the contractions of the myometrium. *European Journal of Obstetrics & Gynecology and Reproductive Biology* 55(1), 7. doi: 10.1016/0028-2243(94)90178-3

37. Tantengco O, Menon R. (2020) Contractile function of the cervix plays a role in normal and pathological pregnancy and parturition. *Medical Hypotheses* 145, 110336. doi: 10.1016/j.mehy.2020.110336

38. Tantengco O, Vink JY, Menon R. (2021) Trends, gaps, and future directions of research in cervical remodeling during pregnancy: A bibliometric analysis. *The Journal of Maternal-Fetal & Neonatal Medicine* 1–9. doi: 10.1080/14767058.2021.1974387

39. Oláh KS, Neilson JP. (1994) Failure to progress in the management of labour. *British Journal of Obstetrics and Gynaecology* 101(1), 1–3. doi: 10.1111/j.1471-0528.1994.tb13000.x

40. Davis E. (2012) *Heart and Hands a Midwife's Guide to Pregnancy and Birth*, 5th edn. Ten Speed Press.

41. Tully G. (2021) *Quick Reference Digital Download *new Edition!**. Spinning Babies. https://www.spinningbabies.com/product/quick-reference-digital-download-2021

42. Shah S, Banh ET, Koury K, Bhatia G, Nandi R, Gulur P. (2015) Pain management in pregnancy: Multimodal approaches. *Pain Research and Treatment* 2015, 987483. doi: 10.1155/2015/987483

43. Calais-Germain B, Parés N. (2012) *Preparing for a Gentle Birth: The Pelvis in Pregnancy*. Healing Arts Press.

44. Phillips CJ. (2001) *Hands of Love: Seven Steps to the Miracle of Birth*. New Dawn Publishing.

45. Alehagen S, Wijma B, Lundberg U, Wijma K. (2005) Fear, pain and stress hormones during childbirth. *Journal of Psychosomatic Obstetrics and Gynaecology* 26(3), 153–165. doi: 10.1080/01443610400023072

46. Buckley S. (2015) *Hormonal Physiology of Childbearing: Evidence and Implications for Women, Babies and Maternity Care*. Childbirth Connection Programs, National Partnership for Women & Families. https://www.nationalpartnership.org/our-work/resources/health-care/maternity/hormonal-physiology-of-childbearing.pdf

47. Clark CJ, Kalanaviciute G, Bartholomew V, Cheyne H, Hundley VA. (2022) Exploring pain characteristics in nulliparous women; A precursor to developing support for women in the latent phase of labour. *Midwifery* 104, 103174. doi: 10.1016/j.midw.2021.103174

48. Waldenström U, Hildingsson I, Ryding EL. (2006) Antenatal fear of childbirth and its association with subsequent caesarean section and experience of childbirth. *BJOG: An International Journal of Obstetrics and Gynaecology* 113(6), 638–646. doi: 10.1111/j.1471-0528.2006.00950.x

49. Alehagen S, Wijma B, Wijma K. (2006) Fear of childbirth before, during, and after childbirth. *Acta Obstetricia Et Gynecologica Scandinavica* 85(1), 56–62. doi: 10.1080/00016340500334844

50. Nieminen K, Stephansson O, Ryding EL (2009) Women's fear of childbirth and preference for cesarean section–a cross-sectional study at various stages of pregnancy in Sweden. *Acta Obstetricia et Gynecologica Scandinavica* 88(7), 807–813. doi: 10.1080/00016340902998436

51. Seng J. (2015). How does traumatic stress affect pregnancy and birth? In: J Seng, J Taylor (eds), *Trauma Informed Care in the Perinatal Period* (pp. 57–73). Dunedin Academic Press.

52. Sydsjö G, Bladh M, Lilliecreutz C, Persson AM, Vyöni H, Josefsson A. (2014) Obstetric outcomes for nulliparous women who received routine individualized treatment for severe fear of childbirth - a retrospective case control study. *BMC Pregnancy and Childbirth* 14, 126. doi: 10.1186/1471-2393-14-126

53. Lowe NK. (2007) A review of factors associated with dystocia and cesarean section in nulliparous women. *Journal of Midwifery & Women's Health* 52(3), 216–228. doi: 10.1016/j.jmwh.2007.03.003

54. Nahaee J, Abbas-Alizadeh F, Mirghafourvand, M, Mohammad-Alizadeh-Charandabi, S (2020) Pre- and during- labour predictors of dystocia in active phase of labour: A case-control study. *BMC Pregnancy and Childbirth* 20(1), 425. doi: 10.1186/s12884-020-03113-5

55. Wuitchik M, Bakal D, Lipshitz J. (1989) The clinical significance of pain and cognitive activity in latent labor. *Obstetrics and Gynecology* 73(1), 35–42.

56. Malvasi A, Barbera A, Di Vagno G, Gimovsky A, Berghella V, Ghi T, Di Renzo GC, Tinelli A. (2015) Asynclitism: A literature review of an often forgotten clinical condition. *The Journal of Maternal-Fetal & Neonatal Medicine* 28(16), 1890–1894. doi: 10.3109/14767058.2014.972925

57. King J. (1993) *Back Labor No More!!: What Every Woman Should Know before Labor*. Plenary Systems.

58. Tully G. (2020) *Abdominal Lift and Tuck*. Spinning Babies. https://www.spinningbabies.com/pregnancy-birth/techniques/abdominal-lift-tuck

59. el Halta V. (1995) Posterior labor: A pain in the back. *Midwifery Today* (36), 19–21.

60. Glavind J, Greve T, de Wolff MG, Hansen MK, Henriksen TB. (2020) Medication used in Denmark in the latent phase of labor - do we know what we are doing? *Sexual & Reproductive Healthcare: Official Journal of the Swedish Association of Midwives* 25, 100515. doi: 10.1016/j.srhc.2020.100515

61. Maykin MM, Ukoha EP, Tilp V, Gaw SL, Lewkowitz AK. (2021) Impact of therapeutic rest in early labor on perinatal outcomes: A prospective study. *American Journal of Obstetrics & Gynecology MFM* 3(3), 100325. doi: 10.1016/j.ajogmf.2021.100325

62. Kavanagh J, Kelly AJ, Thomas J. (2005) Breast stimulation for cervical ripening and induction of labour. *The Cochrane Database of Systematic Reviews* 2005(3), CD003392. doi: 10.1002/14651858.CD003392.pub2

63. Demirel G, Guler H. (2015) The effect of uterine and nipple stimulation on induction with oxytocin and the labor process. *Worldviews on Evidence-Based Nursing* 12(5), 273–280. doi: 10.1111/wvn.12116

64. Razgaitis EJ, Lyvers AN. (2010) Management of protracted active labor with nipple stimulation: A viable tool for midwives? *Journal of Midwifery & Women's Health* 55(1), 65–69. doi: 10.1016/j.jmwh.2009.05.002

65. Stein JL, Bardeguez AD, Verma UL, Tegani N. (1990) Nipple stimulation for labor augmentation. *The Journal of Reproductive Medicine* 35(7), 710–714.

66. Curtis P, Resnick JC, Evens S, Thompson CJ. (1999) A comparison of breast stimulation and intravenous oxytocin for the augmentation of labor. *Birth (Berkeley, Calif.)* 26(2), 115–122. doi: 10.1046/j.1523-536x.1999.00115.x

67. Finucane EM, Murphy DJ, Biesty LM, Gyte GM, Cotter AM, Ryan EM, Boulvain M, Devane D. (2020) Membrane sweeping for induction of labour. *The Cochrane Database of Systematic Reviews* 2(2), CD000451. doi: 10.1002/14651858. CD000451.pub3

68. Smyth RM, Markham C, Dowswell T. (2013) Amniotomy for shortening spontaneous labour. *The Cochrane Database of Systematic Reviews* 6, CD006167. doi: 10.1002/14651858.CD006167.pub4

69. World Health Organization. (2018) *WHO recommendations: Intrapartum care for a positive childbirth experience: Transforming care of women and babies for improved health and well-being: Executive summary.* https://apps.who.int/iris/bitstream/ handle/10665/272447/WHO-RHR-18.12-eng.pdf

70. Petersen A, Poetter U, Michelsen C, Gross MM. (2013) The sequence of intrapartum interventions: A descriptive approach to the cascade of interventions. *Archives of Gynecology and Obstetrics* 288(2), 245–254. doi: 10.1007/s00404-013-2737-8

71. Rossignol M, Chaillet N, Boughrassa F, Moutquin JM. (2014) Interrelations between four antepartum obstetric interventions and cesarean delivery in women at low risk: A systematic review and modeling of the cascade of interventions. *Birth (Berkeley, Calif.)* 41(1), 70–78. doi: 10.1111/birt.12088

72. Ingvarsson S, Schildmeijer K, Oscarsson M. (2020) Swedish midwives' experiences and views of amniotomy: An interview study. *Midwifery* 91, 102840. doi: 10.1016/j.midw.2020.102840

73. Grobman WA, Rice MM, Reddy UM, Tita A, Silver RM, Mallett G, Hill K, Thom EA, El-Sayed YY, Perez-Delboy A, Rouse DJ, Saade GR, Boggess KA, Chauhan SP, Iams JD, Chien EK, Casey BM, Gibbs RS, Srinivas SK, Macones GA. (2018) Labor induction versus expectant management in low-risk nulliparous women. *The New England Journal of Medicine* 379(6), 513–523. doi: 10.1056/NEJMoa1800566

74. Erickson EN, Bailey JM, Colo SD, Carlson NS, Tilden EL. (2021) Induction of labor or expectant management? Birth outcomes for nulliparous individuals choosing midwifery care. *Birth (Berkeley, Calif.)* 48(4), 501–513. doi: 10.1111/birt.12560

75. Schlaeger JM, Gabzdyl EM, Bussell JL, Takakura N, Yajima H, Takayama M, Wilkie DJ. (2017) Acupuncture and acupressure in labor. *Journal of Midwifery & Women's Health* 62(1), 12–28. doi: 10.1111/jmwh.12545

76. Smith CA, Armour M, Dahlen HG. (2017) Acupuncture or acupressure for induction of labour. *The Cochrane Database of Systematic Reviews* 10(10), CD002962. doi: 10.1002/14651858.CD002962.pub4

77. Smith CA, Collins CT, Crowther CA, Levett KM, Armour M, Dahlen HG, Tan AL, Mesgarpour B. (2020) Acupuncture or acupressure for pain management in labour. *The Cochrane Database of Systematic Reviews* (2), CD009232. doi: 10.1002/14651858.CD009232

78. Takahata K, Horiuchi S, Tadokoro Y, Sawano E, Shinohara K. (2019) Oxytocin levels in low-risk primiparas following breast stimulation for spontaneous onset of labor: A quasi-experimental study. *BMC Pregnancy and Childbirth* 19(1), 351. doi: 10.1186/s12884-019-2504-3

79. Carbone L, De Vivo V, Saccone G, D'Antonio F, Mercorio A, Raffone A, Arduino B, D'Alessandro P, Sarno L, Conforti A, Maruotti GM, Alviggi C, Zullo F. (2019) Sexual intercourse for induction of spontaneous onset of labor: A systematic review and meta-analysis of randomized controlled trials. *The Journal of Sexual Medicine* 16(11), 1787–1795. doi: 10.1016/j.jsxm.2019.08.002

80. Smith CA. (2003) Homoeopathy for induction of labour. *Cochrane Database of Systematic Reviews* 4. Art. No.: CD003399. doi: 10.1002/14651858.CD003399

81. Mallory DJ. (2018) *Integrative Medicine, Chapter 53- Postdates Pregnancy* Fourth edn, Elsevier. ISBN 978-0-323-35868-2

82. DeMaria AL, Sundstrom B, Moxley GE, Banks K, Bishop A, Rathbun L. (2018) Castor oil as a natural alternative to labor induction: A retrospective descriptive study. *Women and Birth: Journal of the Australian College of Midwives* 31(2), e99–e104. doi: 10.1016/j.wombi.2017.08.001

83. Gilad R, Hochner H, Savitsky B, Porat S, Hochner-Celnikier D. (2018) Castor oil for induction of labor in post-date pregnancies: A randomized controlled trial. *Women and Birth: Journal of the Australian College of Midwives* 31(1), e26–e31. doi: 10.1016/j.wombi.2017.06.010

84. Tunaru S, Till F, Althoff A, Nusing R, Diener M, Offermanns S. (2012) Castor oil induces relaxation and uterus contraction via ricinoleic acid activating prostaglandin EP3 receptors. *Proceedings of the National Academy of Sciences of the USA* 109(23), 9179–9184.

85. Kalati M, Kashanian M, Jahdi F, Naseri M, Haghani H, Sheikhansari N. (2018) Evening primrose oil and labour, is it effective? A randomised clinical trial. *Journal of Obstetrics and Gynaecology: The Journal of the Institute of Obstetrics and Gynaecology* 38(4), 488–492. doi: 10.1080/01443615.2017.1386165

86. Najafi M, Loripoor M, Saghafi Z, Kazemi M. (2019) The effect of vaginal evening primrose on the Bishop score of term nulliparous women. *Nursing Practice Today* 6(4), 202–211.

87. Bowman R, Taylor J, Muggleton S, Davis D. (2021) Biophysical effects, safety and efficacy of raspberry leaf use in pregnancy: A systematic integrative review. *BMC Complementary Medicine and Therapies* 21(1), 56. doi: 10.1186/s12906-021-03230-4

88. Muñoz Balbontín Y, Stewart D, Shetty A, Fitton CA, McLay JS. (2019) Herbal medicinal product use during pregnancy and the postnatal period: A systematic review. *Obstetrics and Gynecology* 133(5), 920–932. doi: 10.1097/AOG.0000000000003217

89. Nasiri M, Gheibi Z, Miri A, Rahmani J, Asadi M, Sadeghi O, Maleki V, Khodadost M. (2019) Effects of consuming date fruits (Phoenix dactylifera Linn) on gestation, labor, and delivery: An updated systematic review and meta-analysis of clinical trials. *Complementary Therapies in Medicine* 45, 71–84. doi: 10.1016/j.ctim.2019.05.017

Chapter 7

Prolonged Active Phase

Amy Marowitz, DNP, CNM

Simkin's Labor Progress Handbook: Early Interventions to Prevent and Treat Dystocia, Fifth Edition. Edited by Lisa Hanson, Emily Malloy, and Penny Simkin.
© 2024 John Wiley & Sons Ltd. Published 2024 by John Wiley & Sons Ltd.

WHAT IS ACTIVE LABOR? DESCRIPTION, DEFINITION, DIAGNOSIS

Our current understanding of the stages and phases of labor comes primarily from the work of Emmanuel Friedman. Friedman graphed the progress of many labors by plotting rates of dilatation and descent against elapsed time. He observed that the slope of the lines representing dilatation and descent change predictably in most labors, with an initial period of slow cervical dilation followed by a period of more rapid dilation and then fetal descent. This led to a conceptualization of functional divisions of labor with a preparatory phase, a dilation phase, and an expulsive phase. These correspond to latent phase of the first stage, active phase of the first stage, and second stage.[1]

Friedman defined the onset of active labor as the time when there is a sharp rise in the rate of dilation, a consistent finding in the great majority of labors. In his original study, Friedman found that the median dilation at this point of faster progress was about three centimeters.[1] Clinicians and researchers adopted this as the definition of onset of active labor. Contemporary research shows that most people are not in active labor until the cervix is five or six centimeters dilated.[2] The American Congress of Obstetricians and Gynecologists (ACOG), Society for Maternal Fetal Medicine (SMFM), and the World Health Organization (WHO) all support the use of the 5–6 centimeters threshold as the time when most people begin active labor.[3,4]

WHEN IS ACTIVE LABOR PROLONGED OR ARRESTED?

In addition to describing the stages and phases of labor, Friedman also studied labor duration. He developed criteria for normal labor progress by calculating the slowest, fastest, and average rate of progression for each stage and phase of labor. Based on his research he designated the minimum progress in dilation considered normal to be 1.2 centimeters per hour for nulliparas and 1.5 centimeters per hour for multiparas.[5] Labors with slower progress than this were called protracted. In addition, Friedman arbitrarily defined arrested active labor as no cervical change in two hours.[5]

More recent research has resulted in a re-evaluation of these criteria. Of particular significance are two studies using large databases to examine labor progress: the Collaborative Perinatal Project (CPP) from 1959 to 1966 and the Consortium on Safe Labor (CSL) from 2002 to 2008.[2] Analysis of both databases showed that expectations of labor progress based on Friedman's criteria were far too stringent. As a result of these and other studies, suggested thresholds for minimum normal progress are 0.5–0.7 centimeters per hour for nulliparas, and 0.5–1.3 centimeters per hour for multiparas.[2] The range reflects the fact that these data show the rate of dilation increases as labor progresses. Revision of expectations for labor progress are supported by ACOG and SMFM and the World Health Organization.[3,4]

Contemporary studies show that no progress for two hours is a common finding and should not be considered abnormal.[2] Researchers and professional organizations such as ACOG/SMFM recommend defining arrested labor as no cervical change in active labor (dilation of at least 6 cm) for 4 hours.[3,6]

POSSIBLE CAUSES OF PROLONGED ACTIVE LABOR

Fetopelvic factors: a poor fit between the fetal head and birthing pelvis may result from the size of the head in relationship to the pelvis or a discrepancy between the shape of the fetal head and the dimensions and shape of the birthing pelvis. Other factors may be a fetal malpresentation such brow or face presentations, persistent asynclitism, or malpositions such as persistent occiput posterior.

Disruptions to the hormonal physiology of labor: can be caused by environmental factors such as lack of privacy, noise, bright lights, inadequate support, or emotional factors such fear or anxiety.

Hypocontractile uterine activity (inadequate contractions): can be caused by immobility, medications, disruptions to the hormonal physiology of labor, and possibly uterine lactate production in long labors.

Soft tissue (cervix, muscles, ligaments, and fascia) and musculoskeletal factors: cervical stenosis, musculoskeletal problems such as lumbar lordosis combined with lack of lumbar mobility, abdominal weakness, pendulous abdomen, other musculoskeletal problems.

Combination of etiologies or unknown etiology: a delay in progress often results from a combination of interconnected factors. For example, a persistent malposition associated with a large fetus, maternal exhaustion, and inadequate contractions. Sometimes the cause is unclear.

TREATMENT OF PROLONGED LABOR

There is no definitive evidence or expert opinion on the optimal treatment strategy for prolonged labor. There is a continuum of options ranging from risk-free techniques that support the physiologic process of labor and are appropriate in any labor, to higher technology medical and pharmacological interventions with varying associated risks. Starting with less invasive measures and moving toward more invasive as needed is a common-sense approach. However, there is insufficient evidence to determine the best timing and sequencing of various noninvasive approaches to encourage labor progress, and when to transition to more medical and/or pharmacologic treatments such as amniotomy and oxytocin augmentation. Neal and Lowe suggest considering oxytocin augmentation when there has been no cervical change in active labor for more than four hours.[6] ACOG/SMFM simply state that oxytocin augmentation is "commonly recommended" when active labor is protracted or arrested.[3]

Choosing a strategy to address prolonged labor should be done in collaboration with the laboring person using Shared Decision Making. Thorough data collection may identify areas that are the cause of or are contributing to the prolonged labor. Recommendations for interventions should be based on the results of the data collection. Often there is more than one reasonable approach and maternal preference is a critical consideration.

FETOPELVIC FACTORS

Cephalopelvic disproportion (CPD) is the broad term that denotes a poor fit between the fetal head and the birthing pelvis. It is often assumed that this is a result of a smaller pelvis and/or larger head. Size discrepancies can be the sole factor responsible for a delay in progress. However, CPD can also be caused by any factor that affects the presenting diameter of the head or the ease with which the presenting shape of the fetal head and architecture of the maternal pelvis allows the fetus to move through the pelvis.

Position denotes the relationship of the fetal denominator to the pelvis. The denominator is the anatomical reference point on the presenting part of the fetus. When the fetus is cephalic (headfirst) with a well flexed head, the back of the head or occiput is the denominator. When the occiput is facing the front of the pelvis, this is an anterior position-occiput anterior or OA. When the occiput faces the back of the pelvis, this is a posterior position-occiput posterior or OP (Fig. 7.1). Halfway in between these is a traverse position-occiput transverse or OT (Fig. 7.2). The smallest diameter is presented with an occiput anterior position.

Attitude denotes the degree of flexion or extension of the fetal head. The attitude can be flexed (typically termed vertex presentation), neither flexed nor extended (military presentation), partially extended (brow presentation), or fully extended (face presentation). The smallest diameter and best fit present with a fully flexed head.

New figure: attitude

Asynclitism denotes a fetal head that is tilted toward one shoulder. This means the fetal head is angled so that one parietal bone enters the pelvis first, and the fetal biparietal diameter is not parallel to the plane of the inlet of the pelvis (Figs. 7.3 and 7.4). When the head is not tilted in this manner it is synclitic (Fig. 7.5). Asynclitism is

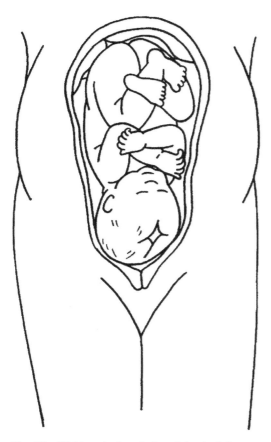

Fig. 7.1.   Right occiput posterior, abdominal view.

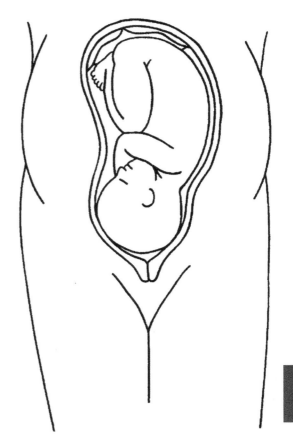

Fig. 7.2.   Left occiput transverse, abdominal view.

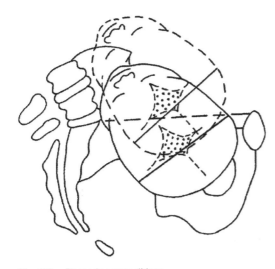

Fig. 7.3.   Posterior asynclitism.

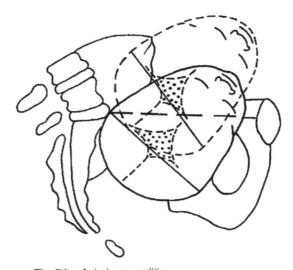

Fig. 7.4.   Anterior asynclitism.

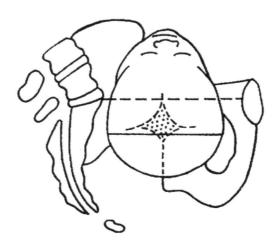

Fig. 7.5. Synclitism.

beneficial as the head enters the pelvis because the presenting diameter is smaller than with synclitism. However, if the head remains asynclitic as the fetal descends lower in the pelvis, rotation is prevented, and labor progress slows or stops.[7,8]

All these factors can affect the fit of the fetus within the pelvis and thus the progress of labor. They can occur individually or together. For example, a fetus in a posterior position can also be asynclitic.

HOW FETAL MALPOSITIONS AND MALPRESENTATION DELAY LABOR PROGRESS

Determining fetopelvic relationships

Malpositions

The available means to identify fetal position include observations of abdominal shape, Leopold's maneuvers, where the fetal heart rate is most easily heard, location of pain, the contraction pattern, and digital vaginal examination to palpate suture lines and fontanels of the fetal skull. However, according to several studies, these diagnostic techniques are not reliable.[8–12] Barros and colleagues[13] studied the effect of simulation-based training on the accuracy of determining fetal head position during labor and found no significant improvement following simulation.

Malpresentations

Diagnosis of attitudes of deflexion and persistent asynclitism are equally challenging. Determination of fetal attitude is theoretically possible via Leopold's maneuver or digital vaginal examination. Palpation of the cephalic prominence of the same side as the fetal back during Leopold's Maneuvers indicates some degree of extension of the fetal head, that is, a brow or face presentation. The cephalic prominence may be subtle and difficult to palpate. Identification of attitude via vaginal exam is possible, especially with the full extension of a face presentation. Partial extension (brow presentation) and a head that is neither flexed nor extended (military position) are more common and may be much more difficult to identify by examination. Asynclitism can theoretically be identified by vaginal exam based on the location of the sagittal suture in relation to the maternal pelvis. As with position and attitude, asynclitism is sometimes difficult to determine. Issues such as the degree of cervical dilation, fetal caput succedaneum and/or molding, and maternal discomfort during the exam impact the caregiver's ability to accurately assess malposition and malpresentation.

Both malpresentation and malposition result in a larger fetal head diameter coming through the pelvis than occurs when the head is in a well-flexed occiput anterior position. Malpresentation and malposition also affect the biomechanics of labor and birth. The pressure of the fetal head or forewaters on the cervix, which normally enhances dilation, may be uneven or generally reduced. Descent may also be delayed until the fetal head rotates, flexes, or aligns with the plane of the pelvis. When rotation or improved alignment is needed, it makes sense that labor will take more time than when the fetus is ideally positioned.

Use of ultrasound

The most accurate way to diagnose malposition or malpresentation is ultrasound by an experienced operator.[11,14,15,16] Proponents of using ultrasound to determine fetal position, attitude, or asynclitism during labor argue that the information allows the caregiver to select the best primary interventions such as positions, movements, or digital or manual techniques to facilitate fetal rotation, and to determine whether they were successful. However, there is no research comparing outcomes when these primary interventions are based on an ultrasound confirmed malposition or malpresentation as compared to a trial-and-error approach of these types of interventions when a malposition of malpresentation is suspected. Maternal positions and movements that may help encourage a more favorable fetopelvic relationship are generally safe for anyone. Without ultrasound confirmation, caregivers should not rule out the possibility of a fetal malposition and/or malpresentation as an etiology when there is a delay in active labor.

Artificial rupture of the membranes (amniotomy) when there is a fetal malposition or malpresentation

When active labor is prolonged, clinicians often rupture the membranes to accelerate progress. Amniotomy is believed to enhance labor progress by increasing pressure on the cervix and lower uterine segment, thus stimulating the release of prostaglandins and oxytocin, and can be successfully used to augment labor.[17] There is some concern over the wisdom of such a practice when there is a fetal malposition or malpresentation due to possibly more difficult rotation to OA after membranes rupture. The explanatory hypothesis is as follows: When the fetus is poorly positioned, intact forewaters may provide some protection and maneuverability for the fetal head. When the forewaters are removed, the malpositioned fetus may be subjected to uneven head compression, excessive molding, more pronounced caput succedaneum, and a greater likelihood of operative delivery than would otherwise occur. There is little evidence on this issue. One study on factors associated with a persistent occiput posterior position included amniotomy and did find a correlation between this malposition and ruptured membranes.[18] A 2013 Cochrane review comparing spontaneous labor with routine amniotomy and intention to keep membranes intact did not examine the incidence of persistent malpositions or malpresentations.[19] This review found no difference on labor duration between the two groups and a possible increase in cesarean births with amniotomy. Further large trials of amniotomy in labors with known OP positions or asynclitism are warranted to establish whether the malposition is more or less likely to self-correct or be corrected with or without intact membranes.

Epidural analgesia and malposition or malpresentation

Several observational studies show a correlation between epidural analgesia and the presence and persistence of malpositions or malpresentations.[10,18,20,21] Other studies show this association between persistent malpositions and epidural analgesia only when the epidural is placed before engagement of the head.[22,23] It is not known if this association is the result of epidurals causing more malpositions and malpresentations, or if laboring people with these conditions are more likely to request epidurals.

MATERNAL POSITIONS AND MOVEMENTS FOR SUSPECTED MALPOSITION, MALPRESENTATION, OR ANY "POOR FIT"

Overview and evidence

The birthing person's positions and movements alter the forces of gravity, pelvic dimensions, and the various pressures within the uterus and on the cervix and pelvic joints.[24,25] In theory, these changing forces improve the biomechanics of labor and positively influence fetopelvic relationships. Use of positions and movements to correct a malposition or malpresentation or encourage progress with prolonged labor is promoted and practiced by many caregivers, especially midwives. For example, midwife and author Gail Tully has written extensively on this topic[26,27] and created "Spinning Babies," a website that describes many principles to promote labor progress with maternal postures and other techniques (Spinning Babies, https://www.spinningbabies.com).[28] Considerable anecdotal evidence exists on the effectiveness of this approach, with reports of correction of malpositions and malpresentations with the use of these techniques followed by rapid labor progress.

Scientific evidence on maternal postures to correct malpositions or malpresentations has shown mixed results. Table 7.1 describes five randomized controlled trials (RCTs) on the use of specific maternal postures to prompt rotation from an OP to OA position. Only one study[29] showed a statistically significant difference between the control and intervention groups. In this study the participants in the intervention group maintained a side-lying position on the same side as the fetal spine for at least 40 minutes every hour until rotation to OA or birth.

In all but one study[30] the epidural rates were over 90% for all participants, and the rate of ruptured membranes at the time of randomization was 100%[29,31,33] or around 90%.[32] Since both ruptured membranes and epidural

Table 7.1.   Scientific evidence on maternal postures for fetal malposition or malpresentation.

Study	Study design	N	Intervention	% Epidural analgesia	% Ruptured membranes at randomization	% Rotation to occiput anterior
				I vs. C[a]	I vs. C[a]	I vs. C[a]
Stremmler[30]	Randomized controlled trial (RCT)	147	Hands and knees for at least 30 minutes	19% vs. 22%	43% vs. 48%	16% vs. 7%[b,e]
Desbriere[31]	Randomized controlled trial (RCT)	220	One of three positions based on fetal station until rotation to OA or birth[d]	93.6% vs. 95.5%	Both 100%	78.2% vs. 76.4%[c,e]
Guittier[32]	Randomized controlled trial (RCT)	439	Hands and knees for at least 10 minutes	94.5% vs. 93.1%	88.6% vs. 93.1%	17.2% vs. 11.5%[b,e]
LeRay[33]	Randomized controlled trial (RCT)	322	Side lying, opposite side of fetal spine for one hour	90% vs. 89.5%	Both 100%	21.9% vs. 21.6%[b,e]
Bueno-Lopez[29]	Randomized controlled trial (RCT)	120	Side Lying, same side as fetal spine, 40 minutes per hour until rotation to OA or birth	Both 100%	Both 100%	50.8% vs. 21.7%[f]

Notes: a. Intervention group vs. control group; b. one hour after randomization; c. at birth; d. −3 to −5 station: hands and knees −2 to 0 station: side lying same side as fetal spine, inferior leg folded, superior leg extended, and within axis of body > 0 station: side lying same side as fetal spine, inferior leg extended, superior leg 90-degree angle with leg support; e. not statistically significant; f. timing of assessment for rotation not specified.

analgesia are associated with a higher rate of malpositions and malpresentations, the results cannot be generalized to all laboring persons with a fetus in a posterior position. In addition, the authors of one study[33] speculate that the short duration of the intervention posture have led to nonsignificant findings in between group comparisons.

In all these studies, the high rate of rotation to occiput anterior for participants in both the control and interventions groups confirms the finding from other studies[15,34] that most fetuses in a posterior position in the earlier part of labor will rotate to an anterior position by the time of birth. In the studies that measured comfort,[30,32] laboring persons reported increased comfort with a hands and knees position.

It is interesting to contrast the results of these studies with those that more broadly examine the activity of laboring persons. A 2013 Cochrane systematic review[35] compared persons who were upright vs. recumbent during labor. The upright groups had shorter labors, fewer cesarean births, and were less likely to use epidural analgesia[36] compared to "active" and "non-active" childbirth. Active childbirth was defined by at least 3 positions changes for least 20 minutes each throughout labor. "Active birth" was associated with a statistically significant decrease in cesarean birth, faster labor, and increased satisfaction. Although determination of fetal position was not part of these studies, greater activity during labor may have optimized fetopelvic relationships.

Given what is known about postures and activity during labor, it is reasonable to recommend keeping active and trying different positions when labor progress is slow, especially if a malposition or malpresentation is known or suspected. Additional interventions may be needed for the small percentage of malposition or malpresentation that do not resolve spontaneously or with these first line measures. More research is needed on specific positions for resolving malpositions and malpresentations, especially for persons with intact membranes and no epidural.

Positions to encourage optimal fetal positioning

Forward-leaning positions

Forward-leaning positions (Fig. 7.6) may help reposition the fetus during labor.[32,37] These positions are vigorously promoted by Tully,[27] Scott,[37] Sutton,[38] and others, for their contributions to optimal fetal positioning.

Side-lying positions

The effects of gravity on the fetus are quite different when a laboring person is in a pure side-lying position versus a semiprone (runner's lunge) position. When the fetus is thought (or known with ultrasound confirmation) to be OP evidence suggests that the best "pure side-lying" position is on the side toward which the occiput is already directed, with the baby's back "toward the bed"[29] (Figs. 7.7 and 7.8). Theoretically this encourages the OP fetus toward OT. If the laboring person is semiprone, they should lie on the side opposite the direction of the occiput, with the fetal back "toward the ceiling"[39] (Fig. 7.9). With the "side-prone lunge" (Figs. 7.9, 7.10a and 7.10b), the laboring person lies semiprone and gentle pressure is applied to the sole of their upper foot, in the direction of their head, to increase hip flexion and abduction. This widens the pelvis, improving the chances of fetal rotation. The side-lying lunge with support provided by another person, pillows, or a peanut-shaped ball is useful for the person with an epidural, who cannot hold their leg in place by themself. The pressure against their foot should be gentle since they will not feel if the stretching of the hip joint is excessive. The peanut ball (Fig. 7.10b) supports the person's upper leg in a position of greater hip abduction without another person providing support.[27,40]

The side-lying release (Fig. 7.10c) passively releases tension or tightness in the pelvis and adjoining soft tissue, with the intention of making room for fetal rotation. Each time the side-lying release is used it should be done on both sides.

Asymmetrical positions and movements

Asymmetrical positions, such as those pictured in Figs. 7.10, 7.11 and 7.12, theoretically result in enlargement of the pelvis on one side. This may promote rotation of a fetal in an OP position or straightening of an asynclitic fetal head. When using these positions, it may help to alternate from side to side.

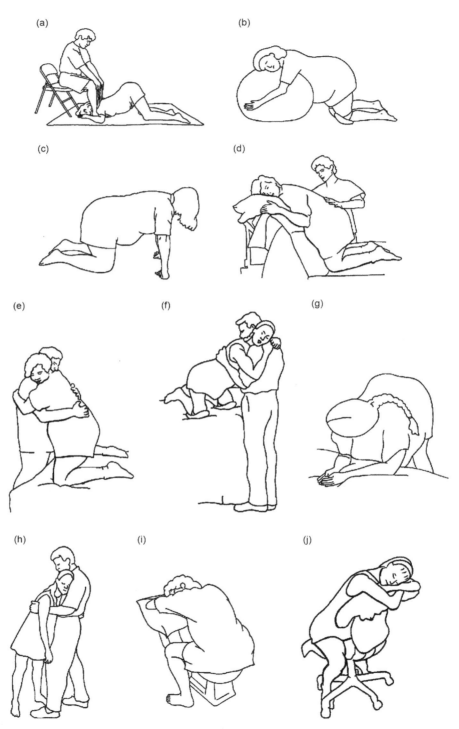

Fig. 7.6. Forward learning positions. (**a**) Open knee–chest, resting shoulders on partner's padded shins. (**b**) Kneeling with ball and knee pads. (**c**) Hands and knees. (**d**) Kneeling over bed back. (**e**) Kneeling, with partner support. (**f**) Kneeling on bed with partner support and knee pads. (**g**) Standing, leaning on bed. (**h**) Standing, leaning forward. (**i**) Straddling a toilet, facing backwards. (**j**) Straddling a chair.

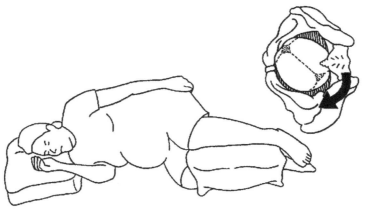

Fig. 7.7. Pregnant person with suspected or known occiput posterior (OP) fetus in pur side-lying on the "correct side" for Right Occiput Posterior (ROP) fetus.

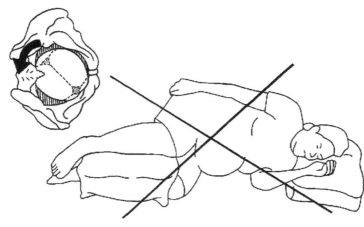

Fig. 7.8. Pregnant person with suspected or known occiput posterior (OP) fetus in pure side-lying on the "wrong" (left). Fetal back is "toward the ceiling." Gravity pulls fetal occiput and trunk towards the direct OP.

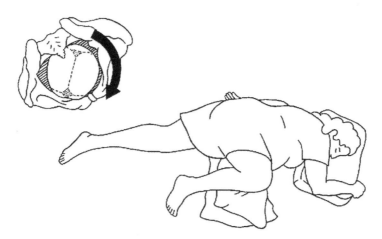

Fig. 7.9. Pregnant person with a suspected or known occiput posterior (OP).

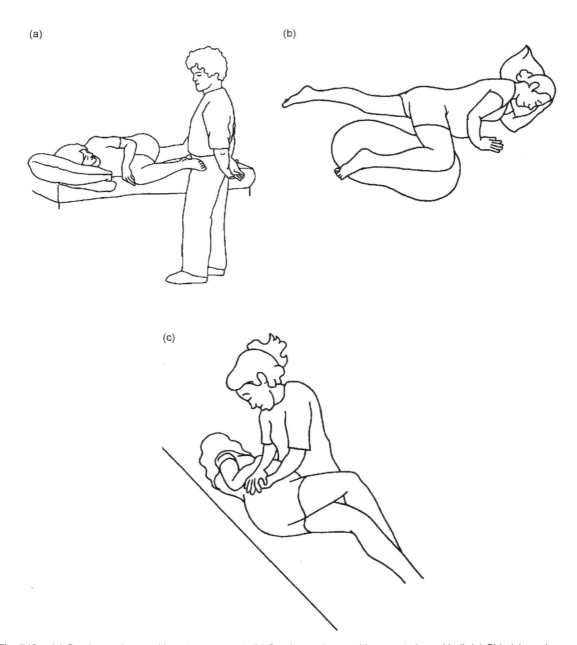

Fig. 7.10.   (**a**) Semiprone lunge with partner support. (**b**) Semiprone lunge with peanut-shaped ball. (**c**) Side-lying release.

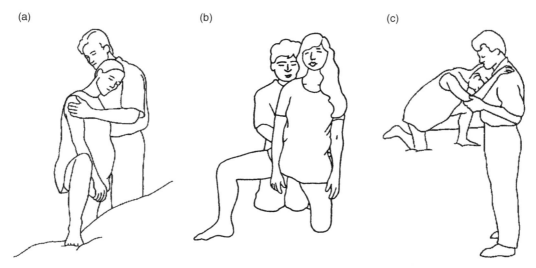

Fig. 7.11. (**a**) Standing with one leg elevated. (**b**) Asymmetrical kneeling. (**c**) Asymmetrical kneeling with partner support.

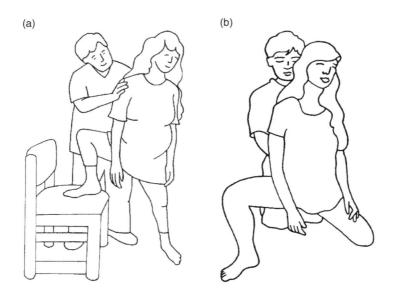

Fig. 7.12. (**a**) Standing lunge. (**b**) Kneeling lunge.

Box 7.1. Supine and semisitting positions for occiput posterior

When a laboring person is fully supine or semisitting, gravity encourages the trunk of the OP fetus to lie next to their spine, increasing the chances of compressing the inferior vena cava and causing supine hypotension but also minimizing the likelihood of rotation to OA. These positions also increase the pressure of the fetal occiput against the sacrum and may increase back pain. There is a greater likelihood of rotation and less back pain with an upright sitting position or leaning forward on hands and knees.[18,32]

  When the laboring person is upright, the uterus tilts forward, thus encouraging flexion of the fetal head into the pelvic basin.

Note: A person with a pendulous abdomen may need to lean back into a semi-reclining position to align the fetal head with the pelvic inlet.

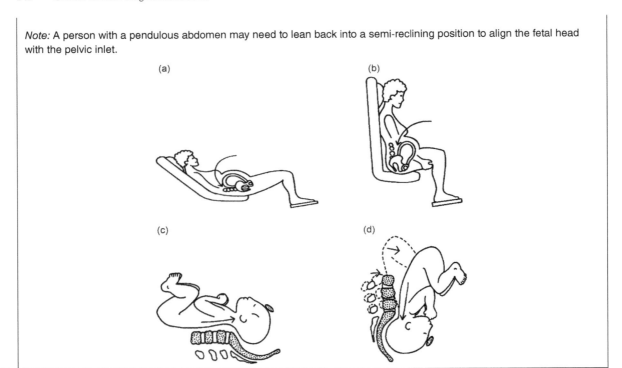

(a)   (b)   (c)   (d)

Abdominal lifting

This maneuver helps improve the alignment of the fetal trunk and head with the axis of the birth canal. During contractions, the laboring person bends their knees to tilt the pelvis, places their hands beneath their abdomen, and lifts their abdomen (Fig. 7.13).[35] Using a rebozo—a woven cloth shawl measuring approximately 45 cm wide (folded to about 15 cm wide) by 150–180 cm long—aids abdominal lifting.[41]

Caution: On rare occasions, the umbilical cord is located low and in front, and there is a possibility that the cord could be compressed with abdominal lifting. It is wise for the midwife or nurse to check the fetal heart rate occasionally during contractions while abdominal lifting is being done. If fetal heart rate decelerations occur, abdominal lifting should be discontinued.

"Walcher's" position

This maneuver may enlarge the pelvic inlet, allowing more room for the fetus to engage.[26] It is recommended when the fetus at a high station, not engaged in the pelvis. It is done by having the laboring person lie on their back and hang their legs over the end of a high bed or table. The weight of the legs moves the symphysis pubis away from the spine and widens the anterior posterior diameter at the inlet. Tully[26] suggested the laboring person maintain this position for a relatively short time-through and between several contractions. (Fig. 7.14) If a high bed or table is not available, the laboring person can lie on the floor on their back with a large roll 15–18 inches in diameter under the trochanter of the femur (right at the top of the thighs).

Flying cowgirl

This is essentially a side-lying variation of Walcher's position. It works well for laboring people with epidurals. The laboring person lies on their side with the knees bent and as far away from the abdomen as possible. The knees are help wide apart with a peanut ball or pillows if a peanut ball is not available (Fig. 7.15).

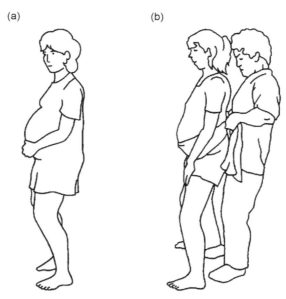

Fig. 7.13.   (**a**) Abdominal lifting. (**b**) Abdominal lifting with a shawl.

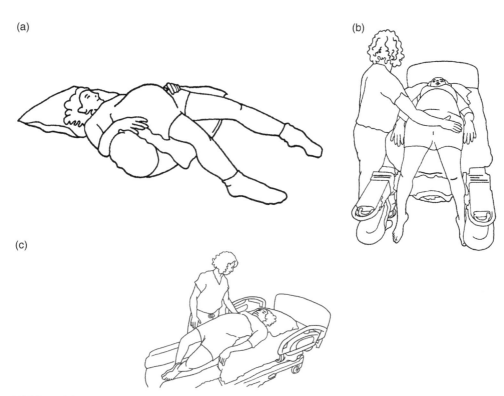

Fig. 7.14.   Walcher's (**a**) With pillows. (**b**) Hospital bed front view. (**c**) Hospital bed side view.

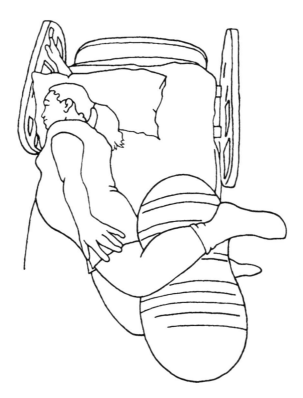

Fig. 7.15. Flying cowgirl.

Low technology clinical approaches to alter fetal position

If labor progress seems particularly slow during active phase, there are several strategies that can be used if the situation warrants. The strategies that will be described are warm water immersion, artificial rupture of the membranes, manual reduction of a persistent cervical lip, and digital or manual rotation of the fetal head.

Digital or manual rotation of the fetal head

Half of multiparas and at least one-fourth of nulliparas who experience labor with a fetus in a persistent OP or OT position will deliver spontaneously. However, when progress does not continue and the interventions suggested in earlier chapters are not successful, the midwife or physician can attempt to rotate the OP or OT fetus digitally or manually to an occiput anterior (OA) position with only a small risk of complications. Complications of both manual and digital rotation are rare but include prolapse of the umbilical cord or fetal small parts, and cervical laceration (with manual rotation only).[42] Bedside ultrasound is increasingly available and may be used to identify the location of the fetal back and eyes prior to rotation.[14,43] Elmore et al.[42] note that although more study is needed, the use of ultrasound may be beneficial when attempting to rotate a fetus from OP or OT, although it is not mandatory. It is important to ensure fetal wellbeing before, during, and after rotation attempts. It has been suggested in the literature that an indeterminate fetal heart tracing is an indication to attempt manual or digital rotation of an OP fetus, to expedite birth. However, the development of category 3 fetal heart tones during the procedure would be an indication to stop the rotation attempt immediately.[44]

While digital and manual rotation are described in obstetric and midwifery textbooks and have been the subject of recent research studies, they are not mainstream clinical interventions in the United States and elsewhere. However, according to Cargill et al., the Society of Obstetricians and Gynecologists of Canada recommends their use "alone or in conjunction with instrumental birth with little or no increased risk to the pregnant woman or to the fetus,"[45] (p. 749). Therefore, practitioners who would like to attempt these in clinical practice are encouraged to practice with models and then ideally conduct initial rotations under the guidance of a caregiver who is experienced with the procedure.

To accomplish a digital or manual rotation, the midwife or doctor must be skilled in identifying the landmarks on the fetal skull. Further, careful abdominal palpation to fully assess fetal position should be done prior to the attempt. While some caregivers recommend ultrasound visualization of the location of the fetal head position prior to the procedure, it is not mandatory.[45] With the increasing availability of affordable portable ultrasound units at the bedside, practitioners may become more willing and able to safely attempt these procedures. It has been suggested that digital or manual rotation is best attempted when cervical dilatation is 7 cm or greater.[44]

Reichman and colleagues studied the outcomes of 61 participants who entered the second stage of labor with the fetus in an OP position.[46] Half received no intervention and served as controls; half were managed using digital or manual rotation. Digital or manual rotation resulted in a significant increase in spontaneous vaginal birth in an OA position and a significant reduction in the length of the second stage of labor, use of episiotomy, incidence of cesarean birth, and length of hospital stay.

The choice of digital versus manual rotation is not discussed in the clinical or scientific literature. Digital rotation may be easier than manual at higher stations because only two fingers are necessary to accomplish the maneuver. Manual rotation may be best accomplished when the station is lower and the fetal head can be more easily reached using the whole hand, during late first or early second stage labor. In either approach, preliminary steps consist of informed consent, with discussion of the potential benefits, risks, and discomfort associated with the maneuver, as well as alternatives. Birthing person comfort measures should be used, including positions that increase the pelvic diameters and pain relief measures as needed including IV medication, nitrous oxide, pudendal block, or epidural to optimize relaxation.[42] The birthing person's bladder should be emptied (via catheter if needed), and they should be assisted to the dorsal recumbent position with adequate physical and emotional support for the rotation. Continuous fetal monitoring is recommended during the procedure to monitor fetal tolerance.[47] Both techniques are described and illustrated later. The doula can assist during this procedure by providing reassurance and coaching the birthing person to bear down when contractions start, as instructed by the midwife or doctor.

Digital rotation

Digital rotation is accomplished by using the tips of the index and middle fingers of one hand. The fingers are inserted into the vagina to palpate the lambdoid sutures located at the posterior most aspect of the parietal bone at its juncture with the posterior fontanelle where it overlaps the occipital bone.[46] Upward pressure is exerted to

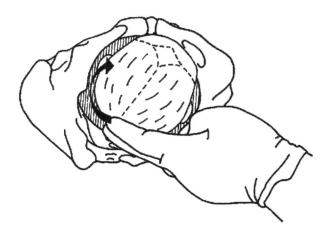

Fig. 7.16. Digital rotation.

rotate the posterior fontanelle toward the symphysis pubis via rotation of the examiner's hand and forearm in a dialing motion.[46] Cargill and colleagues[45] suggested holding the fetal head in the rotated position for several contractions to avoid spontaneous return to the OP (Fig. 7.16). Masturzo and colleagues[43] found that identifying the alignment of the fetal head and spine after the procedure increased the odds of successful rotation.

Manual rotation

There is no specific recommendation that manual rotation requires analgesia; however, since the procedure may be associated with significant discomfort, and relaxation will facilitate manual rotation, epidural analgesia or nitrous oxide may be considered. In fact, many caregivers are unwilling to perform manual rotation without analgesia for the birthing person.[45]

When performing a manual rotation, the midwife or doctor uses the hand opposite the fetal head position. For example, if the fetus is in the left OP position or left OT position, the caregiver uses her or his right hand. Following a contraction, the clinician places the entire hand (palm up) behind the fetal ear, slightly dislodging the fetal head while encouraging flexion.[45] The fingers are placed under the posterior parietal bone with the thumb positioned on the anterior parietal bone (Fig. 7.17). During the next contraction while the birthing person bears down, the caregiver rotates the baby's occiput to an anterior position. Depending on the situation, this may involve rotating one's hand at the wrist or rotating with the entire forearm. As was suggested for digital rotation, the fetal head can be held in the rotated position for several contractions to prevent spontaneous return to the OP position.[45] If this procedure is unsuccessful and the fetal heart rate is reassuring, manual rotation can be reattempted assuming the associated discomfort is well tolerated.[47]

Researchers evaluated the outcomes of manual rotation.[47] Multiparity—greater than or equal to 2, maternal age less than 35, and BMI less than 28 at the time of procedure were associated with successful rotations to the OA position. Rotations done in first-stage labor were three times more likely to be unsuccessful than those done after complete dilation. Prophylactic rotation, not surprisingly, was more successful than rotation done for failure to progress.[47,48] Following successful rotation, the cesarean rate was 2%, compared with 34% when rotation failed.[48] In a more recent examination of the outcomes of the same retrospective cohort (fetus in persistent OP position), researchers found that manual rotation significantly reduced the risk of cesarean, severe perineal laceration, postpartum hemorrhage, and chorioamnionitis compared with those managed expectantly.[44]

Manual and digital rotation procedures offer a lower-technology option to promote progress when the fetus is in an OP or OT position. The use of these rotations may promote successful vaginal birth and should be more widely researched, taught, and used.

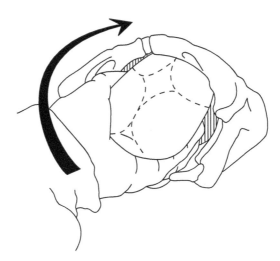

Fig. 7.17.   Manual rotation.

EARLY URGE TO PUSH, CERVICAL EDEMA, AND PERSISTENT CERVICAL LIP

The urge to push, also called Ferguson's reflex, is caused by pressure of the presenting part on the cervix and vagina. This pressure stimulates nerves that cause a surge of oxytocin and lead to an involuntary urge to push. It is not uncommon for laboring persons to experience a compelling urge to push before complete cervical dilation is achieved. Many caregivers believe that pushing before complete dilation is associated with complications such as cervical edema and cervical lacerations. There is no evidence to support a cause-and-effect relationship between these complications and early pushing.

Only one small study has examined this issue.[49] Thirty-one women without formal childbirth education were supported and observed in their involuntary pushing efforts but given no instruction on pushing. They found that the average dilation at the onset of the urge to push was 9 cm, with a range of 5–10 cm. In the great majority of the women, the presenting part was at +1 station or lower when the urge began. Of these 31 women, 20 had the urge to push prior to complete dilation. There was a total of 3 cervical lacerations in the 31 women. Two were in the group that started pushing after complete dilation. The third began pushing at 6.5 cm and had a forceps-assisted vaginal birth. Given that the use of forceps is associated with an increased risk of cervical laceration, it is not possible to know if the timing of onset of pushing was a causative factor.

There are many anecdotal reports of an early urge to push and cervical edema when there is a malposition or malpresentation.[50] The malposition or malpresentation may be the causative factor for the occurrence of both the early pushing urge and cervical edema in some situations. Differences in the way the head is positioned in the pelvis with these variations and the resulting pressure on the vagina and cervix could explain the early urge to push. Uneven pressure on the cervix by the presenting part could lead to edema in the area which receives less pressure. Caregivers may inadvertently believe that the cervical edema is causing a slowing or cessation of labor progress, when in fact the cause is the malposition or malpresentation.

Often the laboring person cannot stop pushing when there is a strong urge. If admonished to stop a reflex that is beyond their control, the laboring person may feel upset. Position changes such as hands and knees (Fig. 7.18), semiprone (exaggerated runners lunge, Fig. 7.19), or open knee–chest (Fig. 7.20) may help resolve the malposition or malpresentation or lessen the urge to push by using gravity to move the head away from the cervix and ease pressure on the posterior vaginal wall.

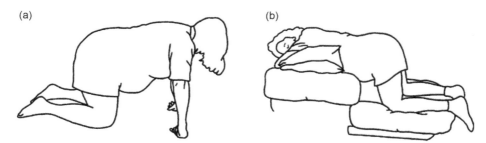

Fig. 7.18. (**a**) Hands and knees. (**b**) Kneeling on foot of bed.

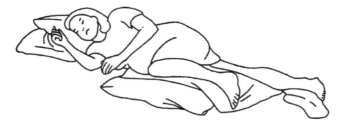

Fig. 7.19. Semiprone (exaggerated runner's lunge).

(a)   (b)

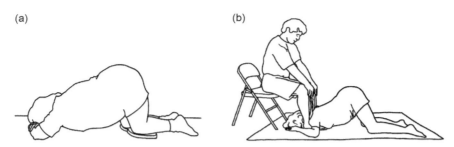

Fig. 7.20. (**a**) Open knee–chest position. (**b**) Open knee–chest position—shoulders resting on partner's padded shins.

The same approach can be used to reduce a persistent cervical lip or reduce a swollen cervix. Side-lying, semi-prone, or standing positions (Fig. 7.22) redistribute the pressure on the cervix and may reduce a lip. Immersion in deep water is another option. The weightlessness and buoyancy reduce the effects of gravity and may relieve pressure on the cervix. If patience, position changes, and water immersion do not resolve a persistent cervical lip, manual reduction is another option.

Manual reduction of a persistent cervical lip

The presence of an anterior cervical lip sometimes indicates that the fetus is in an OP or asynclitic position. If patience, position changes, or warm water immersion fail to reduce the cervical lip, manual reduction may be warranted. This is of particular use if there are concerns about the fetal heart rate or involuntary bearing-down efforts begin before complete or nearly complete dilation and are strong and uncoordinated. The manual reduction technique, used by midwives and physicians, is explained next:

- Explain the procedure, including the discomfort that the birthing person may experience along with the expected benefit of shortening the time until complete dilation and/or improved ability to push and obtain informed consent. Emphasize the need for cooperation with the clinician for the procedure to be successful.
- Using water-soluble lubricant, place two fingers slightly separated at the 11 and 1 o'clock positions between the head and the lip of cervix before the onset of a contraction.[51]
- Instruct the birthing person (who may or may not be experiencing a spontaneous urge to push) not to push until you tell her/them to do so.
- As you feel the contraction begin, push the anterior cervix over the baby's head (as if you were pushing up your upper lip to make your teeth visible).

If the cervical lip moves easily, instruct the birthing person to push to help the head advance, leaving the cervical lip behind it and pushing your fingers out of the vagina.

- Check after the contraction to be sure that the lip has not reappeared.
- Repeat if necessary and if the birthing person can tolerate it.
- It is prudent to repeat the cervical exam if, after a few more contractions, progress is not obvious to ensure that the cervix remained completely dilated and is not becoming trapped and swollen.

Reducing swelling of the cervix or anterior lip

Swelling of the cervix or cervical lip is an additional deterrent to continued labor progress. To reduce swelling of the cervix, homeopathic Arnica 12C to 30C can be administered orally, evening primrose oil or ice can be directly applied and held in place,[51] although these approaches have not be studied scientifically.

Another option that is used in practice with only anecdotal evidence is IV Benadryl. Some birth attendants use a low dose of IV Benadryl (12.5–25 mg) if there is an edematous cervix or swollen anterior lip stalling labor. Common practice is to give IV Benadryl, and then allow the person 1–2 hours to rest in hands and knees or side-lying position.

(a)

(b)

(c)

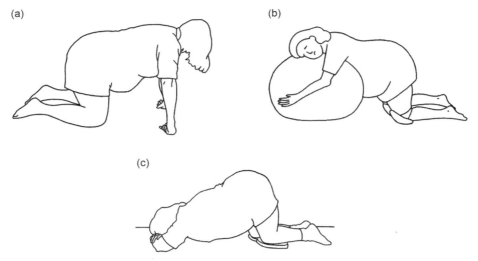

Fig. 7.21. (**a**) Hands and knees. (**b**) Kneeling with ball and knee pads. (**c**) Open knee–chest position.

(a)

(b)

(c)

(d)

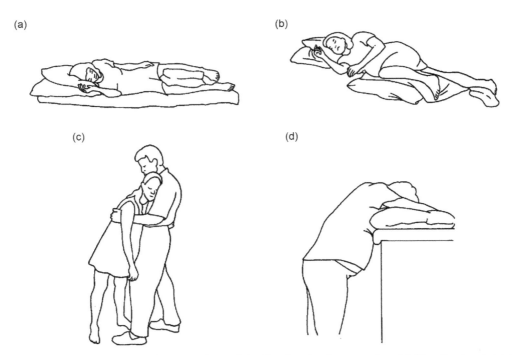

Fig. 7.22. (**a**) Side-lying. (**b**) Semiprone, lower arm forward. (**c**) Standing, leaning on partner. (**d**) Standing, leaning on counter.

DISRUPTIONS TO THE HORMONAL PHYSIOLOGY OF LABOR

Overview

The neurobiological processes that result in the onset and progress of labor and birth are referred to as the hormonal physiology of labor. This involves complex interactions between several hormonal systems: oxytocin; beta-endorphins; and stress hormones such as epinephrine, norepinephrine. These processes have evolved over millions of years to optimize birth outcomes and are shared by all mammals.[52,53]

The delicate interplay between the hormonal systems is an important consideration in prolonged labor. For example, endogenous oxytocin is required for uterine contractions but also decreases fear, anxiety, and pain. When events or stimuli occur that cause fear, anxiety, and increased pain, stress hormones are overproduced. This decreases oxytocin and can disrupt labor. This in turn reduces the protective effects of oxytocin in decreasing fear, anxiety, and pain which can further increase stress hormone production and decrease oxytocin. Overstimulation of the neocortex is also theorized to inhibit the "primitive" part of the brain which is responsible for the cascade of hormones required for effective labor.[54,55]

In today's maternity care settings, many practices can overstimulate the neocortex, interfere with a laboring person's sense of safety and relaxation, increase stress, and potentially disrupt labor.

Environmental factors that may disrupt the hormonal physiology of labor:

- noise
- bright lights
- lack of privacy
- interaction with strangers
- painful procedures (IV insertions, vaginal exams)
- restricted activity
- food and drink restrictions
- lack of support
- conversation
- asking the laboring person many questions
- a hectic environment[54,55]

Understanding what makes laboring people vulnerable to disruptions of the hormonal physiology of labor allows caregivers to counteract these factors and create an environment optimal for the necessary hormonal milieu.

Strategies to optimize oxytocin, beta-endorphins and minimize stress hormone production:

- touch
- support
- privacy
- small spaces
- low lighting
- quiet
- calm demeanor of caregivers and others present
- unrestricted activity
- warm water immersion (see discussion below)

IF EMOTIONAL DYSTOCIA IS SUSPECTED

Some caregivers use the term "emotional dystocia" to denote an increase in fear, anxiety, or other emotions that disrupts labor. This can be caused by environmental factors such as those listed above, but theoretically can also result from pre-existing factors that contribute to the laboring person's emotional state.

Predisposing factors theorized to contribute to emotional dystocia

- previous difficult births; injury or death of the baby
- previous traumatic hospitalizations
- a history of childhood abuse or neglect: physical, sexual, or emotional[56]
- dysfunctional family of origin (mental illness, substance abuse, fighting by parents, or other family problems)
- fears about current serious health problems for one's self or one's baby
- domestic violence (previous or present)
- cultural factors, including beliefs leading to extreme shame when viewed nude or when viewed in labor by men or when behaving in a way that is contrary to cultural expectations
- language barriers, or inability to hear or understand what is happening or being done
- death of one's own mother (especially in childbirth or when the laboring person was very young)
- fear of childbirth

Possible indicators of emotional dystocia during active labor

- expression or display of fear, anxiety, or exhaustion
- lack of rhythm and ritual in responses to contractions
- asking many questions, or remaining very alert to surroundings
- exhibiting unusually needy behavior
- displaying extreme modesty
- exhibiting strong reactions to mild contractions or to examinations
- an unusually high degree of muscle tension
- appearing demanding, distrustful, angry, or resentful toward staff
- seeming hypervigilant, highly alert, or easily startled
- exhibiting a strong need for control over caregivers' actions
- extreme reaction to contractions such as writhing, panicked, screaming, being unresponsive to suggestions or questions intended to help
- expressing fear of loss of control as labor becomes more intense

It is important to acknowledge that most people have some fear or anxiety about labor, birth, and the impact of a new child on their lives. This does not necessarily lead to prolonged labor. However, for some people emotional issues are powerful enough to interfere with an efficient labor pattern. This is not always manifested by visible struggle. People experiencing this can be silent and still, afraid to move or express their distress. The questions stated above may help identify some whose obvious behavior does not indicate extreme distress. Being able to recognize and help these people may reduce the negative impact of emotional distress. Sensitivity and attentiveness from a caregiver will contribute to a laboring person's sense of being cared for and cared about.

Measures to help cope with expressed fears

- Restate what the laboring person has said to confirm understanding.
- Validate the fear, rather than dismissing it. "Yes, others have told me they worried about that, too" or "That must be frightening. We're also concerned about babies during labor and that's why we check your baby's heartbeat frequently."
- Provide reassuring information (but not empty promises): "As I listen to the heartbeat, the baby sounds just fine right now. Would you like to know how babies adapt to contractions during labor? They have some really amazing coping mechanisms."
- Between contractions, let them know that after the baby is born, there are helpful resources available. For example, if the fear or worry is about being an inadequate mother, it may help to know there are parenting classes and support groups and a hotline for help at any time, day or night. Sometimes calming a laboring

person's conscious fears will lead to a more relaxed state in which the "primitive" parts of the brain will predominate and promote the labor process.

- Provide ideas (non-judgmentally) that can be used to alter the situation. For example, if the person feels helpless lying down, they might feel stronger if standing up and active.
- If intense, frequent, and unmanageable contractions make conversation impossible, the goal becomes getting through the difficult time by simplifying what needs to be done: "Right now, all that matters is that you keep your rhythm through the contraction. Let me help you. Follow my moving hand with your breathing or moaning and keep that rhythm. We will get through this together."

HYPOCONTRACTILE UTERINE ACTIVITY

Factors that can contribute to contractions of inadequate intensity and/or frequency

- immobility
- emotional and environmental factors
- uterine lactate production in long labors
- BMI >30
- Epidural

Immobility

Activity and upright positions results in labor shorter labors, fewer cesarean births, and less use of epidural analgesia.[35,36,57] If labor is slow, increasing activity and position changes are a reasonable intervention. Changing positions may trigger stronger contractions, either by shifting the fetus's weight or by improving circulation to the uterus. Upright positions and movements, including walking, may intensify contractions. The supine position, by contrast, seems to be correlated with weaker contractions when compared with other positions.[57]

Laboring persons who are restricted to bed (e.g., for hypertension, analgesia or anesthesia, indeterminate or non-reassuring fetal heart rate responses, or institutional custom) may still be able to use position changes to improve labor progress. If the person has back pain or other indicators of malposition, the side-lying position is recommended. If there are no indicators of malposition or if it is difficult to determine which side the fetal back is on, it is appropriate to try the "rollover." In the "rollover," shown in Fig. 7.23, the laboring person spends 20–30 minutes in each of the following positions: semisitting, left side-lying, left semiprone, hands and knees, right semiprone, right side-lying, and back to semisitting.

Environmental and emotional factors

Many factors can disrupt the hormonal physiology of labor. Attention to these environmental and emotional factors can increase oxytocin production and decrease the overproduction of stress hormones. This can be an effective way to promote stronger and more frequent contractions. A private, quiet, and calm space with low lighting is optimal. Some laboring persons respond well to small spaces such as a bathroom. Being in the shower or bath can provide the protective atmosphere of a small space in addition to the soothing nature of warm water. The presence of too many people can be disruptive, though some laboring individuals find it comforting to be surrounded by a group of people they know. Support and physical touch also promote the release of oxytocin. Helping the laboring person deal with emotions such as fear and anxiety can decrease the production of stress hormones that can lead to inadequate contractions.

Uterine lactate production in long labors

Lactate is a substance produced when there is anaerobic metabolism in muscle (muscle contraction without using oxygen for energy). Anaerobic metabolism generally results from strenuous or prolonged exercise. Accumulation of lactate is thought to cause muscle fatigue leading to weaker and less efficient muscle contractions.[58]

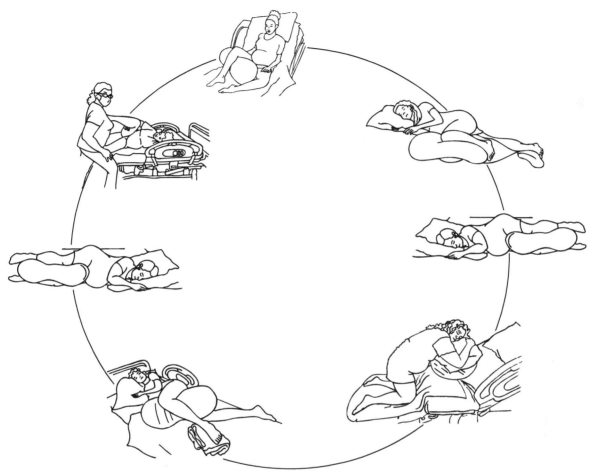

Fig. 7.23. The "rollover sequence" for use—there are no indication of malposition, or when it is difficult to determine the location of the fetal back.

Lactate is produced in the myometrium (uterine muscle) and can be measured in the amniotic fluid. This prompted researchers to study the relationship between amniotic fluid lactate and cesarean birth for prolonged labor. Some degree of lactate production in the uterus is apparently normal due to the unique function of the myometrium. However, research shows a relationship between higher levels of uterine lactate and cesarean birth for prolonged labor.[59,60] In addition, laboratory studies using rats show that lactate decreases uterine contractility.[61] Evidence is currently insufficient to conclude with certainty that uterine lactate is a cause of prolonged labor. Nevertheless, this is an idea worthy of consideration and may explain why contractions are slow in long labors.[59,62]

Sodium bicarbonate

One low-cost and low-intervention option that clinicians can consider during a prolonged first stage of labor is a dose of sodium bicarbonate. Some athletes take a mixture of baking soda dissolved in water (bicarbonate 0.3 g/kg of weight) prior to expected lactic acidosis one hour before exercise.[63] Because the uterus is a large muscle, and labor involves intense physical exertion by the uterus, sodium bicarbonate may be helpful during dysfunctional labor. Wiberg-Itzel, Wray, and Akerud[63] randomized 200 primiparas with dysfunctional labor and the need to start oxytocin to either starting oxytocin immediately or a dose of sodium bicarbonate ("SamarinVR" which contains sodium bicarbonate 2.13 gm, tartic acid, citric acid, sodium, potassium, and silica mixed with 200 mL of water) followed by one hour of rest and then starting oxytocin. Of the laboring people in the sodium bicarbonate 84% had a vaginal birth, compared to 67% in the immediate oxytocin group (p =.007). Further, newborns in the sodium bicarbonate group had better outcomes at birth (higher arterial pH (p = <.01), no Apgar scores below 7 at 5 minutes.[63] However, it is possible that the sodium bicarbonate group benefited from the hour of rest in addition to the sodium bicarbonate. An additional study of 142 primiparous laboring people who were being induced found that oral sodium bicarbonate may shorten labor duration and decrease instrumental deliveries.[64]

Calcium carbonate

In some areas, 1000 mg of oral Tums or calcium carbonate are used for dysfunctional labors, although this has not been scientifically studied. It is thought that the calcium improves uterine muscle contractility.

Sodium bicarbonate or calcium carbonate are low-cost interventions with no known potential harms that may be considered for those with dysfunctional labor. Further study is needed to fully understand the relationship between uterine lactate, calcium carbonate, and prolonged labor, and what approach is best suited to address this condition.

When the cause of inadequate contractions is unknown

When the cause of inadequate contractions is unknown, the following measures may lead to stronger contractions:

Breast stimulation

Used for centuries to start or augment labor, breast stimulation is frequently employed by caregivers in out-of-hospital settings. The laboring person or partner lightly strokes one or both nipples or massages the breasts to increase oxytocin release which augments contractions. Alternatively, a breast pump is used.[65]

Only two small trials have been conducted in the past three decades comparing breast stimulation and oxytocin for labor augmentation.[65,66] Methodological problems in both prevent reliable conclusions regarding effectiveness.[67] Other studies of breast stimulation were investigations of its use as a method of conducting the Contraction Stress Test or as a method of inducing labor.[68] A Cochrane review comparing breast stimulation with no treatment for labor induction found that for persons with a favorable cervix, breast stimulation increased the chances they would go into labor within 3 days.[65] Compared with oxytocin, breast stimulation had similar success rates for starting labor. These findings suggest a role for breast stimulation in labor augmentation.

Case reports of nipple stimulation by high-risk women as part of a contraction stress test (CSTs) described tetanic contractions.[66] CSTs have been replaced by Biophical Profiles in contemporary practice. Uterine tachysystole did not occur in the low-risk women in the trials in the Cochrane review.[65] When nipple stimulation is used, it is important to monitor for fetal wellbeing and tachysystole.

Walking and changes in position

Walking and position changes, including upright positions, improve the effectiveness of contractions and reduce the length of the first stage of labor by 1–1½ hours, without increasing intervention use or negative effects. The freedom to move improves laboring person's satisfaction with the birth experience,[69] and for many this apparently harmless practice also improves comfort and sense of control. Walking and position changes are discussed further in this chapter.

Acupressure or acupuncture

These traditional Eastern healing approaches may be used to stimulate more frequent contractions. Acupressure has been studied scientifically for its effects on labor pain and for its effects on labor progress. A Cochrane review

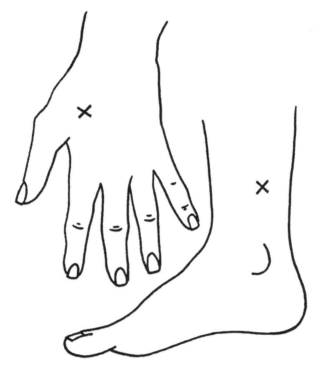

Fig. 7.24. Accupuncture points.

of 13 trials of acupuncture and acupressure during labor found that although there is need for more research, the trials of acupressure (compared to usual care) indicated that acupressure reduced labor pain intensity.[70] A more recent trial found that acupuncture also reduced pain intensity, to a greater degree than acupressure, and reduced the use of analgesic drugs and instrumental deliveries[71] (see Fig. 7.24). It also increased the laboring person's satisfaction with pain relief. No harmful effects have been reported when these techniques are used properly.[70] The use of acupuncture during labor requires specialized training for the midwife or consultation with a qualified acupuncturist.

COPING AND COMFORT ISSUES

Regardless of the cause of prolonged labor, attention to comfort and coping is critical. In addition to the importance of prevent suffering among laboring people, effective comfort and coping measures optimize the hormonal physiology of labor.[52] This may itself promote labor progress.

Individual coping styles

Childbirth education programs first emerged in the 1940s, when much less was known about the powerful, multisensory ways in which people spontaneously cope with labor. Much has been learned since then, but older ideas have left their stamp on Western culture and seem to be reiterated endlessly in the popular media. Many people still think that coping well means that the laboring person remains silent and does not move during contractions. There is a common belief that those who are physically active and vocal are coping poorly, and caregivers and support people may encourage that the birthing person remain quiet. However, we know now that people with kinesthetic and vocal coping styles often derive much more effective relief from pain and stress when they move and make sounds than when they try to be quiet and still.

Simkin's 3 Rs: Relaxation, rhythm, and ritual: The essence of coping during the first stage of labor

Simkin wrote extensively on the "3 Rs."[72] When we look closely at active vocal people in labor, we notice that some follow a rhythm and others vocalize irregularly and move jerkily, without rhythm. Those whose activities are rhythmic and repetitious are generally coping well, even though they may be loud and active.

Rhythm is the common element in coping during the first stage of labor, just as it is the key to success in physical endurance events and some kinds of meditation, yoga, and self-calming techniques. Rhythmic breathing, vocalizing, swaying, tapping, self-stroking—even rhythmic mental activities, such as counting breaths through a contraction, repeating a mantra or verse, or singing a song aloud or silently to themselves—are all examples of using rhythm as a coping technique. Usually, by the time a person is in active labor, they are no longer using the exact techniques they were taught in prenatal classes, although these may have been helpful earlier. Rhythmic activities in active labor are unique and unplanned. They emerge spontaneously when laboring people are not afraid and are not disturbed or restricted in their behavior. When these spontaneous rhythmic behaviors develop, the cognitive parts of the brains are less active, and behavior becomes more instinctual. In fact, people often express surprise and pleasure later at the repetitive rhythmic behaviors they discovered during labor and at how effective they were.

Other spontaneous coping behaviors exhibited include relaxation during and/or between contractions and routines, or rituals, which are the repetition of the same rhythmic activities for many contractions in a row. Coping rituals often involve other people (the partner, doula, or someone else). The laboring person may want them to continue doing the same comforting behaviors with each contraction. They may hold them, stroke or sway with them, speak to them or moan softly in their rhythm, and help them regain their rhythm if they lose it. These three coping mechanisms—relaxation, rhythm, and ritual—are referred to as the 3 Rs. They constitute the essence of coping during the first stage of labor.

The caregiver, in assessing wellbeing during labor, should observe the person's coping behavior. If there is rhythm in whatever they are doing, they are coping. If the rhythm is lost, she needs help to regain it. In summary, coping well during labor and birth often includes instinctive vocalization, movement, and self-comforting behavior. During the first stage, relaxation, rhythm, and ritual (the 3 Rs) represent good signs of coping.

Hydrotherapy: Warm water immersion or warm shower

Warm water immersion or hydrotherapy during the first stage of labor is a low-technology intervention that can be used for pain relief during labor, to decrease anxiety, and promote maternal satisfaction. Birthing people may enter the warm water at any time in the first stage.

Studies comparing warm water immersion during labor with usual care show that this non-pharmacologic comfort measure is associated with less epidural and other pain medication use, reports of less pain and anxiety and higher satisfaction scores.[73,74] Buoyancy, hydrostatic pressure, warmth, skin stimulation, and other factors induce relaxation, temporarily reduce pain awareness, and may reduce production of stress hormones. Warm showers may be effective as well, although without the buoyancy and hydrostatic pressure provided by immersion in a tub of water. (See Fig. 7.25) The inherent increases in privacy and small space of a shower or tub may be additional factors that optimize labor hormones. Some caregivers recommend aiming the shower at the nipples for breast stimulation if contractions are inadequate.

Comfort measures for back pain

Baths and showers, back pressure and massage, the knee press, kneeling and swaying on the birth ball, transcutaneous electrical nerve stimulation, cold or warm compresses, and intracutaneous or subcutaneous sterile water injections are effective in relieving back pain.

(a)   (b)

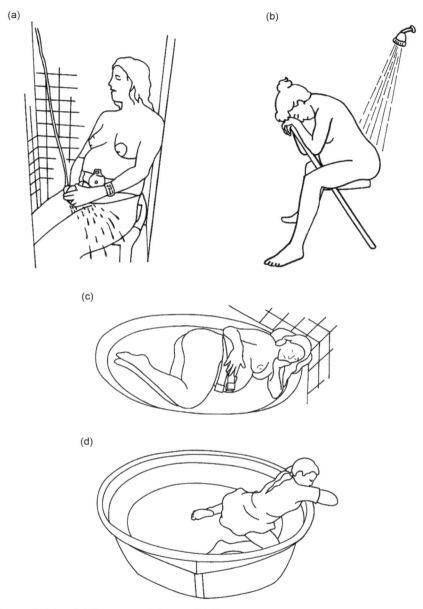

(c)

(d)

Fig. 7.25. Hydrotherapy in labor. (**a**) Shower on abdomen. (**b**) Shower on back. (**c**) Laboring in bath with continuous fetal monitoring. (**d**) Laboring in birthing pool.

Exhaustion

Fatigue or exhaustion, especially if combined with fear or distress, is a major concern for people experiencing long labors. Massage, music, dim light, aromatherapy, guided imagery, a bath, or whatever the person finds soothing may help with relaxation and acceptance of the slow pace of labor. Reassurance from a patient and empathic

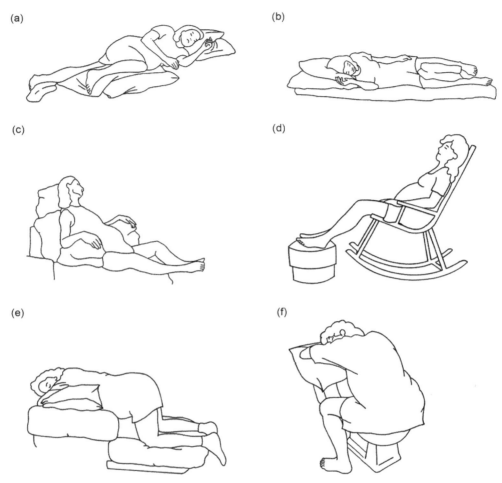

Fig. 7.26.   Positions for tired people. (**a**) Semiprone. (**b**) Side-lying. (**c**) Semisitting. (**d**) Sitting in a rocking chair. (**e**) Kneeling on foot of bed. (**f**) Straddling a toilet.

caregiver and/or doula can ease worry. Positions for tired people, shown in Fig. 7.26, are more restful than others and may provide a welcome change.

Sterile water injections

When the baby is in an OP position, the laboring person often experiences significant lower back pain, sometimes referred to as "back labor." Back labor, no matter what the cause, can be severely painful. Intradermal or intracutaneous sterile water injections injected into four specific points on the laboring person's back can be used as a non-pharmacologic approach for relief of back pain in labor. The mechanism of action is not fully understood but appears to be linked to the Gate Control Theory of pain relief.[75,76] More specifically, it appears that the sterile water acts as a mild irritant stimulating localized discomfort. The use of sterile water injections does not preclude the use of epidural anesthesia. Therefore, for those who would like to avoid epidural anesthesia, sterile water injections may be used in a stepwise attempt to address overwhelming back pain. Formerly, the sterile water injections were administered intracutaneously (0.05–0.1 mL) and were considered to cause significant acute pain that lasted about 30 seconds, followed by 60–90 minutes of back pain relief.[75,76] A single intradermal sterile water injection is an alternative approach using the same technique. The laboring person identifies the place of the most pain, to determine the injection site. Lee and colleagues conducted a randomized clinical trial comparing the single to the four intradermal injection techniques with 305 laboring people with lower back pain.[77] While injection pain was significantly less with the single-site technique, those who experienced the injections at four sites experienced significantly greater pain relief at 30 minutes.

Subcutaneous injections (0.5 mL) have been studied in comparison to intracutaneous injections. A randomized controlled trial compared 0.5 mL of sterile water injected subcutaneously in each of the four sites to 0.1 mL injected intracutaneously in each site and 1 mL of placebo (saline solution) in each site. The subcutaneous injections were found to be as effective as intracutaneous injections in relieving back pain and significantly less painful during administration.[75] A more recent study confirmed this finding.[78] Therefore, experts now recommend giving subcutaneous sterile water injections rather than intradermal injections for back pain relief in labor.[75] Hutton and colleagues[79] conducted a meta-analysis of sterile water injections that included eight randomized controlled trials. They found that those who received the sterile water injections had a significant reduction in cesarean birth. This finding suggests broader benefits of sterile water injections and warrants further study. A randomized control trial by Genc and colleagues[80] found laboring people who received sterile water injections had both less back pain and higher maternal satisfaction scores than the control group.

Procedure for subcutaneous sterile water injections

Saline cannot be used for this procedure as it will have no effect.[75] Sterile water is drawn up into one or more tuberculin syringes (in an amount sufficient to allow for four injections of 0.5 mL each).[81] The skin is cleansed with isopropyl alcohol, and the water is injected subcutaneously into four points located in the sacral region of the back (Fig. 7.27). Even though subcutaneous injections are less painful than the intracutaneous injections, the discomfort

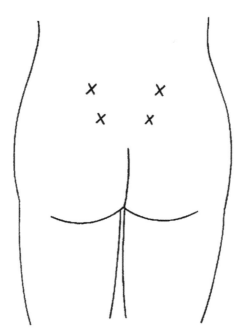

Fig. 7.27.   Sterile water injection points.

of the procedure can be further reduced if two health professionals administer the injections simultaneously and administer them during, rather than between, contractions. Pain relief is often noticed within minutes.

Hydration and nutrition

It is well known that pregnancy, labor and intrapartum analgesia slow gastrointestinal motility. Surprisingly little is known about fluid and energy needs of laboring people. Common sense, application of research on nutritional needs during strenuous exercise, and some recent studies on energy utilization in labor reasonably lead to the conclusion that labor is an event that requires calories and hydration.[82]

Nevertheless, a policy of withholding food and fluids during labor that became widespread in North America and the United Kingdom in the 1940s and 1950s remains in many places.[83] This policy was based on concerns about the dangers of general anesthesia for laboring people who had food in their stomachs, because they were more likely to vomit and aspirate food particles and gastric acid while under general anesthesia. Fasting has not been proven to solve such problems; in fact, pure gastric secretions that are not mixed with food are more acidic and thus more damaging if aspirated.[82] Safe anesthesia techniques appear to be the best safeguard against aspiration. Furthermore, the use of general anesthesia for cesareans has been almost entirely replaced by epidural and spinal anesthesia. The risk of aspiration from general anesthesia in labor is extremely low.[84]

Evidence on the best approach to meeting fluid and energy needs in labor is mixed. Intravenous fluids can theoretically meet both fluid and energy needs in labor. There is some evidence that 250 mL/hour of IV fluids as compared to 125 mL/hour or only fluids by mouth results in shorter labors of about 30 minutes.[85] However, the authors of this Cochrane review point out that IV fluids are not risk free and can lead to fluid overload in the laboring person and excess weight loss in the newborn in the first few days of life. In addition, the discomfort and decrease mobility that an intravenous line can cause can negatively impact labor as well.

A meta-analysis of unrestrictive food intake during labor found that this approach also resulted in shorter labors of about 30 minutes.[86] Though no studies on satisfaction with various oral intake policies during labor have been done, it is reasonable to assume that restrictions on food and especially fluids can be stressful and uncomfortable. The World Health Organization (WHO), American College of Nurse-Midwives (ACNM), and Society of Obstetricians and Gynecologist of Canada[87] recommend that laboring people without risk factors for aspiration should determine their own oral intake. The simplest practice to prevent dehydration and provide nourishment is to encourage drinking to thirst with water, electrolyte-balanced beverages, broth, or fruit juice and eating as desired. This is especially important during long labors.

CONCLUSION

Labor progress may slow in active labor for a variety of reasons. Determining the possible cause or causes is a good first step. When the laboring person and fetus are faring well, interventions or actions specific to the cause may be used to address the problem. Slow progress is often caused by more than one issue and several measures may be appropriate.

REFERENCES

1. Friedman E. (1954) The graphic analysis of labor. *American Journal of Obstetrics & Gynecology* 68, 1568–1575.
2. Zhang J, Troendle J, Mikolajczyk R, Sundaram R, Beaver J, Fraser W. (2010) The natural history of the normal first stage of labor. *Obstetrics and Gynecology* 115(4), 705–710. doi: 10.1097/AOG.0b013e3181d55925
3. American College of Obstetricians and Gynecologists and Society for Maternal Fetal Medicine. (2014) Obstetric care consensus no. 1: Safe prevention of the primary cesarean delivery. *Obstetrics and Gynecology* 123(3), 693–711. doi: 10.1097/01.AOG.0000444441.04111.1d
4. World Health Organization. (2018) *WHO Recommendations: Intrapartum Care for a Positive Childbirth Experience*. Geneva: World Health Organization. 2018. License: CC BY-NC-SA 3.0 IGO. ISBN 978-92-4-155021-5.
5. Friedman E. (1978) *Labor: Clinical Evaluation and Management*, 2nd edn. New York: Appleton-Century-Crofts.

6. Neal JL, Lowe NK. (2012) Physiologic partograph to improve birth safety and outcomes among low-risk, nulliparous women with spontaneous labor onset. *Medical Hypotheses* 78(2), 319–326. doi: 10.1016/j.mehy.2011.11.012

7. Malvasi A. (ed.) (2012) *Intrapartum Ultrasonography for Labor Management.* Berlin: Springer Science & Business Media.

8. Malvasi A, Tinelli A, Barbera A, Eggebø, TM, Mynbaev OA, Bochicchio M, Pacella E, Di Renzo GC. (2014c) Occiput posterior position diagnosis: Vaginal examination or intrapartum sonography? A clinical review. *The Journal of Maternal-Fetal & Neonatal Medicine: The Official Journal of the European Association of Perinatal Medicine, The Federation of Asia and Oceania Perinatal Societies, The International Society of Perinatal Obstetricians* 27(5), 520–526. doi: 10.3109/14767058.2013.82559

9. Gardberg M, Laakkonen E, Sälevaara M. (1998) Intrapartum sonography and persistent occiput posterior position: A study of 408 deliveries. *Obstetrics and Gynecology* 91(5 Pt 1), 746–749. doi: 10.1016/s0029-7844(98)00074-x

10. Lieberman E, Davidson K, Lee-Parritz A, Shearer E. (2005) Changes in fetal position during labor and their association with epidural analgesia. *Obstetrics and Gynecology* 105(5 Pt 1), 974–982. doi: 10.1097/01.AOG.0000158861.43593.49

11. Malvasi A, Bochicchio M, Vaira L, Longo A, Pacella E, Tinelli A. (2014b) The fetal head evaluation during labor in the occiput posterior position: The ESA (evaluation by simulation algorithm) approach. *The Journal of Maternal-fetal & Neonatal Medicine: The Official Journal of the European Association of Perinatal Medicine, the Federation of Asia and Oceania Perinatal Societies, the International Society of Perinatal Obstetricians* 27(11), 1151–1157. doi: 10.3109/14767058.2013.851188

12. Simkin P. (2010) The fetal occiput posterior position: State of the science and a new perspective. *Birth (Berkeley, Calif.)* 37(1), 61–71. doi: 10.1111/j.1523-536X.2009.00380.x

13. Barros JG, Gomes-da-costa A, Afonso M, Carita AI, Ayres-de-campos D, Graça LM, Clode N. (2019) Effect of simulation-based training on the accuracy of fetal head position determination in labor. *European Journal of Obstetrics, Gynecology, and Reproductive Biology* 242, 68–70. doi: 10.1016/j.ejogrb.2019.09.019

14. Bellussi F, Ghi T, Youssef A, et al. (2017a) The use of intrapartum ultrasound to diagnose malpositions and cephalic malpresentations. *American Journal of Obstetrics and Gynecology* 217(6), 633–641. doi: 10.1016/j.ajog.2017.07.025

15. Hjartardóttir H, Lund SH, Benediktsdóttir S, Geirsson RT, Eggebø TM. (2021) When does fetal head rotation occur in spontaneous labor at term: Results of an ultrasound-based longitudinal study in nulliparous women. *American Journal of Obstetrics and Gynecology* 224(5), 514.e1–514.e9. doi: 10.1016/j.ajog.2020.10.054

16. Malvasi A, Barbera A, Di Vagno G, et al. (2014a) Asynclitism: A literature review of an often-forgotten clinical condition. *Journal of Maternal-Fetal & Neonatal Medicine* 28(16).

17. Penfield CA, Wing DA. (2017) Labor induction techniques: Which is the best? *Obstetrics and Gynecology Clinics of North America* 44(4), 567–582. doi: 10.1016/j.ogc.2017.08.011

18. Cheng YW, Shaffer BL, Caughey AB. (2006) Associated factors and outcomes of persistent occiput posterior position: A retrospective cohort study from 1976 to 2001. *The Journal of Maternal-fetal & Neonatal Medicine: The Official Journal of the European Association of Perinatal Medicine, the Federation of Asia and Oceania Perinatal Societies, the International Society of Perinatal Obstetricians* 19(9), 563–568. doi: 10.1080/14767050600682487

19. Smyth RM, Markham C, Dowswell T. (2013) Amniotomy for shortening spontaneous labour. *The Cochrane Database of Systematic Reviews* (6), CD006167. doi: 10.1002/14651858.CD006167.pub4

20. Menichini D, Mazzaro N, Minniti S, Ricchi A, Molinazzi MT, Facchinetti F, Neri I. (2022) Fetal head malposition and epidural analgesia in labor: A case-control study. *The Journal of Maternal-fetal & Neonatal Medicine: The Official Journal of the European Association of Perinatal Medicine, the Federation of Asia and Oceania Perinatal Societies, the International Society of Perinatal Obstetricians* 35(25), 5691–5696. doi: 10.1080/14767058.2021.1890018

21. Sizer AR, Nirmal DM. (2000) Occipitoposterior position: Associated factors and obstetric outcome in nulliparas. *Obstetrics and Gynecology* 96(5 Pt 1), 749–752. doi: 10.1016/s0029-7844(00)01030-9

22. Le Ray C, Carayol M, Jaquemin S, Mignon A, Cabrol D, Goffinet F. (2005) Is epidural analgesia a risk factor for occiput posterior or transverse positions during labour? *European Journal of Obstetrics, Gynecology, and Reproductive Biology* 123(1), 22–26. doi: 10.1016/j.ejogrb.2005.02.009

23. Robinson CA, Macones GA, Roth NW, Morgan MA. (1996) Does station of the fetal head at epidural placement affect the position of the fetal vertex at delivery? *American Journal of Obstetrics and Gynecology* 175(4 Pt 1), 991–994. doi: 10.1016/s0002-9378(96)80039-1

24. Siccardi M, Valle C, Di Matteo F. (2021) Dynamic external pelvimetry test in third trimester pregnant women: Shifting positions affect pelvic biomechanics and create more room in obstetric diameters. *Cureus* 13(3), e13631. doi: 10.7759/cureus.13631

25. Siccardi M, Valle C, Di Matteo F, Angius V. (2019) A postural approach to the pelvic diameters of obstetrics: The dynamic external pelvimetry test. *Cureus* 11(11), e6111. doi: 10.7759/cureus.6111

26. Tully G. (2016) Opening the pelvic brim with Walcher's position. *Midwifery Today with International Midwife* (117), 26–27.

27. Tully G. (2020) *Changing Birth on Earth: A Midwife and Nurse's Guide to Using Physiology to Avoid Another Unnecessary Cesarean.* Bloomington, MN: Maternity House Publishing. ISBN 10: 1735748994.

28. Spinning Babies. (2023). https://www.spinningbabies.com

29. Bueno-Lopez V, Fuentelsaz-Gallego C, Casellas-Caro M, Falgueras-Serrano AM, Crespo-Berros S, Silvano-Cocinero AM, Alcaine-Guisado C, Zamoro Fuentes M, Carreras E, Terré-Rull C. (2018) Efficiency of the modified Sims maternal position in the rotation of persistent occiput posterior position during labor: A randomized clinical trial. *Birth (Berkeley, Calif.)* 45(4), 385–392. doi: 10.1111/birt.12347

30. Stremler R, Hodnett E, Petryshen P, Stevens B, Weston J, Willan AR. (2005) Randomized controlled trial of hands-and-knees positioning for occipitoposterior position in labor. *Birth (Berkeley, Calif.)* 32(4), 243–251. doi: 10.1111/j.0730-7659.2005.00382.x

31. Desbriere R, Blanc J, Le Dû R, Renner JP, Carcopino X, Loundou A, d'Ercole C. (2013) Is maternal posturing during labor efficient in preventing persistent occiput posterior position? A randomized controlled trial. *American Journal of Obstetrics and Gynecology* 208(1), 60.e1–60.e608. doi: 10.1016/j.ajog.2012.10.882

32. Guittier MJ, Othenin-Girard V, de Gasquet B, Irion O, Boulvain M. (2016) Maternal positioning to correct occiput posterior fetal position during the first stage of labour: A randomised controlled trial. *BJOG: An International Journal of Obstetrics and Gynaecology* 123(13), 2199–2207. doi: 10.1111/1471-0528.13855

33. Le Ray C, Lepleux F, De La Calle A, Guerin J, Sellam N, Dreyfus M, Chantry AA. (2016) Lateral asymmetric decubitus position for the rotation of occipito-posterior positions: Multicenter randomized controlled trial EVADELA. *American Journal of Obstetrics and Gynecology* 215(4), 511.e1–511.e5117. doi: 10.1016/j.ajog.2016.05.033

34. Blanc-Petitjean P, Le Ray C, Lepleux F, De La Calle A, Dreyfus M, Chantry AA. (2018) Factors affecting rotation of occiput posterior position during the first stage of labor. *Journal of Gynecology Obstetrics and Human Reproduction* 47(3), 119–125. doi: 10.1016/j.jogoh.2017.12.006

35. Lawrence A, Lewis L, Hofmeyr GJ, Styles C. (2013) Maternal positions and mobility during first stage labour. *The Cochrane Database of Systematic Reviews* (10), CD003934. doi: 10.1002/14651858.CD003934.pub4

36. Lepleux F, Hue B, Dugué AE, Six T, Riou C, Dreyfus M. (2014 Sep). Données obstétricales dans une population bénéficiant de variations posturales en cours de travail et d'accouchement [Obstetric data in a population with postural changes during labor and delivery]. *Journal of Obstetrics Biology Reproductive (Paris)* 43(7), 504–513. French. doi: 10.1016/j.jgyn.2013.06.013. Epub 2013 Aug 22. PMID: 23972772.

37. Scott P. (2003) *Sit up and Take Notice! Positioning Yourself for a Better Birth.* Tauranga, New Zealand: Great Scott Publications.

38. Sutton J. (2001) *Let Birth Be Born Again: Rediscovering and Reclaiming Our Midwifery Heritage.* Bedfont, Middlesex, UK: Birth Concepts.

39. Grant CH. (2014) *Peanut Ball Positions.* Tulsa: M & W Productions.

40. Tussey CM, Botsios E, Gerkin RD, Kelly LA, Gamez J, Mensik J. (2015) Reducing length of labor and cesarean surgery rate using a peanut ball for women laboring with an epidural. *The Journal of Perinatal Education* 24(1), 16–24. doi: 10.1891/1058-1243.24.1.16

41. Cohen SR, Thomas CR. (2015 Jul-Aug). Rebozo technique for Fetal Malposition in labor. *Journal of Midwifery Women's Health* 60(4), 445–451. doi: 10.1111/jmwh.12352. PMID: 26255805.

42. Elmore C, McBroom K, Ellis J. (2020) Digital and manual rotation of the persistent occiput posterior fetus. *Journal of Midwifery & Women's Health* 65(3), 387–394. doi: 10.1111/jmwh.13118

43. Masturzo B, Farina A, Attamante L, et al. (2017) Sonographic evaluation of the fetal spine position and success rate of manual rotation of the fetus in occiput posterior position: A randomized controlled trial. *Journal of Clinical Ultrasound* 45(8), 472–476.

44. Shaffer BL, Cheng YW, Vargas JE, Caughey AB. (2011) Manual rotation to reduce caesarean delivery in persistent occiput posterior or transverse position. *The Journal of Maternal-Fetal & Neonatal Medicine: The Official Journal of the European Association of Perinatal Medicine, The Federation of Asia and Oceania Perinatal Societies, The International Society of Perinatal Obstetricians* 24(1), 65–72. doi: 10.3109/14767051003710276

45. Cargill YM, MacKinnon CJ, Arsenault MY, Bartellas E, Daniels S, Gleason T, Iglesias S, Klein MC, Lane CA, Martel MJ, Sprague AE, Roggensack A, Wilson AK, Clinical Practice Obstetrics Committee. (2004) Guidelines for operative vaginal birth. *Journal of Obstetrics and Gynaecology Canada: JOGC = Journal D'obstetrique Et Gynecologie du Canada: JOGC* 26(8), 747–761. doi: 10.1016/s1701-2163(16)30647-8

46. Reichman O, Gdansky E, Latinsky B, Labi S, Samueloff A. (2008) Digital rotation from occipito-posterior to occipito-anterior decreases the need for cesarean section. *European Journal of Obstetrics, Gynecology, and Reproductive Biology* 136(1), 25–28. doi: 10.1016/j.ejogrb.2006.12.025

47. Le Ray C, Serres P, Schmitz T, Cabrol D, Goffinet F. (2007) Manual rotation in occiput posterior or transverse positions: Risk factors and consequences on the cesarean delivery rate. *Obstetrics and Gynecology* 110(4), 873–879. doi: 10.1097/01.AOG.0000281666.04924.be

48. Phipps H, de Vries B, Hyett J, Osborn DA. (2014) Prophylactic manual rotation for fetal malposition to reduce operative delivery. *The Cochrane Database of Systematic Reviews* (12), CD009298. doi: 10.1002/14651858.CD009298.pub2

49. Roberts JE, Goldstein SA, Gruener JS, Maggio M, Mendez-Bauer C. (1987 Jan-Feb) A descriptive analysis of involuntary bearing-down efforts during the expulsive phase of labor. *Journal of Obstetric, Gynecologic, & Neonatal Nursing* 16(1), 48–55. doi: 10.1111/j.1552-6909.1987.tb01438.x. PMID: 3643994.

50. Perez-Bortella M, Downe S. (2006) Stories as evidence: The premature urge to push. *British Journal of Midwifery* 14(11), 636–642.

51. Frye A. (2013) *Healing Passage*, 6th edn. Portland OR: Labrys Press.

52. Buckley SJ. (2015) *Hormonal Physiology of Childbearing: Evidence and Implications for Women, Babies, and Maternity Care*. Washington, D.C.: Childbirth Connection Programs, National Partnership for Women & Families.

53. Olza I, Uvnas-Moberg K, Ekström-Bergström A, Leahy-Warren P, Karlsdottir SI, Nieuwenhuijze M, Villarmea S, Hadjigeorgiou E, Kazmierczak M, Spyridou A, Buckley S. (2020 Jul 28) Birth as a neuro-psycho-social event: An integrative model of maternal experiences and their relation to neurohormonal events during childbirth. *PLoS One* 15(7), e0230992. doi: 10.1371/journal.pone.0230992. PMID: 32722725; PMCID: PMC7386571.

54. Odent M. (1999) *The Scientification of Love*. London: Free Association Press. Chapter 6.

55. Wuitchik M, Bakal D, Lipshitz J. (1989 Jan) The clinical significance of pain and cognitive activity in latent labor. *Obstetrics & Gynecology* 73(1), 35–42. PMID: 2909041.

56. Simkin P, Klaus P. (2004) *When Survivors Give Birth: Understanding and Healing the Effects of Early Sexual Abuse on the Childbearing Woman*. Seattle: Classic Day Publishing.

57. Kibuka M, Price A, Onakpoya I, Tierney S, Clarke M. (2021) Evaluating the effects of maternal positions in childbirth: An overview of cochrane systematic reviews. *European Journal of Midwifery* 5, 57. doi: 10.18332/ejm/142781

58. Westerblad H, Allen DG, Lännergren J. (2002 Feb) Muscle fatigue: Lactic acid or inorganic phosphate the major cause? *News in Physiological Sciences* 17, 17–21. doi: 10.1152/physiologyonline.2002.17.1.17. PMID: 11821531.

59. Murphy M, Butler M, Coughlan B, Brennan D, O'Herlihy C, Robson M. (2015 Nov) Elevated amniotic fluid lactate predicts labor disorders and cesarean delivery in nulliparous women at term. *American Journal of Obstetrics and Gynecology* 213(5), 673.e1–8. doi: 10.1016/j.ajog.2015.06.035. Epub 2015 Jun 25. PMID: 26116871.

60. Wiberg-Itzel E, Pembe AB, Järnbert-Pettersson H, Norman M, Wihlbäck AC, Hoesli I, Todesco Bernasconi M, Azria E, Åkerud H, Darj E. (2016) Lactate in amniotic fluid: Predictor of labor outcome in oxytocin-augmented primiparas' deliveries. *PloS One* 11(10), e0161546. doi: 10.1371/journal.pone.0161546

61. Hanley JA, Weeks A, Wray S. (2015 Oct 15). Physiological increases in lactate inhibit intracellular calcium transients, acidify myocytes and decrease force in term pregnant rat myometrium. *Journal of Physiological* 593(20), 4603–4614. doi: 10.1113/JP270631. Epub 2015 Sep 3. PMID: 26223765; PMCID: PMC4606541.

62. Quenby S, Pierce SJ, Brigham S, Wray S. (2004 Apr) Dysfunctional labor and myometrial lactic acidosis. *Obstetrics & Gynecology* 103(4), 718–723. doi: 10.1097/01.AOG.0000118306.82556.43. Erratum in: *Obstet Gynecol. 2004 Jun;103*(6):1344. PMID: 15051564.

63. Wiberg-Itzel E, Wray S, Åkerud H. (2018) A randomized controlled trial of a new treatment for labor dystocia. *The Journal of Maternal-fetal & Neonatal Medicine: The Official Journal of the European Association of Perinatal Medicine, the Federation of Asia and Oceania Perinatal Societies, the International Society of Perinatal Obstetricians* 31(17), 2237–2244. doi: 10.1080/14767058.2017.1339268

7

64. Seyedi M, Ghorashi Z, Sedighi Darijani T. (2021) Randomized controlled trial of oral bicarbonate treatment for labor stagnation. *The Journal of Obstetrics and Gynaecology Research* 47(1), 114–118. doi: 10.1111/jog.14438

65. Stein JL, Bardeguez AD, Verma UL, Tegani N. (1990) Nipple stimulation for labor augmentation. *The Journal of Reproductive Medicine* 35(7), 710–714.

66. Curtis P, Resnick JC, Evens S, Thompson CJ. (1999) A comparison of breast stimulation and intravenous oxytocin for the augmentation of labor. *Birth (Berkeley, Calif.)* 26(2), 115–122. doi: 10.1046/j.1523-536x.1999.00115.x

67. Razgaitis EJ, Lyvers AN. (2010) Management of protracted active labor with nipple stimulation: A viable tool for midwives? *Journal of Midwifery & Women's Health* 55(1), 65–69. doi: 10.1016/j.jmwh.2010.05.002

68. Mozurkewich EL, Chilimigras JL, Berman DR, Perni UC, Romero VC, King VJ, Keeton KL. (2011 Oct 27) Methods of induction of labour: A systematic review. *BMC Pregnancy Childbirth* 11, 84. doi: 10.1186/1471-2393-11-84. PMID: 22032440; PMCID: PMC3224350.

69. Simkin PP, O'Hara M. (2002) Nonpharmacologic relief of pain during labor: Systematic reviews of five methods. *American Journal of Obstetrics and Gynecology* 186(5), S131–S159. doi: 10.1016/s0002-9378(02)70188-9

70. Smith C, Collins C, Crowther C, Levett K. (2011) Acupuncture or acupressure for pain management in labour (review). *Cochrane Database of Systematic Reviews* (7), Art. No.: CD009232. doi: 10.1002/14651858.CD009232

71. Yesilcicek Calik K, Komurcu N. (2014) Effects of SP6 acupuncture point stimulation on labor pain and duration of labor. *Iranian Red Crescent Medical Journal* 16(10), e16461. doi: 10.5812/ircmj.16461

72. Simkin P. (2016) The 3 Rx in childbirth preparation: Relaxation, rhythm, and ritual. https://www.pennysimkin.com/project/three-rs-of-labor

73. Cluett ER, Burns E. (2009 Apr 15) Immersion in water in labour and birth. *Cochrane Database of Systematic Reviews* (2), CD000111. doi: 10.1002/14651858.CD000111.pub3. Update in: Cochrane Database Syst Rev. 2018 May 16;5:CD000111. PMID: 19370552; PMCID: PMC3982045.

74. Shaw-Battista J. (2017 Oct/Dec) Systematic review of hydrotherapy research: Does a warm bath in labor promote normal physiologic childbirth? *Journal of Perinatal and Neonatal Nursing* 31(4), 303–316. doi: 10.1097/JPN.0000000000000260. PMID: 28520654.

75. Martensson L, Nyberg K, Wallin G. (2000) Subcutaneous versus intracutaneous injections of sterile water for labour analgesia: A comparison of perceived pain during administration. *British Journal of Obstetrics and Gynaecology* 107, 1248–1251.

76. Simkin P, Klein MC. (2015) Nonpharmacological approaches to management of labor pain. *UpToDate* 17(3), 1–14.

77. Lee N, Webster J, Beckmann M, et al. (2013) Comparison of a single vs. a four intra dermal sterile water injection for relief of lower back pain for women in labour: A randomized controlled trial. *Midwifery* 29, 585–591.

78. Bahasadri S, Ahmadi-Abhari S, Dehghani-Nik M, Habibi GR. (2006) Subcutaneous sterile water injections for labour pain: A randomised controlled trial. *Australian and New Zealand Journal of Obstetrics and Gynaecology* 46(2), 102–106. doi: 10.1111/j.1479-828X.2006.0053

79. Hutton EK, Kasperink M, Rutten M, Reitzma A, Wainman B. (2009) Sterile water injection for labour pain: A systematic review and meta-analysis of randomised controlled trials. *British Journal of Obstetrics and Gynaecology* 116, 1158–1166. doi: 10.1111/j.1471

80. Genç Koyucu R, Demirci N, Ender Yumru A, et al. (2018) Effects of intradermal sterile water injections in women with low back pain in labor: A randomized, controlled, clinical trial. *Balkan Medical Journal* 35(2), 148–154. doi: 10.4274/balkanmedj.2016.0879

81. Martensson L, Wallin, G. (1999) Labour pain treated with cutaneous injections of sterile water: A randomised controlled trial. *British Journal of Obstetrics and Gynaecology* 106, 633–637.

82. American College of Nurse-Midwives. (2016) Providing oral nutrition to women in labor. *Journal of Midwifery Women's Health* 61(4), 528–534. doi: 10.1111/jmwh.12515.

83. Declercq ER, Sakala C, Corry MP, Applebaum S, Herrlich A. (2013 May). *Listening to Mothers III: Pregnancy and Birth*. New York: Childbirth Connection.

84. Singata M, Tranmer J, Gyte GM. (2013 Aug 22) Restricting oral fluid and food intake during labour. *Cochrane Database of Systematic Reviews* 2013(8), CD003930. doi: 10.1002/14651858.CD003930.pub3. PMID: 23966209; PMCID: PMC7104541.

85. Dawood F, Dowswell T, Quenby S. (2013 Jun 18) Intravenous fluids for reducing the duration of labour in low-risk nulliparous women. *Cochrane Database of Systematic Reviews* (6), CD007715. doi: 10.1002/14651858.CD007715.pub2. PMID: 23780639.

86. Ciardulli A, Saccone G, Anastasio H, Berghella V. (2017 Mar) Less-restrictive food intake during labor in low-risk singleton pregnancies: A systematic review and Meta-analysis. *Obstetrics & Gynecology* 129(3), 473–480. doi: 10.1097/AOG.0000000000001898. PMID: 28178059.

87. Lee L, Dy J, Azzam H. (2016 Sep) Management of spontaneous labour at term in healthy women. *Journal of Obstetrics and Gynaecology Canada* 38(9), 843–865. doi: 10.1016/j.jogc.2016.04.093. Epub 2016 Jun 25. PMID: 27670710.

Chapter 8

Prevention and Treatment of Prolonged Second Stage of Labor

Kathryn Osborne, PhD, CNM, FACNM, Lisa Hanson, PhD, CNM, FACNM, FAAN, and Emily Malloy, PhD, CNM

Simkin's Labor Progress Handbook: Early Interventions to Prevent and Treat Dystocia, Fifth Edition. Edited by Lisa Hanson, Emily Malloy, and Penny Simkin.
© 2024 John Wiley & Sons Ltd. Published 2024 by John Wiley & Sons Ltd.

8

DEFINITIONS OF THE SECOND STAGE OF LABOR

Anatomically, the second stage of labor begins with complete dilation of the cervix and ends with the birth of the baby. The clinical significance of complete dilation is controversial. There are two basic schools of thought regarding the conduct of the second stage. One, which is centered on the needs of the health care provider and has dominated North American and other areas where labor speeding is valued, obstetrics for decades. Using this approach, the birth giver is asked to commence maximal breath-holding and bearing-down (pushing) efforts when she is discovered to be fully dilated, regardless of whether she feels an urge to push. If the urge to push occurs before complete dilation, the birth giver is told to resist pushing by panting or blowing throughout each contraction. If the urge to push is not present when the birth giver is completely dilated, the desire for a speedy delivery may lead the caregiver to direct the birth giver to begin pushing with instructions to take in a deep breath—hold it, and push—while others in the room count; this is repeated several times for the duration of each contraction. Although commonly used, prolonged breathing holding, also known as Valsalva pushing, may have a deleterious effect on the birthing person and fetus. Therefore, in instances when directed pushing is desired to expedite delivery, the birthing person should be encouraged to limit breath holding to 6 seconds or less.[1]

A preferred approach with a stable birthing person and fetus is less hurried management, where complete dilatation alone is not sufficient reason to begin pushing. A physiologic approach to second stage labor care is based on the normal course of second stage and the recognition that contractions may decrease temporarily around the time of full dilation. As a result, not everyone who gives birth feels an urge to push immediately upon complete cervical dilation. Physiologic management has long been followed in Europe and much of the world, especially by midwives. Using this person-centered approach to second stage labor care often results in later onset and shorter duration of active pushing than occurs with the directive approach.

PHASES OF THE SECOND STAGE OF LABOR

Similar to the first stage of labor, the second stage of labor can be divided into two phases (the latent phase and the active phase). Each phase represents different maternal behaviors and different physiologic accomplishments.

The latent phase of the second stage

An apparent lull in uterine activity around the time of complete dilation has long been observed and is referred to as the "latent phase of the second stage," or the "resting phase," or "the lull."[2–4] There are no reports of the frequency with which a noticeable lull actually occurs, although it is a phenomenon widely recognized by health care providers and researchers. How and why it occurs are not fully understood, but experts have suggested that onset of the maternal urge to push may be related to the station and disposition of the fetal head.

During most of the first stage, the uterus is tightly wrapped around the fetus. Uterine contractions in the first stage not only dilate the cervix but also shorten the uterine muscle fibers, and these actions gradually reduce the intrauterine space and press the fetus down. The last 2 cm of dilation are accompanied by cervical retraction around the head (or presenting part) and the beginnings of descent of the head into the vaginal canal (Fig. 8.1).[5,6] Simkin[5] suggested that when the head (representing one-fourth of the contents of the uterus) slips through the cervix, the uterine muscle slackens because it is no longer tightly stretched around the entire fetus, and the intrauterine space must now shrink to "catch up" with the fetus. This "catching up" consists of shortening of the uterine muscle fibers (as happened gradually in the first stage), further reducing the intrauterine space until once again the uterine muscle is tightly wrapped around the fetal trunk.

This may take minutes or longer, during which the birth giver's contractions are weak or unnoticeable, allowing them time to rest. The contractions resume and the birth giver experiences an increasingly powerful urge to push, accompanied by a documented spurt in oxytocin release.[7,8,9] However, not all laboring people experience a noticeable lull or latent phase. Fetal position and station may be two of the factors that determine whether, when, and for how long the birth giver will experience a resting phase.

A slightly different hypothesis to explain the period of rest early in the second stage is offered by Roberts.[10] During the latent phase, contractions that are measurable with electronic monitoring continue, although they may be below the threshold of the birth giver's awareness. These cause fetal rotation, alignment, and descent. During

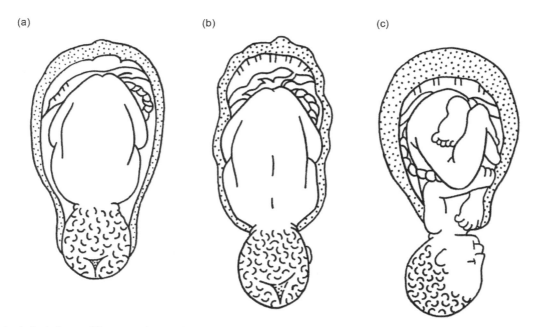

(a)   (b)   (c)

Fig. 8.1.   Latent phase of the second stage. Fetal head slips through the cervix, and uterine muscles slacken. Uterine muscle fibers shorten until the uterus is once again tightly wrapped around the fetal trunk. (**a**) Fetus in uterus at full dilation. (**b**) Head out of uterus which slackens. (**c**) Uterus shortened and thickened around fetal torso.

this time laboring people exhibit less pain and distress than earlier in labor because of the retraction of the cervix around the descending fetal head, as described by Friedman.[11] Birth givers begin to experience involuntary bearing-down efforts once the fetal head is at a +1 station and has rotated to occiput anterior and the contractions have achieved and maintained an intensity of 30 mm Hg. Therefore, the urge to push signals the "physiologic" onset of the second stage of labor.[10,12] Both of these hypotheses are consistent with our knowledge of uterine physiology in labor, with Friedman's classic observations of normal labor progress, and with the numerous observational studies of maternal spontaneous bearing-down efforts that document an increasing urge to push and greater spontaneous bearing-down efforts with time and descent of the presenting part.[13,14]

Evidence-based support during the latent phase of second stage labor

During the latent phase, when uterine activity is markedly reduced, the fetal heart tones usually remain reassuring. Although the exact duration of the latent phase of second stage labor varies, investigators have identified that with no interventions, powerful contractions accompanied by an urge to bear down usually resume within 15–45 minutes.[11] The latent phase of labor provides an opportunity to rest while the fetus descends spontaneously and the urge to bear down strengthens.[12]

Caregivers who believe that women need to be directed about when and how to push may misinterpret the latent phase to mean labor has slowed down and intervene to speed the second stage. Two interventions commonly used to hasten second stage are the use of directive pushing, where laboring people are instructed to hold their breath and push for long periods—often in the absence of adequate contractions or an urge to push, and initiating the administration of intravenous oxytocin (Pitocin) to augment uterine contractions. Although widely used to augment labor, oxytocin is not free from potential adverse effects, such as tetanic contractions and fetal intolerance of labor, leading to increased reliance on cesarean deliveries.[15,16]

In contrast, care providers who recognize the distinct phases of second stage labor use a person-centered physiologic approach, where birth givers are encouraged to push in response to the normal sensations, they experience in second stage.[17] These care providers are unlikely to provide direction about when and how to begin pushing. Instead, they wait for the birth giver to experience an urge to bear down and then support their spontaneous pushing efforts.[17] In an unanesthetized birth giver with an uncomplicated labor, an uncontrollable urge to push is usually the best indicator of when they should begin bearing down spontaneously.[18]

What if the latent phase of the second stage persists?

If the lull in uterine activity persists for more than 20 or 30 minutes, the clinician may continue monitoring and waiting or may initiate measures to bring on contractions and an urge to push. These measures may include a change in the birth giver's position to sitting upright (in bed or on the toilet), squatting, or walking; "trial" expulsive efforts (gentle grunting) by the birth giver; acupressure; and nipple stimulation. Given the many studies conducted of "laboring down" with epidurals, a delay in pushing until there is at minimum an urge to push, in caring for healthy laboring people without epidurals is a reasonable strategy.[18,19]

Birth attendants who honor this resting phase await evidence of an urge to push before checking the birth giver's cervix.[17] Rather than defining the onset of second stage as the moment a birth giver's cervix is fully dilated, this allows use of the two-fold definition of second stage: complete dilation plus spontaneous expulsive efforts. It may be necessary for birth attendants who promote spontaneous pushing to make their management plans clear to nursing staff in order to assure that long-standing patterns of directed pushing are not followed out of habit.

The active phase of the second stage

The active phase of the second stage is usually characterized by an involuntary urge to push and descent of the fetus. It is sometimes referred to as the "pelvic division" of labor,[11] the "press period,"[18] or the descent phase.[3] The forces that bring about delivery include the birth giver's contractions, their expulsive efforts, their body positions, and fetal efforts.

Archaeological evidence suggests that traditionally, birthing people in labor were active, powerful participants in birth. They gave birth in upright positions, standing and squatting as they pushed, likely in response to the physiologic urges they experienced.[20] It wasn't until childbirth moved from individual homes to the hospital that evidence (in artwork, early textbooks, and medical supplies) of birthing people in a passive role during childbirth, in supine positions and often unconscious began to emerge.[20,21] It is unclear when or why second stage labor management began to include what is referred to as directive pushing; commands for the birth giver in labor to take a deep breath and hold it to the count of ten. Some have theorized that it may have been introduced by early natural childbirth advocates as a way to hasten birth in order to avoid an instrumental (forceps) delivery or other interventions.[22] Despite concerns about the safety of directive pushing, first raised over half a century ago it is a commonly used practice that persists today in birth rooms across the United States and in other areas where efforts to hasten labor have become the norm.[7,22]

For the remainder of this chapter readers will see references to two distinct approaches to care during the second stage of labor. The directive approach includes commands from a care provider for a birth giver in labor, usually in supine positions, to take a deep breath and hold it while they push to the count of 10; these sustained pushes are repeated until the contraction ends. In contrast, care providers who use the spontaneous approach support a birth giver's actions and behavior in response to physiologic urges and sensations. This includes supporting spontaneous bearing down in response to an urge to push and encouraging the birth giver to move about the room, periodically changing positions to promote fetal descent and maternal comfort.

Physiologic effects of prolonged breath-holding and straining

Research regarding expulsive efforts (positions, breathing, bearing down) for second stage has resulted in differing opinions about how women should push and the role of clinical personnel in assisting the birth giver in the active phase of second stage labor. Prolonged breath-holding and straining, also known as closed-glottis pushing or the Valsalva maneuver, has multiple physiologic effects on the birth giver and the fetus. Moreover, this form of directive pushing may not result in a clinical significant shortening of the second stage of labor or duration of active bearing down.[14,23]

Effects on the birth giver

Prolonged breath-holding and straining lead to a closed pressure system in the birth giver's chest with increased intrathoracic and intra-abdominal pressure, which leads to the following chain of events in laboring people:

- decreases in venous return to the heart and increased venous pressure
- lower arterial blood pressure and increased heart rate
- a decrease in maternal blood oxygen levels and blood flow to the placenta
- an increase in carbon dioxide levels
- discontinued straining and gasp for air reverses physiologic changes that occurred with straining and results in bradycardia before blood pressure and heart rate return to base-line
- Lactic acidosis that may result in changes in fetal heart rate, newborn acidemia, and poor Apgar scores
- rapid distention of the vaginal canal and pelvic musculature, along with stretching of supportive ligaments, leading to perineal trauma and possible urinary stress incontinence
- exhaustion
- longer pushing time[18]

Effects on the fetus

Indeterminate fetal heart rate patterns may occur when the laboring people pushes using the Valsalva maneuver. The prolonged pressure caused by straining may increase fetal head compression. If such bearing-down efforts are combined with a dorsal position, supine hypotension may lead to more serious fetal heart rate patterns. The decreases in blood pressure, blood oxygen content, and placental blood flow cause a decrease in the oxygen available to the fetus (fetal hypoxia and acidosis).[24,25] These effects are generally well tolerated by a healthy, well-nourished term fetus but may distress the fetus who is pre-term, small for gestational age, previously compromised, or experiencing cord compression. Furthermore, directive pushing during second stage is not associated with better neonatal outcomes.[24,25]

Spontaneous expulsive efforts

Observational studies of laboring people's behavior in the second stage reveal that laboring people who push spontaneously, without direction, take more frequent breaths and bear down less during second stage contractions than those who are directed to use prolonged maximal bearing-down efforts.[9,12] Also, undirected laboring people change positions more frequently.[18] The undesirable side effects of directive pushing with the Valsalva maneuver in the supine position generally do not occur with spontaneous bearing down.

When supported to spontaneously bear down, most laboring people experience an involuntary urge to push that comes and goes several times during each contraction. Their spontaneous bearing-down efforts last approximately 5–7 seconds, with several breaths between bearing-down efforts.[15,18] As the second stage progresses and the fetus descends, spontaneous bearing-down efforts usually become more forceful and more frequent.[18] With support and encouragement, a number of positions (side-lying, semi-reclining, standing, a supported squat, hands and knees, kneeling on one or both knees, or squatting) can be used to facilitate comfort, bearing-down efforts, and progress.

The caregiver's role is different when the laboring people push spontaneously in physiologic positions than when they push with direction in a supine position. In the former, the caregiver encourages and praises the efforts and reassures the birth giver that their sensations are normal. The caregiver emphasizes the value of relaxing the perineum rather than breath-holding or pushing to a count of 10. Chart 8.1 illustrates the caregiver's step-by-step approach to bearing-down (pushing) efforts once dilation is complete.

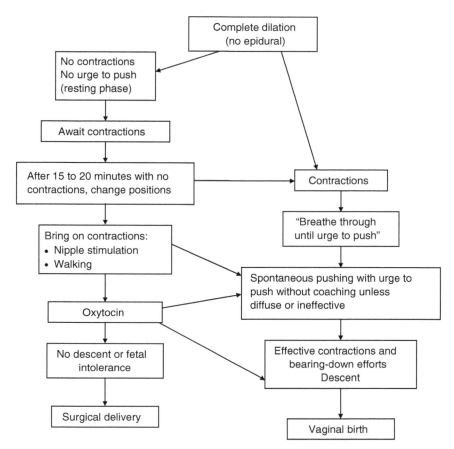

Chart 8.1. Spontaneous bearing down.

This approach has also been called "self-directed pushing," because the caregiver is helping the birth giver to direct their own bearing-down efforts. This type of direction, offered by birth care providers that promote spontaneous pushing, has been viewed as an intervention aimed at avoiding potential problems.[1,18] These simple measures often result in progress without fetal distress or serious perineal damage.

The support of spontaneous bearing down requires patience and presents a useful alternative to the ritualistic practice of counting to 10 with each push that has been done with women in labor for decades. Support of spontaneous bearing down offers a more physiologic approach. It is often tempting for providers to begin directing bearing down. If the caregiver believes they need to provide directions to push, they should remember that the fetus usually tolerates the second stage better when the birth giver holds their breath and strains for less than 6 seconds at a time.[10,24,26] If these measures are ineffective, consider emotional distress as a possible underlying cause.

Diffuse pushing

Sometimes the birth giver has an irresistible urge to bear down but their spontaneous pushing is unfocused, or "diffuse," and may result in little progress (Chart 8.2). It is almost as if all their effort has no single direction. Such diffuse pushing seems to occur when the birth giver's eyes are tightly closed, and there may be little or no apparent progress after 20 or 30 minutes. This may be a sign that conditions are not yet conducive to fetal descent.[10,18] For example, fetal malposition or compound presentation (hand by face) may be an underlying factor in diffuse pushing. If

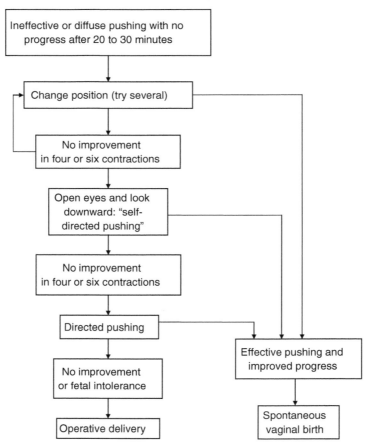

Chart 8.2.   Diffuse pushing without progress.

progress is made with diffuse pushing, there is no reason to intervene, unless the birth giver seems distressed. If there appears to be no progress or if the birth giver asks for more direction, caregivers may encourage position changes or a period of rest for a few contractions. These actions may provide time to rest as the urge to push builds. If not, encouraging the birth giver to open their eyes and direct their bearing-down efforts toward their vagina while they think about moving the baby down may help focus the bearing down efforts so that they are more effective. It may also help to remind them that the pushing efforts are moving the baby down and out of their body.

Second stage time limits

Second stage labor duration limits were proposed by the American College of Obstetricians and Gynecologists (ACOG) in 2003, but raised controversy because they were based on time, not progress of individual laboring women.[27,28] Zhang et al.[29] identified the upper limits of normal for second stage duration for women in spontaneous labor. The 95th percentile for second stage duration for nulliparous women with an epidural is 3.6 hours, and 2.8 hours without. For multiparas the 95th percentile is 1.6 with epidural, and 1.1 without. In 2012, ACOG and the Society for Maternal-Fetal Medicine (SMFM) collaborated in a workshop aimed at preventing first cesarean sections.[30] In the resulting publication, this workgroup adopted new more liberal guidelines defining second stage labor arrest. These guidelines are consistent with the Ottowa protocol described by Oppenheimer and Black.[28] In 2014, ACOG and the SMFM[31] published a consensus statement that was consistent with these findings and recommendations.[28,30]

The Ottowa protocol (presented in Table 8.1) helps translate contemporary evidence and recommendations into practice, including the recognition that the acceptable duration of second stage labor is longer than previously understood for women with and without an epidural.[1] Until recently this protocol was consistent with the recommendations of ACOG with regard to the period of rest allowed at the onset of second stage labor. However, in 2019 ACOG published an updated Committee Opinion on Approaches to Limit Interventions During Labor and Birth.[32] While the opinion included recommendations for many of the practices used to support spontaneous second stage described in this handbook, the authors modified the previously held position on delayed pushing for nulliparous women giving birth under epidural anesthesia. This decision appears to have been made based on the findings of a single randomized controlled trial that found an increased risk for chorioamnionitis, postpartum hemorrhage, and neonatal acidemia in nulliparous women with epidural anesthesia who were allowed to delay pushing for 60 minutes. The committee's revised opinion is that nulliparous women with epidural anesthesia should begin pushing at the start of the second stage of labor; the risks of delayed pushing should be shared with those who request to use that approach.[32]

Table 8.1. The Ottawa Hospital Second Stage Protocol.

	Recommended Care Approach				Recommended maximum SSL duration
	1st hour	**2nd hour**	**3rd hour**	**4th hour**	
Primigravida, epidural	Labor down	Labor down	Labor down/support spontaneous pushing*	Support spontaneous pushing	4 hours
Primigravida, no epidural	Labor down	Labor down	Support spontaneous pushing		3 hours
Multigravida, epidural	Labor down	Labor down	Support spontaneous pushing		3 hours
Multigravida without epidural	Labor down	Labor down			2 hours

*A third hour of waiting may be appropriate in the presence of continued progress during latent second stage labor (SSL).
Source: Adapted from Osborne and Hansen (2012); Openheimer and Black (2013).[17,33]

8

More recently, a systematic review and meta-analysis of randomized controlled trials found that when compared to immediate pushing, delayed pushing resulted in a slightly longer second stage of labor but a shorter duration of total time pushing.[19] Researchers also found a significant improvement in maternal fatigue scores and no adverse maternal or fetal outcomes with delayed pushing.[19] It appears as though questions and controversy about when and how to push during second stage labor are likely to continue. Shared decision-making offers an opportunity for patients and practitioners to discuss the risks and benefits of options for care during labor and birth. Using this process, the care provider reviews the risks and benefits of all available options. Decision-making about how to proceed is shared between the birth giver in labor and the care provider, taking into consideration all available evidence about the options as well as the birth giver's preferences and beliefs. Most researchers did not specify the approach by pushing and/or positioning used with study participants. Therefore it is possible these outcomes are the result supine positions and/or directed pushing rather than delayed bearing down and longer second stage duration.

There is evidence that allowing a longer duration for second stage in women with an epidural improves the likelihood of a spontaneous delivery without risking the wellbeing of the neonate. As long as the fetus and birth giver are tolerating second stage labor well, many caregivers see no clinical indication to intervene, even if rotation and descent are slow.[1,18,33] In addition, changing maternal positions every 20–30 minutes often improves progress. Figure 8.2 illustrates pushing positions that may be used by women with epidural anesthesia, depending on the density of the block.

POSSIBLE CAUSES AND PHYSIOLOGIC SOLUTIONS FOR SECOND STAGE DYSTOCIA

The challenge for caregivers during a long second stage is to identify reasons for the slow progress and institute appropriate corrective measures. The choice of early interventions depends, to an extent, on the presumed etiology, although a trial-and-error approach is sometimes warranted.

Position changes and other strategies for suspected occiput posterior or persistent occiput transverse fetuses

The optimal position for fetal descent occurs when the fetal head is in the occiput anterior position. Although the fetal head is capable of navigating the pelvis in other positions, the occiput posterior (OP) and occiput transverse (OT) positions may cause increased discomfort and a delay in progress during second stage labor. Figure 8.3 illustrates abdominal and vaginal views of the occiput posterior (OP) and occiput transverse (OT) positions. Changing the position of the birth giver in labor can result in rotation and descent of the fetal head. As long as the birth giver is well supported and she has no musculoskeletal or medical problems and the fetus is monitored, a wide variety of positions may be used to promote rotation and descent.

The use of supine positions

Supine positions are routinely used during the second stage in the United States and throughout the world. This is based on comfort of the birth attendant rather than the preference of the birthing person.[34] Supine positions do not take advantage of gravity and movement to facilitate the birth.[35] We do not recommend the routine use of supine positions for laboring people.

Why not the supine position?

Supine positions tend to exacerbate fetal malposition and deny the effects of gravity. In some specific situations, however, the advantages of exaggerated lithotomy may outweigh the risks. For most laboring people, the positions shown in Fig. 8.4 are more effective in promoting fetal rotation and descent and may be more comfortable for the birth giver than supine positions. Changing positions every 20 minutes (every five or six contractions) when progress is slow may help solve the problem. Even if the fetus cannot be rotated, these same measures may make a vaginal birth possible in a persistent OP or OT position.

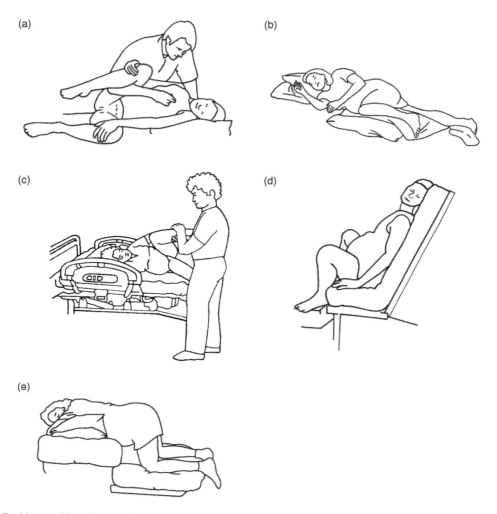

Fig. 8.2. Pushing positions that may be used with epidural anesthesia. (**a**) Side-lying. (**b**) Semiprone. (**c**) Semiprone lunge. (**d**) Semisitting. (**e**) Kneeling on foot of bed.

The effects of gravity in promoting descent are lost with supine or any recumbent positions as seen in the comparison of Figs. 8.4a and 8.4b. In addition, supine hypotension is caused by the weight of the uterus on the inferior vena cava and aorta, which leads to a reduction in venous return and cardiac output. Subsequently, the fetus may experience hypoxia due to the concomitant decrease in blood flow to the placenta and resulting reduction in oxygen supply to the fetus, especially if combined with prolonged breath-holding and maximal straining.[18] Besides supine hypotension, the weight of the uterus along the spinal column reduces the angle of the uterus with the spine, resulting in poor alignment of the fetus with the pelvis (Fig. 6.36a).[34,36] Use of the supine position is also associated with increased risk of severe perineal injury.[37]

With persistent OP, persistent asynclitism, or other malpositions, the birth giver should be encouraged to push in nonsupine positions. It is ironic that two widely prescribed practices for second stage—prolonged breath-holding with straining, and the supine position—are at least partly responsible for the frequently observed fetal

(a)   (c)

(b)   (d)

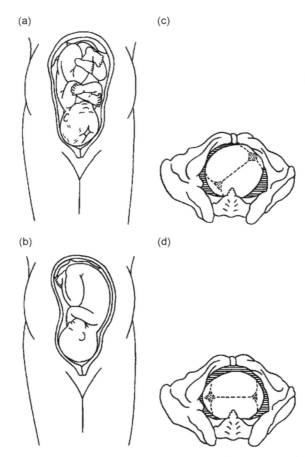

Fig. 8.3.   (**a**) Right occiput posterior fetus, abdominal view. (**b**) Left occiput transverse fetus, abdominal view. (**c**) Right occiput posterior, fetus in synclitism, vaginal view. (**d**) Left occiput transverse fetus, vaginal view.

bradycardias and prolonged second stage that have led caregivers to believe that the duration of the second stage must be curtailed. The further irony is that if laboring people were encouraged to behave instinctually, they would rarely lie on their backs, nor would they use prolonged breath-holding and straining.[38] Last, the long-term pelvic floor damage, widely attributed to vaginal birth, is likely to be largely caused by these two entrenched practices and the widespread use of episiotomy.[18,39] Misguided efforts to improve birth outcomes have not only made outcomes worse, but the harmful practices have been extremely difficult to change, so the problems persist.

Use of the exaggerated lithotomy (McRobert's) position

Although lithotomy and other supine positions are not recommended as a routine, midwives reported using the lithotomy position with birthing people only rarely (<1% of the time) and as an intervention.[40,41] The most common example of this is the exaggerated lithotomy (McRoberts') position. Use of exaggerated lithotomy may succeed in promoting descent when other positions do not. It can be useful when the birth giver has been unable to bring the fetus beneath the pubic symphysis in any other position. To achieve this position, the birth giver lies flat on their back with their knees drawn back (by themselves or others) so that their buttocks are lifted slightly off

(a)

(b)

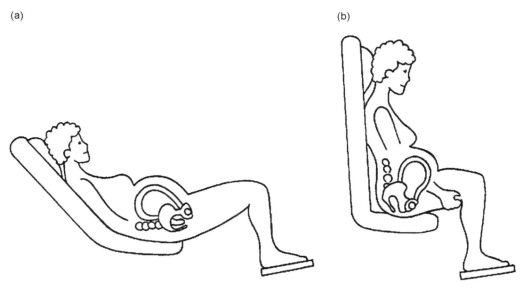

Fig. 8.4. Drive angle. (**a**) Supine. (**b**) Sitting upright. Adapted from Fenwick L., Simkin P.[39] Position to prevent or alleviate dystocia in labor.

(a)

(b)

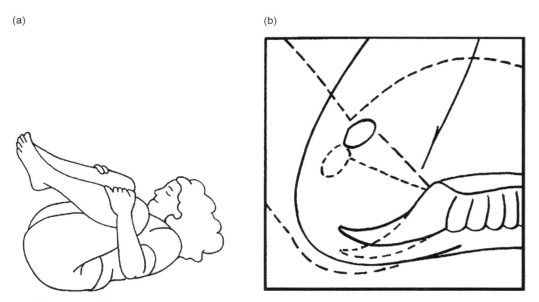

Fig. 8.5. (**a**) Exaggerated lithotomy position. (**b**) Exaggerated lithotomy (detail). Dotted line shows pelvic position when the birth giver's feet are on the bed; solid line, when the birth giver's legs are drawn up.

the bed and hips very flexed, in an abducted position (Fig. 8.5). This position passively rotates the pubic arch upward toward the birth giver's head and brings the pelvic inlet perpendicular to the maximum expulsive force.[42,43]

The exaggerated lithotomy position, combined with bearing down efforts, may facilitate the passage of the fetal head beneath the pubic arch. With a persistent delay in descent, this benefit may outweigh the disadvantages of supine hypotension and loss of any gravity advantage. A note of caution: Those who are supporting the birth giver's legs in the exaggerated lithotomy position must exercise particular caution not to pull their legs into extreme abduction and/or flexion. This can cause damage to the pubic symphysis, sacroiliac joints, or hip joints and may cause nerve damage.[44] The use of the exaggerated lithotomy position (or the McRoberts' position) with women who have epidurals can lead to lumbar-sacral nerve injury[44] and therefore is not recommended. Moreover, due to the risk of supine hypotension, the use of exaggerated lithotomy for more than a few contractions is not recommended.

Differentiating between pushing positions and birth positions

As shown in Fig. 8.6, some positions used to enhance progress might be awkward or impractical for caregivers during the actual birth. It may help to think of these as "pushing positions" and to distinguish them from "birth positions." Midwives readily distinguished the two[40] and reported that their patients used several positions for both pushing and birth. The birth giver may use a variety of pushing positions to bring the baby down, then when the birth is imminent, assume a position that allows the attendant to see adequately, support the perineum, and "catch" the baby without awkwardness or back strain.

Sitting and semi-sitting

Sitting and semisitting positions take advantage of gravity and allow the birth giver to see and interact with the birth attendant. Sitting and semisitting do not require physical excursion and therefore may be useful for those laboring with an epidural or who are fatigued. During pushing, caregivers gently holding one or more legs, may facilitate progress. Relaxed legs for crowning and birth create less tension on the perineum and may diminish lacerations.

Positions to Improve [or promote] Sacral Mobility

When laboring people assume the sitting position the sacrum becomes less mobile or may move anteriorly, thereby reducing the pelvic outlet. As second stage progresses, creating more space in the outlet is optimal to faciliate fetal head crowning and birth. Sacrum flexible positions include positions where the sacrum can move freely (e.g. side-lying, standing, kneeling, hands and knees, and squatting). Berta and colleagues[45] conducted a systematic review on birth positions and second stage labor duration (P<000). The researcher found that sacrum flexible positions significantly reduced second stage [21 minutes(CI:11.839-30.396;).

Knees together pushing

Recently, Tully and others have suggested the use of knees together pushing (Figure 8.7). The laboring person puts knees together and heels apart. Suggested uses are for early second stage or situations where progress has stalled. Knees together pushing appears to increase the distance between the ischial tuberosities, thereby enlarging the pelvic outlet.

Leaning forward while kneeling, standing, or sitting

These positions (see Fig. 8.6(a–f)) take advantage of gravity to encourage rotation of the fetal trunk from posterior to anterior. Back pain, common with OP, is also relieved because the pressure of the fetal head on the sacrum is relieved.

Squatting positions

Squatting positions use weight-bearing with hip abduction to widen the pelvic outlet, which may enlarge the space in the pelvic basin enough to promote rotation and descent (Fig. 8.8).

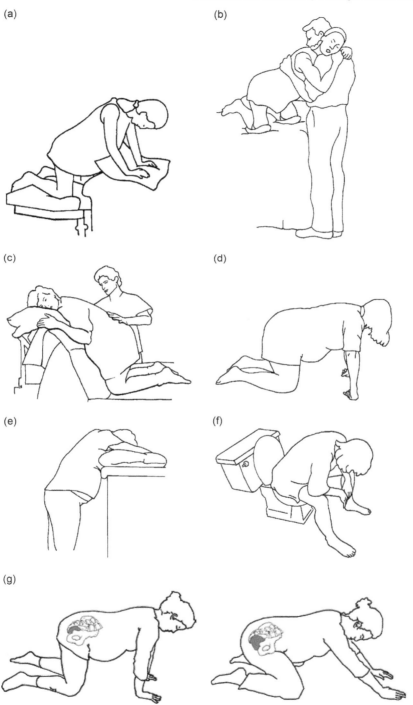

Fig. 8.6. Pushing positions to promote rotation and descent. (**a**) Kneeling on foot of bed. (**b**) Kneeling on partner to push. (**c**) Kneeling, leaning on the raised head of the bed. (**d**) Hands and knees. (**e**) Standing, leaning on counter. (**f**) Sitting forward on toilet. (**g**) Flexion and rocking on hands and knees. Starting position (left), hips and knees fully flexed (right).

(a)   (b)

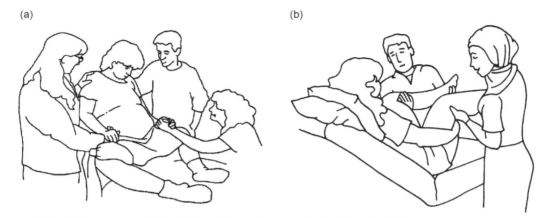

Fig. 8.7. (**a**) Semisitting to push. (**b**) Semisitting with people supporting the birth giver's legs.

(a)   (b)   (c)

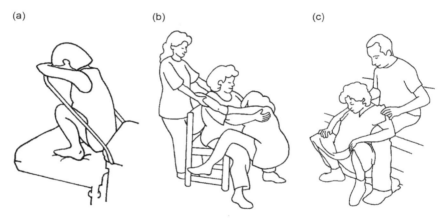

Fig. 8.8. (**a**) Squatting with bar. (**b**) Lap squatting. (**c**) Squatting, supported by seated partner's legs.

Asymmetrical positions

In asymmetrical positions (Figures 8.9), the birth giver's legs are in different positions (e.g., one knee up and one knee down). This changes the shape of the pelvis in ways that are different from "symmetrical" positions such as squatting, and hands and knees. The pelvic joints on one side of the pelvis widen more than the joints on the other side. Sometimes the fetus is more likely to rotate with asymmetrical positions. If the fetal position is known with a degree of certainty, then the birth giver should be in a position to widen the side of their pelvis toward which the occiput is directed. If the position is uncertain, the birth giver should alternate knees, raising one during several contractions and then the other. If raising one knee clearly feels better than the other, we think it makes sense for them to remain longer on that side. Our rationale, supported by clinical experience, is that when the birth giver's position provides space for the fetus to rotate or descend, the birth giver is likely to feel less pain. This is an area where further study would be useful.

(a)   (b)

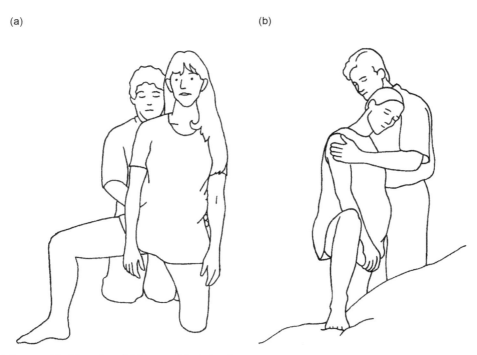

Fig. 8.9. (**a**) Asymmetrical kneeling. (**b**) Asymmetrical standing.

Lateral positions

For the birth giver who is exhausted or restricted to bed, side-lying (Fig. 8.10a) and the semiprone (side-lying runner's lunge, Fig. 8.10b) positions are good alternatives to the dorsal or semisitting positions. If the fetus is known with some certainty to be OP, the birth giver should lie on the same side as the posterior occiput if side-lying, and the side opposite the posterior or transverse occiput if in semiprone (exaggerated runner's lunge) (Fig. 8.10b).

If the fetal position is uncertain then it is best to alternate between the two sides on a trial-and-error basis, since theoretically, at least, remaining for a long duration in what might be the "wrong" position could do more harm than good.

Supported squat or "dangle" positions

In a "dangle position," the birth giver is supported under their arms, with minimal or no weight-bearing by their legs or feet (Fig. 8.11). These unique positions are the only ones in which the birth giver is supported from their upper body. We propose the following mechanisms to explain how the dangle positions enhance the fetal position.

The birth giver's own body weight lengthens their trunk by providing traction to their spinal column. This provides more vertical space for the fetus to maneuver. Most second-stage positions require that the birth giver flex their trunk and neck, to add pressure to the fundus and promote descent of the fetus.

However, this added pressure may not help if the head will not fit because it is asynclitic or deflexed. The dangle positions offer room for the head to reposition itself.

Furthermore, the dangle positions are free from external pressures on the pelvis, such as those that occur when the birth giver is sitting or lying down, or when their joints are stretched (e.g., when squatting or with legs pulled back). An absence of such external pressures, in cases where the fetal head appears to be "stuck," may allow the pressure from the descending fetal head (and, presumably, fetal head movements) to change the shape of the pelvic basin as needed for the fetus to find the path of least resistance through the pelvis.

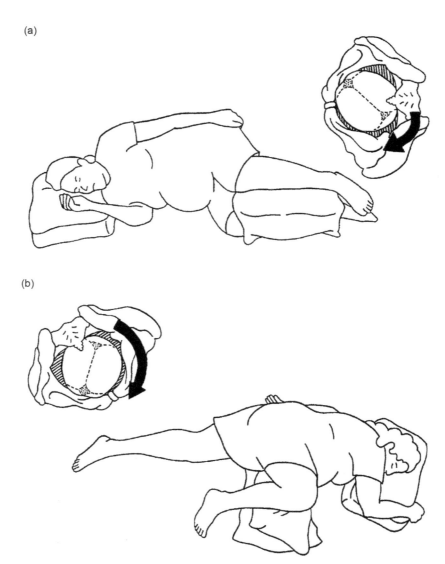

Fig. 8.10. (**a**) Pregnant person with suspected or known occiput posterior (OP) fetus in pure side-lying on the "correct side" with fetal back "toward the bed". If the fetus is Right Occiput Posterior (ROP), the person lies on their right side. Gravity pulls the fetal occiput and the trunk towards the right occiput transverse (ROT) position. (**b**) Pregnant person with suspected or known occiput posterior (OP) semiprone on the "correct side," with fetal back "toward the ceiling." If fetus is ROP, the semiprone person lies on their left side. Gravity pulls fetal occiput and trunk towards the ROT, then right occiput anterior (ROA). If position is uncertain, laboring people should alternate sides after a few contractions.

Other strategies for malposition and back pain

The pelvic press may help in cases of deep transverse arrest, occiput posterior, or a "tight fit" in the second stage, to increase mid-pelvic and outlet dimensions and make room for fetal rotation and descent.[46] Please note that the pelvic press is not the same as the "double hip squeeze" (Table 8.2 and Fig. 8.10). The main difference between

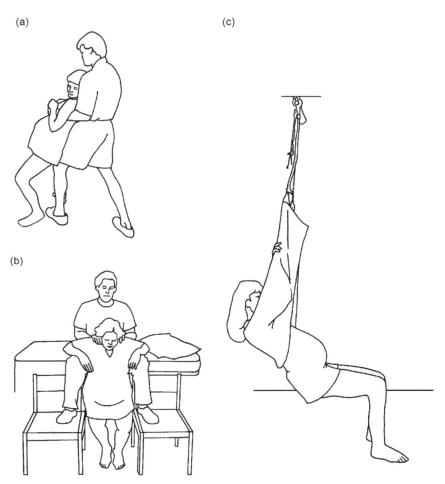

Fig. 8.11. Positions in which the birth giver is supported from their upper body. (**a**) Supported squat. (**b**) Dangle. (**c**) Dangle with birth sling.

the two is the placement of the hands. In the pelvic press (Fig. 8.12), the helper's hands are placed on the iliac crests; in the double hip squeeze, they are placed lower over the gluteal muscles on the buttocks (Fig. 8.13). The pelvic press is used to enlarge the pelvic outlet in the second stage; the double hip squeeze is used to relieve back pain at any time in labor.

In addition to assisting with fetal positioning, a variety of positions can also ease discomfort. Some fetal positions, including OP or OT, asynclitism, nuchal hand or hands and some spinal or pelvic variations are accompanied by severe back pain. Measures to relieve this pain should be used as needed (Figs. 8.15 through 8.24). If the back pain remains tolerable, the birth giver may be more willing and able to endure contractions while awaiting fetal repositioning and descent.

Table 8.2.   Difference between pelvic press and the double hip squeeze.

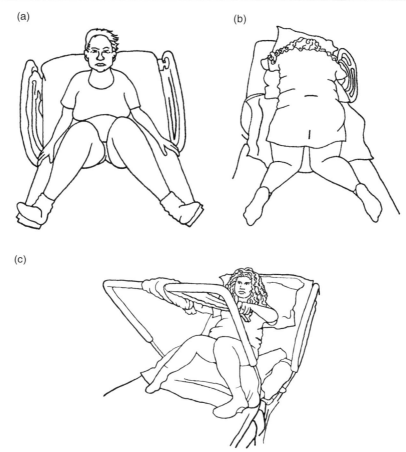

(a)

(b)

(c)

Fig. 8.12.   (**a**) Closed knee pushing. (**b**) Closed knee pushing in hands and knees. (**c**) Closed knee pushing/tug of war.

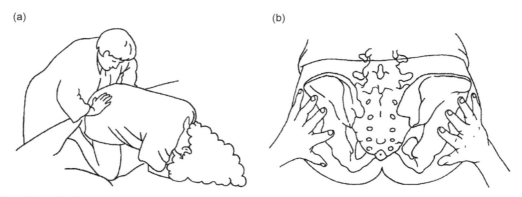

(a)

(b)

Fig. 8.13.   (**a**) Double hip squeeze. (**b**) Double hip squeeze (detail, seen from rear; a comfort measure for back pain).

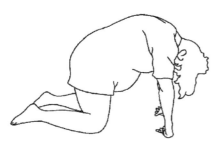

Fig. 8.14. Pelvic rocking, back rounded in flexion.

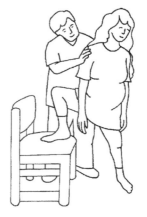

Fig. 8.15. Standing lunge.

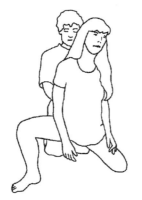

Fig. 8.16. Kneeling lunge.

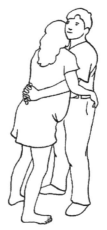

Fig. 8.17. Slow dancing.

(a)   (b)

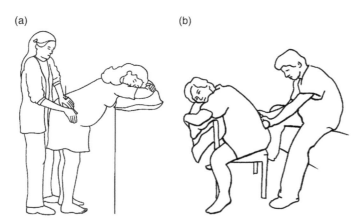

Fig. 8.18. (**a**) Counterpressure. (**b**) Counterpressure with tennis balls.

8

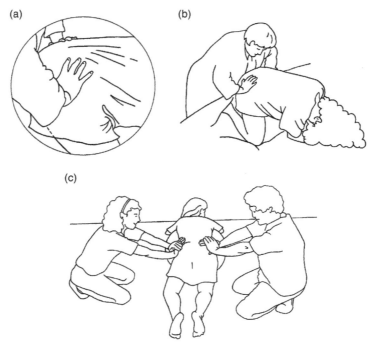

Fig. 8.19   More strategies for malposition and back pain. (**a**) Detail of double hip squeeze. (**b**) Double hip squeeze. (**c**) Double hip squeeze with two support people.

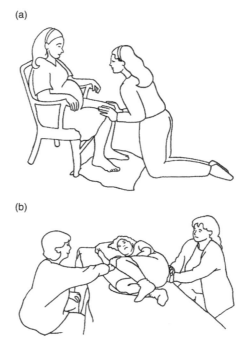

Fig. 8.20.   (**a**) Knee press, laboring person seated. (**b**) Knee press, laboring person on their side.

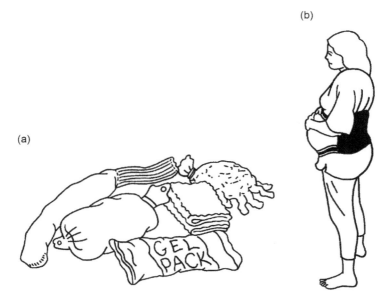

Fig. 8.21. (**a**) Objects for heat and cold. (**b**) Strap-on cold pack.

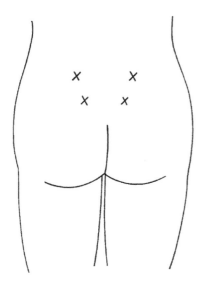

Fig. 8.22. Intradermal sterile water injection sites for back pain.

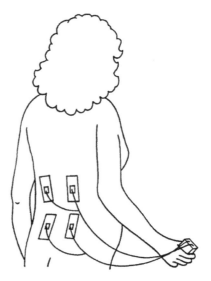

Fig. 8.23. Transcutaneous nerve stimulation (TENS) in use.

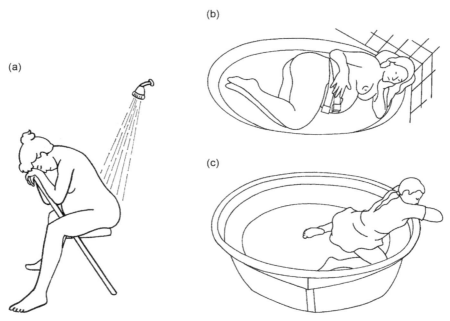

Fig. 8.24.   Hydrotherapy for back pain. (**a**) Shower on laboring persons back. (**b**) Side-lying in bath. (**c**) Kneeling, leaning forward in birthing pool.

Early interventions for suspected persistent asynclitism

Normally, at the onset of labor the fetal head is asynclitic (angled so that one parietal bone—located above the ear—is presenting), which facilitates entry of the head into the pelvic basin. This usually resolves spontaneously to synclitism as the fetus moves lower in the pelvis. Figs. 8.25 and 8.26 show vaginal views of asynclitic and synclitic fetuses in OA, OP, and OT positions. However, persistent asynclitism in the second stage may interfere with flexion, rotation, molding, and descent of the fetal head. A caput (swelling of soft tissue) often forms over one parietal bone.

Extra time, a variety of measures to alter the space within the pelvis, and some specific movements are thought to encourage the fetus to shift into a more synclitic position. Chart 8.3 provides an overview of measures to help in cases of occiput posterior and asynclitism in second stage. If the caregiver suspects persistent asynclitism, changing the birth giver's position may assist labor progress in three ways:

1. Shifting the birth giver may shift the fetus's weight so its position resolves.
2. Changing the birth giver's position may alter the shape of their pelvis slightly, allowing more room for the angle of the fetal head to shift.
3. Having the birth giver take a position that elongates the torso and relieves pressure on the pelvis (i.e., the dangle .and supported squat) may give the fetus room enough to "wiggle" out of asynclitism or mold the pelvis for a better fit.

Positions and movements for persistent asynclitism in second stage

In general, the same positions and movements that relieve back pain and are used for "suspected malposition, cephalopelvic disproportion, or macrosomia," for persistent OP/OT are also useful when the fetus seems to be in a persistent asynclitic position. Specifically, pelvic press and the dangle and supported squat positions may be especially helpful when the fetus is thought to be asynclitic during the second stage. Success with these positions

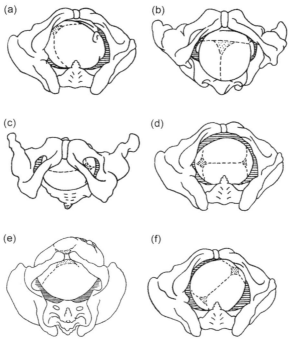

Fig. 8.25. (**a**) Asynclitic fetus in OA. (**b**) OA fetus in synclitisim. (**c**) Asynclitic fetus in OT. (**d**) OT in synlitism. (**e**) Asynclitic fetus in right occiput posterior. (**f**) ROP in synclitism.

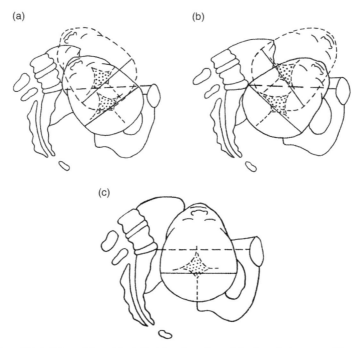

Fig. 8.26. (**a**) Posterior asynclitism (fetus pictured in dotted lines) and persistent posterior asynclitism which indicates that the fetus is at a low station and asynclitism (fetus pictured in solid lines). (**b**) Anterior asynclitism (fetus pictured in dotted lines) and persistent asynclitism (fetus pictured in solid lines). (**c**) Synclitism at a low station.

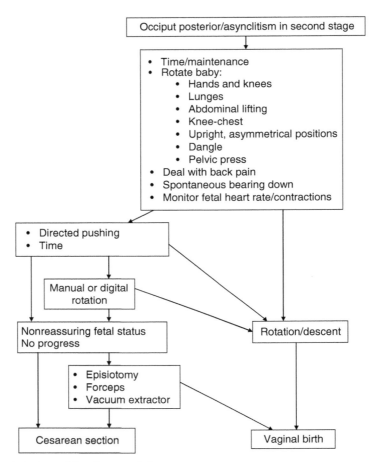

Chart 8.3. Occiput posterior/asynclitism in second stage.

is influenced by the degree of engagement of the fetal head and the fit between the fetal head and the birth giver's pelvis. These techniques merit further study, since the advantages ascribed to them are theoretical and observational.[47]

Nuchal hand or hands at vertex delivery

A search of the obstetric and midwifery literature on nuchal hands (i.e., one or both of the baby's hands at the baby's neck or face) at birth retrieved only scanty anecdotal advice, yet a nuchal hand is a well-known and troublesome deterrent to spontaneous vaginal birth (Fig. 8.27). Anecdotally, birthing people's descriptions of their experience with a "hand-by-face" delivery (as seen on social media) include a common theme of difficult, painful births, and perineal lacerations. The authors have observed that some birthing people who have intractable unrelenting back pain during labor give birth to babies with one or both nuchal hands tucked beneath their chins or alongside their heads. Yet this situation is not easily diagnosed during labor. Therefore, the same measures used for other conditions causing back pain and slow progress should also be used when a nuchal hand is suspected. During birth, the midwife or physician supports the hand against the head and gently allows spontaneous birth of both.

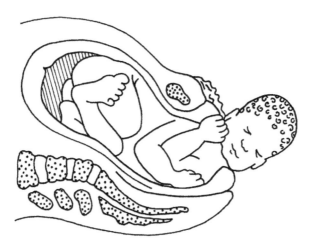

Fig. 8.27   Fetus emerging with a nuchal hand ("hand by face"). (Adapted from Fuchs et al. 1991.)

If cephalopelvic disproportion or macrosomia ("poor fit") is suspected

A variety of factors may contribute to a slow second stage and create doubt regarding whether the baby will fit through the birth giver's pelvis. These factors include the size and shape of the fetal head, the size and shape of the birth giver's pelvis, the position of the fetus, the strength and frequency of contractions, and the birth giver's ability to move around during labor.

Note: Ultrasound measurements of fetal weight and head size are not always reliable. For babies weighing over 4000 g (8 lb 13 oz), ultrasound estimates can vary by up to 10% (almost a pound) or more in either direction. Furthermore, even accurate estimates of fetal head size and weight do not predict the capacity of the fetal head or the pelvis to mold to accommodate safe passage of the fetus.[48,49]

The influence of time on cephalopelvic disproportion

Many suspected cases of cephalopelvic disproportion actually involve fetuses who are subtly malpositioned (asynclitic, deflexed, occiput transverse, or posterior), but who will fit well through the pelvis once the malposition has been resolved. The shape of the birth giver's pelvis also contributes to fetal rotation and descent. The birth giver may need to try pushing in a variety of positions to find the ones that optimize descent. Resolving problems of position or fit often requires extra time.

Many large fetal heads will mold and fit safely through the pelvis, but molding takes time. When heart tones are reassuring and the birth giver's condition is good, time can be an ally, not an enemy, in allowing labor progress to take place.

Fetal head descent

Some birth attendants have strict expectations for an acceptable rate of progress in descent, yet guidelines for normal descent had previously been elusive. Fetal descent has been defined by abnormalities rather than normal or expected progress.[1,50] The results of a retrospective cohort study including 4618 women, serve to inform an improved understanding of the parameter of normal fetal descent in a contemporary population who delivered vaginally.[46] Fetal descent was measured by vaginal exam, most often performed by resident physicians. The researchers found that each centimeter of descent took less than 2 hours, with significant differences in the time to descend one centimeter for nulliparas versus multiparas.[46] Among nulliparas and multiparas the rate of descent increased as labor progressed. At complete dilation, the fetal head station for both primiparas and multiparas was +2, with a range of 0 to +3.[46] More research on normal fetal descent is needed, particularly in those experiencing spontaneous labor.

If fetal descent does not continue, interventions such as amniotomy, oxytocin, episiotomy, forceps, vacuum extraction, or cesarean delivery may be indicated. This is another time when shared decision-making may be used to determine whether or not (or how) to intervene, as long as the fetus appears to be doing well and the birth giver is willing and able to continue. Reviewing the risks and benefits of all available options allows the birth attendant and the birth giver in labor to individualize the care and together, determine the best approach for a specific situation.

Verbal support of spontaneous bearing-down efforts

In 2018 the World Health Organization (WHO) published a statement recommending that birthing people be supported to push according to their own urges. The most appropriate verbal support for the birthing person who is bearing down spontaneously is to offer words of approval and encouragement, along with reminders to relax the legs and perineum. Verbal support and encouragement done in a natural speaking voice can replace the use of outdated, loud directions to "count to 10" that are still heard in many birth rooms today.[51]

Examples of supportive phrases include:

"Listen to your body. Your body knows what to do."
"That's the way; just like that. There is plenty of room for this baby."
"Your perineum is starting to stretch. That's a very good sign."
"Good job."
"I can see the head."
"Would you like to feel your baby's head?"
"You are moving your baby with every push."
"Let yourself rest between contractions. Good."
"That burning you feel is normal. It's your body telling you that the stretching is happening. Feel free to ease off a bit on the push until it starts to go away."

Guiding the birthing person through crowning of the fetal head

In a study of second stage care practices, midwives reported being supportive of spontaneous bearing down, but indicated that they often or always provided more direction as the fetal head emerges to foster perineal integrity.[17] It is recommended that the birth attendants guide the birthing person through intense sensations of burning and stretching. Slow delivery of the fetal head over the perineum allows perineal tissues to stretch more gradually.[18] Instead of using prolonged, closed glottis pushing, many midwives encourage the birthing person to "breathe" the head out as it crowns. Others prefer to deliver the fetal head between contractions.

These approaches require the caregiver to give specific directions to avoid pushing during contractions when the head is crowning. It is important that the birthing person not hear a variety of voices giving conflicting instructions. For this reason, it is helpful when all personnel are familiar with spontaneous bearing down and ways to provide appropriate verbal support, as described earlier. If other people are speaking, they should provide quiet, unobtrusive encouragement. If the birthing person appears distracted, the nurse or doula may say quietly in their ear, "Listen to your midwife or physician. They will guide you through this part." The midwife or physician can speak to everyone in the room at the same time in a calm, assertive voice, using statements like: "Everything is going well. Both the person and baby are doing fine. There is no need to rush. I need [the birthing person's name] to hear my voice as I guide them through this part of the process. There is no need to count or tell them how to push. They know how to give birth and are doing that beautifully."

Hand skills to protect the perineum

Methods of managing the delivery of the fetal head appear to impact perineal outcomes. However, this is not well addressed in the current scientific literature. Midwives use a variety of techniques to direct the head as it emerges and vary approaches to meet birthing person's individual needs. If the fetal head is emerging rapidly, gentle counterpressure can be used to slow the birth and protect the perineum from damage. For example, pressure with three fingers on the vertex can offer both support and control. Some midwives gently squeeze the perineum to avoid sudden overstretching of the delicate tissues. The gentle use of a gloved hand can offer mild counterpressure on the tissues of the perineum while allowing visualization of crowning.

If the fetus is in an OA position, the midwife or physician may give downward pressure to keep the fetal head flexed. If the fetus is in an OP position, upward pressure is used to maintain flexion. However, the use of this manual flexion technique has been criticized because it counters the extension mechanism of labor that is essential for the fetus to negotiate the curve of the birth canal. More research is needed in this area.

Huang and colleagues conducted a systematic review and meta-analysis of "hands-on" to "hands-poised/off" approaches to protect the perineum during birth.[52] Hands-on is when the midwife maintained flexion during crowning, while simultaneously supporting the perineum (Fig. 8.28), and then used lateral flexion to deliberately and gently deliver the fetal shoulders. Hands-poised/off care was operationally defined as keeping hands near the perineum (in case of a rapid birth) but otherwise not touching the head or the perineum, and allowing the shoulders to deliver spontaneously. A total of nine RCTs (7112 participants) and eight non-RCTs (37,786 participants) were included with no difference in perineal tearing, second stage duration, or postpartum hemorrhage in the RCT group and among the non-RCTs less incidence of second degree perineal tears in the hands-poised/off group.[52]

Albers and colleagues[57] studied three techniques commonly used to reduce perineal damage, including:

- Applying warm compresses continuously to the perineum.
- Gently massaging the perineum with lubricated fingers in the vagina using gentle side-to-side motions and downward pressure.
- Using a "hands-off" approach until the fetal head crowns.

Albers et al.[53] found no difference in perineal outcomes between groups . A systematic review of eight randomized controlled trials of perineal management was conducted to determine the effectiveness of various approaches to perineal management in relationship to perineal outcomes.[54] The use of warm compresses and perineal massage versus hands-off was associated with significantly fewer third- and fourth-degree lacerations. However, the hands poised/off approach was significantly associated with a reduced rate of episiotomy.[54] A study

(a)   (b)

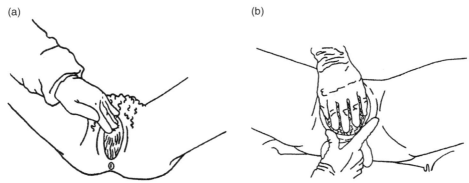

Fig. 8.28. Supported crowning.

by Edqvist and colleagues[55] showed that midwifery management of the second stage of labor using the following three techniques was protective against second degree lacerations:

- encourage spontaneous pushing by the birthing person,
- encourage positions with flexibility in the sacroiliac joints such as hands and knees, kneeling, and standing,
- use a two-step delivery technique (described below) in which the fetal head is born with one contraction and the shoulders and body are born with the next contraction.

Perineal management during second stage

Midwives and other low-intervention birth attendants favor strategies that minimize perineal damage including perineal massage, warm or cool compresses, hands-off or hands-on, and other techniques to reduce perineal trauma.[54] Scientific evidence does not support the routine use of episiotomy.[56] Additionally, support of spontaneous bearing down, rather than prolonged forceful Valsalva pushing, sometimes called "purple pushing" encourages the pregnant person to bear down with their own urges.[23] Spontaneous bearing-down efforts are associated with improved perineal[23] and fetal outcomes compared to outcomes of directed Valsalva bearing down.[18]

Topical anesthetic applied to the perineum

Lidocaine gel, a topical anesthetic, has been studied and found to be safe and effective for perineal pain management during second stage labor.[57] When a laboring person experiences excessive burning that is disruptive to spontaneous pushing efforts and warm compresses do not seem to help, the birth attendant can apply the gel to the internal and external tissues of the outer vagina and perineum. Studies of the use of lidocaine gel indicate that it is safe for both birth giver and fetus.[57] Similar topical anesthetics can be used to supplement injectable anesthetics administered after birth if perineal suturing is needed.

Intrapartum perineal massage

Birth attendants can perform perineal massage during second stage labor by using gloved hand and water-soluble lubricant. The index or middle finger is used to gently massage the perineal tissues between contractions. Perineal massage during contractions should be used with caution as it may add to discomfort and edema. The comfort of the birth giver should guide the use of perineal massage. Intrapartum perineal massage has been shown to significantly reduce the risk of severe perineal trauma (third and fourth degree lacerations).[58]

The term "perineal massage" during labor has sometimes been incorrectly used to describe other more forceful techniques that have not been found to reduce perineal damage. These are done in an attempt to hasten the birth and include pressing vigorously against the posterior vaginal wall (to "show the birthgiver where to push"). Used along with directed closed glottis (Valsalva) pushing, this may have a detrimental impact on perineal outcomes. This combination of interventions is quite different in technique and outcome than the gentle intrapartum massage described earlier.

Waterbirth

Waterbirth is the process of laboring and giving birth in a tub of warm water (Figs. 8.29 – 8.31d). Birth outside of water is referred to as conventional birth, land birth, and bed birth. Waterbirth is used for pain relief. Water immersion has been used for pain relief in many countries worldwide, and the first case of birth in water was reported over 200 years ago.[59] The benefits of waterbirth include high levels of birth giver satisfaction, increased perception of control,[60–62] shorter labor duration,[63,64] fewer perineal lacerations, increased buoyancy, mobility, upright position for birth, and decreased blood pressure.[62,63,65,66] Laboring and giving birth in water has been referred to as a "liquid epidural" or an "aqua-dural" in a comparison to the analgesic effects of epidural anesthesia.[67]

The safety of waterbirth in the home or birth center setting is supported by a study by Bovbjerg et al.[68] of over 6000 waterbirths compared to 10,000 land births. Some countries with greater midwifery presence such as the

(a)

(b)

(c)

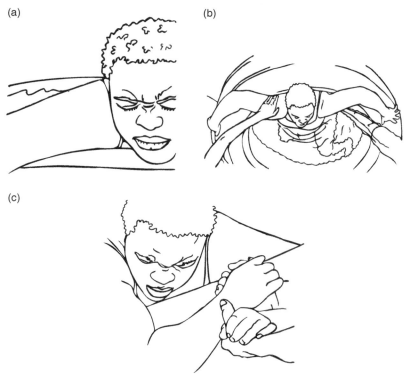

Fig. 8.29. (**a**) Laboring person in the water. (**b**) Laboring person in water with support. (**c**) Pushing in the water.

(a)

(b)

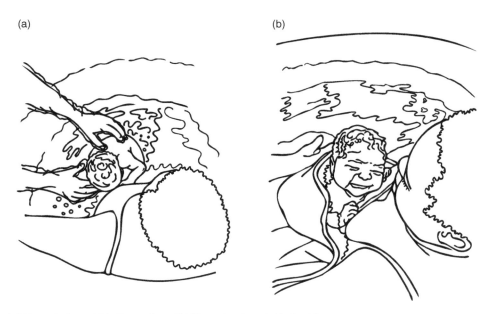

Fig. 8.30. (**a**) Neonate brought to the surface. (**b**) Neonate placed skin to skin.

(a)

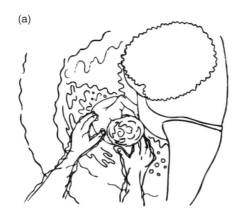

Fig. 8.31a. Birth giver with neonate partially submerged in tub and skin to skin.

(b)

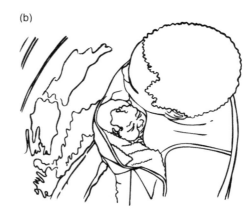

Fig. 8.31b. Skin to skin.

(c)

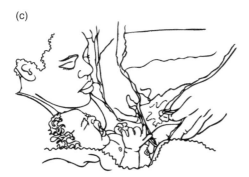

Fig. 8.31c. Cutting the cord.

(d)

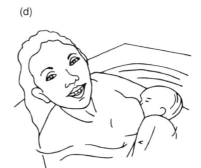

Fig. 8.31d. Breastfeeding in tub.

UK offer routine waterbirth to low-risk, healthy pregnant people, while in other countries it remains controversial.[69] Recent studies of hospital waterbirth have been published and demonstrated benefits for low-risk pregnant people and their neonates.[69–75] A large retrospective cohort study of 6264 waterbirths in England found no increase in maternal or neonatal adverse events.[69] However, Aughey and colleagues[69] did find that health disparities in water use exist, and that birthing people of color and from lower socioeconomic neighborhoods were less likely to have waterbirth. Bailey and colleagues[70] conducted a retrospective observational matched cohort study of two large hospital midwifery practices who offer waterbirth. There were 397 waterbirths compared to 2025 land births with no between-group differences in neonatal Apgar scores or neonatal intensive care (NICU) admissions, and fewer first and second degree lacerations in the waterbirth group.[70] A retrospective matched cohort study of US hospital waterbirths by Sidebottom and colleagues[74] included 314 waterbirths at eight hospitals. The researchers found no differences in maternal or neonatal outcomes and fewer NICU admission and maternal perineal lacerations in the waterbirth group. A small retrospective study by Neiman and colleagues[73] compared three groups: those who gave birth in water (n = 58), those who labored in water (n = 61), and those who did not use water "[n = 111). Neiman et al.[73] found that nulliparas in the waterbirth group had a shorter second stage of labor (P = .03]" and all those in the waterbirth group had a higher risk of hemorrhage (P = .45) but no difference in other outcomes. There were no differences in outcomes for neonates.[73] Ulfsdottir and colleagues[75] found a decrease in perineal tears and interventions, although they caution care providers to be mindful of the possibility of umbilical cord avulsion.

Some experts have voiced concern about neonatal outcomes associated with waterbirth. Vanderlaan and colleagues[76] conducted a systematic review and meta-analysis of neonatal outcomes for neonatal hospital waterbirths. The authors included 39 studies and found no increased risk of adverse neonatal outcomes with waterbirth compared to land birth and found the analysis to be stable for multiple outcomes.[76] In 2020, Vanderlaan and Hall published a systematic review of the case studies, and included 47 cases derived from 35 articles. The authors found that case studies do not offer a rationale to restrict waterbirth for low-risk healthy women, and that concerns of water aspiration and cord rupture are unfounded. However the authors did identify important neonatal safety considerations including the importance of infection prevention with a clean water source, management of compromised infants after the birth, and hyponatremia.

Pregnant people who are offered waterbirth should be healthy and low-risk with full term, uncompromised fetuses and normal vital signs. Pregnant people who choose to labor and birth in water should be offered informed consent, and assessed and managed the same as any other laboring person and their fetus in the same setting including fetal monitoring and routine vital signs. Vigorous hospital protocols for tub maintenance, infection control, and correct water temperature should be in place. Midwives, physicians, and nurses who participate in waterbirths must have protocols in place to handle emergency situations and deviations from normal such as tight nuchal cord, shoulder dystocia, hemorrhage, umbilical cord avulsion, loss of birth giver consciousness, and birth of a compromised neonate. Waterbirth is a safe and desirable option for pain relief for healthy lower risk pregnant people.

Positions for suspected "cephalopelvic disproportion" (CPD) in second stage

In addition to increased birth giver pain and delayed descent, fetal malposition may also signal a care provider to "suspect CPD." For all of these reasons it makes sense to encourage laboring people to try a variety of positions and movements that might resolve an OP, OT, or asynclitic position (Figs. 8.32–8.40).

Toilet-sitting and hydrotherapy may also enhance progress (Figs. 8.38 and 8.39).

Encouraging movements that alter pelvic size and shape also promotes fetal descent (Figs. 8.37 and 8.38). As shown in Fig. 8.14 and 8.41, "pelvic rocking" (also called pelvic tilt) may also change pelvic dimensions.

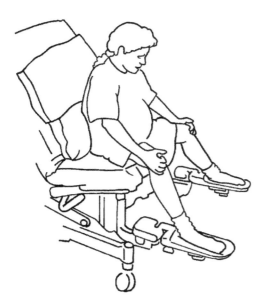

Fig. 8.32. Sitting upright to push.

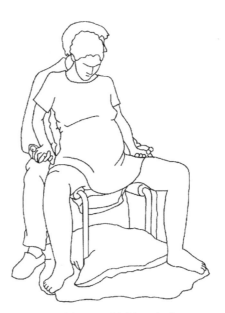

Fig. 8.33. Pushing on a birthing stool (adapted from a photograph of the DeBY Birth Support).

(a)

(b)

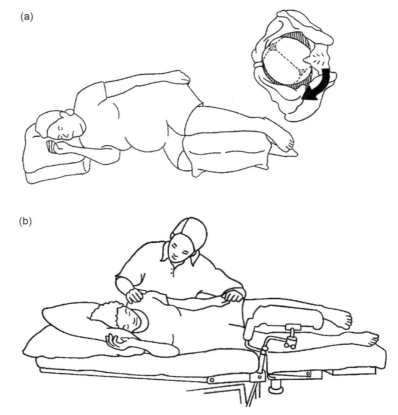

Fig. 8.34. (a) and (b) Pregnant person with known or suspected or known occiput posterior (OP) fetus in pure side-lying on the "correct side" with fetal back "toward the bed". With the fetus is Right Occiput Posterior (ROP), the person lies on their right side. Gravity pulls the fetal occiput and the trunk towards the occiput transverse (OT) position.

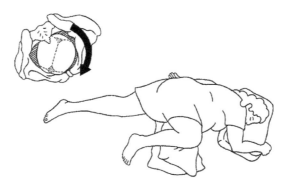

Fig. 8.35. Pregnant person with suspected or known right occiput posterior (ROP) semiprone on the "correct side," with fetal back "toward the ceiling." If fetus is ROP, the semiprone person lies on their left side. Gravity pulls fetal occiput and trunk towards the ROT, then right occiput anterior (ROA). If position is uncertain, laboring people should alternate sides after a few contractions.

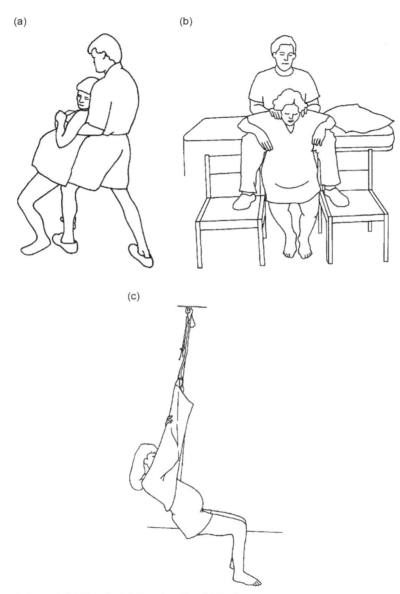

Fig. 8.36.   (**a**) Supported squat. (**b**) Dangle. (**c**) Dangle with a birth sling.

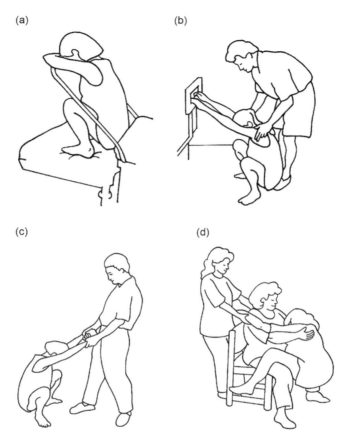

Fig. 8.37. (**a**) Squatting with a bar. (**b**) Squatting with bed rail. (**c**) Partner squat. (**d**) Lap squat, with three people.

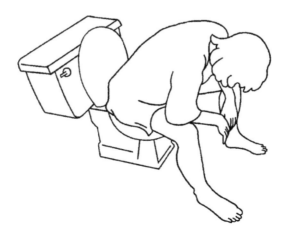

Fig. 8.38.   Sitting, leaning forward on toilet.

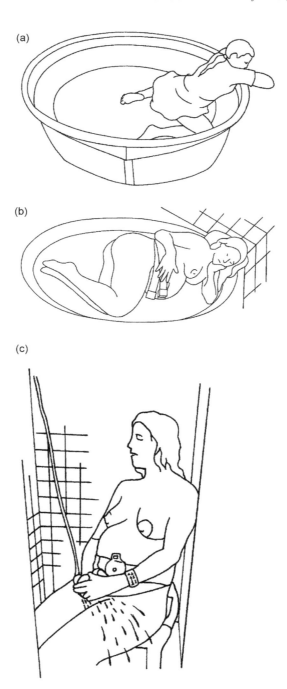

(a)

(b)

(c)

Fig. 8.39. Laboring person (**a**) In birthing pool. (**b**) Bath with telemetry monitors. (**c**) In shower with telemetry monitors.

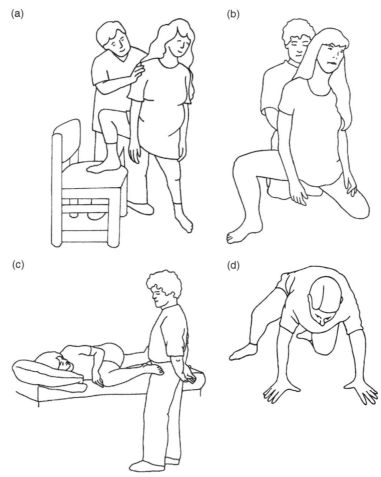

Fig. 8.40.   (**a**) Standing lunge. (**b**) Kneeling lunge. (**c**) Side-lying lunge used to view the perineum easily and/or perform vaginal exams. (**d**) Runner's lung (Front view).

Shoulder dystocia

Shoulder dystocia is defined as a birth requiring extra maneuvers to deliver the fetus after the head is born.[52] One shoulder is behind the symphysis pubis, which prevents the delivery of the shoulders. Shoulder dystocia is an emergency that every birth attend must be prepared to manage effectively. The specific maneuvers for shoulder dystocia require knowledge and skill. It is important for the birth attendant to remain calm so that birth giver and everyone else in the room can work together to resolve the problem. Most cases resolve quickly with appropriate actions.

The overall incidence of shoulder dystocia is 0.2–3% of births.[77] A study by Beta et al.[78] found that the incidence of shoulder dystocia was 0.6% in normally grown infants, 6% in those over 4000 grams, and 14% over 4500 grams. While the risk of shoulder dystocia is higher overall in large babies, approximately half occur when babies weigh less than 4000 grams.[79] Pregravid obesity and/or large prenatal weight gain are thought to increase the incidence of shoulder dystocia. The risk of shoulder dystocia for pregnant people with diabetes is increased by 30–70%.[79,80] Infants of mothers with diabetes have a broader than average chest circumference regardless of birth weight, greater body fat percentage, and a higher distribution of fat in the upper extremities.[79]

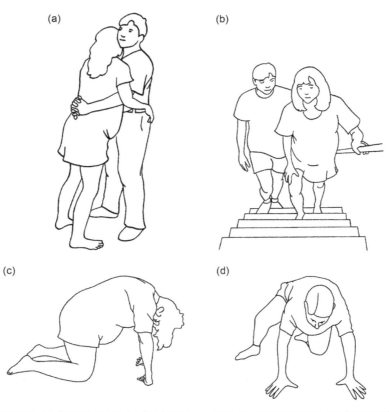

Fig. 8.41. (**a**) Slow dancing. (**b**) Stair climbing. (**c**) Pelvic rocking, back rounded in flexion. (**d**) Runners Lunge (front view).

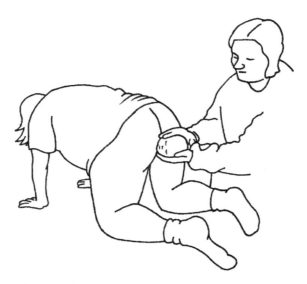

Fig. 8.42. Hands and knees position for birth.

Some authors have identified a relationship between shoulder dystocia and prolonged labor, but findings are not consistent between studies due to the presence of other risk factors such as fetal macrosomia.[79] An obstetric history of a prior shoulder dystocia increases the risk of shoulder dystocia ten-fold.[79] Forceps or vacuum assisted vaginal birth is also associated with a significant risk of shoulder dystocia.[79,80]

A combination of the risk factors previously described may further increase the risk of shoulder dystocia and fetal injury.[79] Rapid fetal descent is also associated with shoulder dystocia, presumably because the fetal shoulders do not have time to rotate properly.[81] Risks of shoulder dystocia include damage to the fetus such as brachial plexus injury, Erb's palsy, broken clavicle, and anoxia—if the situation is unresolved, even death.[82] Therefore, rapid attention and appropriate interventions are necessary to prevent or minimize these negative outcomes.

Precautionary measures

When a large baby is anticipated, midwives may encourage the use of a side-lying or hands-and-knees position for the birth (Fig. 8.42). In these positions, the birthing person's weight is off the sacrum. This maximizes the dimensions of the pelvic outlet, allowing more room for both the fetus and the caregiver to maneuver and for the fetus to be delivered. When the birthing person is in a semi-sitting position, similar expansion of the pelvic outlet can be achieved by providing support for the legs (Fig. 8.43).

Anticipating shoulder dystocia is an important strategy that allows the caregiver to assemble additional health professionals to help in case shoulder dystocia does occur. When a large baby is anticipated, many midwives request an additional nurse to provide suprapubic pressure (see Fig. 8.45 if necessary), and a stool to give the nurse optimal access and maximal downward pressure. The caregiver should also ensure that the birthing person's bladder is empty prior to birth, to promote as much room for the baby as possible.

Two step delivery of the fetal head

Another preventive strategy that some midwives and physicians use is to allow time for the fetal shoulders to rotate spontaneously. This is often called "two-step delivery." After delivery of the fetal head, the caregiver waits for another contraction to deliver the shoulders. Those who use this technique believe that rushing the delivery of the anterior shoulder may contribute to its entrapment and increase the risk of shoulder dystocia. Other caregivers believe that if they wait for a contraction, they have lost valuable minutes that may be needed to resolve a shoulder dystocia if it does occur. The practice of "one-step delivery" results from the belief that a longer time between the birth of the head and body will result in fetal harm. However, recent studies have not shown this. In a two-step delivery, the fetal head is born during or between contractions, and then the fetal shoulders and body are born with the next contraction. This allows the fetus to restitute and be re-oxygenated between contractions. Locatelli and colleagues[83] conducted a

(a)   (b)

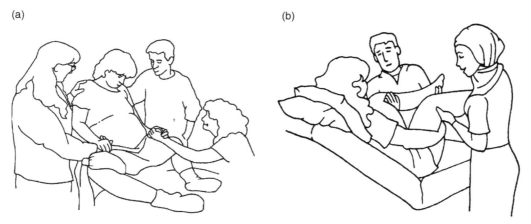

Fig. 8.43. (**a**) Semisitting to push. (**b**) Semisitting with people supporting the birthing person's legs.

prospective observational trial of 789 births and found no differences in fetal outcomes of umbilical arterial pH, operative vaginal delivery, or shoulder dystocia when using the two-step method. Hishikawa and colleagues[84] conducted a prospective observational trial of 262 low risk pregnant people and found two step delivery improves fetal circulation and prevents shoulder dystocia. Several authors have noted that downward traction on the fetal head is unnecessary and possibly harmful and that waiting for the next contraction after the birth of the fetal head protects uncompromised fetuses. This is an example of how a caregiver's philosophy guides clinical practice.

Shoulder dystocia warning signs

Shoulder dystocia may not be evident until the anterior shoulder does not deliver with the next contraction or the midwife or physician is not successful using the usual hand maneuvers. However, there are some warning signs that may indicate that a shoulder dystocia is about to occur. They include:

- the need for the caregiver to "milk the perineum," by pushing perineal tissues manually over the fetal head as it emerges
- the "turtle sign," in which, after the head is born, it recoils against the perineum and turns cyanotic (blue). This signals that a shoulder is caught behind the pubic symphysis.

Shoulder dystocia maneuvers

Caregivers manage shoulder dystocia using a series of maneuvers that are listed in Table 8.3. The key to successful management is for the caregiver efficiently to continue to try different appropriate maneuvers until successful delivery of the baby is achieved. It is important to avoid using the same maneuvers repeatedly without resolution. HELPERR is a mnemonic device that can assist providers to remember the management in a series of steps to relieve shoulder dystocia, where each letter stands for a step in the process:

- H, call for help
- E, evaluate for episiotomy
- L, move legs to McRoberts' position

Table 8.3. Shoulder dystocia maneuvers.

Name of maneuver	Action and notes
McRoberts' maneuver	Birthgiver's knees are flexed onto her abdomen, helping to lift the pubic symphysis and free the fetal shoulder
Gentle downward traction on the fetal head	May be repeated following the use of additional maneuvers to aid the birth
Suprapubic pressure (not fundal pressure)	An assistant presses down firmly behind the symphysis pubis in an attempt to free the anterior shoulder. Used with downward traction and McRoberts' maneuver
Hands and knees (Gaskin maneuver)	Laboring person is quickly moved to the hands-and-knees position. (The caregiver may attempt to deliver the posterior shoulder first.)
Rubin maneuver	Two fingers are inserted into the vagina behind the uppermost shoulder. Caregiver attempts to rotate the fetus to an oblique pelvic diameter
Woods corkscrew	With two fingers positioned as in the Rubin maneuver, caregiver places two fingers of the opposite hand in front of the lower fetal shoulder. Caregiver uses both hands to rotate the fetus to an oblique pelvic diameter
Reverse Woods corkscrew	Similar to the Woods corkscrew, but fetal shoulders are directed in the opposite direction. Used if the Woods corkscrew maneuver is unsuccessful
Delivery of the posterior arm	The caregiver reaches in to grasp the fetal hand of the anterior arm and sweeps it across the chest and out through the vagina

- P, suprapubic pressure
- E, enter maneuvers like internal rotations
- R, remove the posterior arm
- R, roll onto all-fours

Because these steps are so important, checklists, protocols, and simulations may enhance health care team performance.[85] Hoffman and colleagues[86] analyzed the medical records of 132,098 women who gave birth vaginally and found 2018 cases (1.5%) that included shoulder dystocia. Of these, 101 (5.2%) were associated with a neonatal injury. Delivery of the posterior arm was associated with the highest rate of resolution and similar rates of neonatal injuries.[85] Although more research is needed, these authors suggest that delivery of the posterior arm should be considered following McRoberts and suprapubic pressure.[85] It remains prudent to recommend that good clinical judgment should guide decision-making in the management of shoulder dystocia. Historically, shoulder dystocia management involved an early routine (and often large) episiotomy. More recently, clinicians have questioned its utility since shoulder dystocia is not a soft tissue obstruction. Fourteen clinical trials including 9769 cases of shoulder dystocia were systematically reviewed to determine the effectiveness of episiotomy as a management strategy.[87] The authors found that episiotomy increased the risk of significant perineal tears.

The reviewers found no evidence to support its use in the management of shoulder dystocia.[87]

The McRoberts' maneuver

The McRoberts' maneuver (Fig. 8.44) is most often used first and leads to resolution in 40–60% of cases.[88] In this maneuver, the birthing person's legs are flexed against the abdomen into an exaggerated lithotomy position. The McRoberts' maneuver (Fig. 8.6) appears to increase the expulsive force of contractions[89] as well as flattening the sacrum and aligning the pelvic inlet into a perpendicular plan to maximize pushing effort and force, although it does not seem to change the pelvic dimensions.[90]

The assistance of several nurses, and even an additional caregiver, is optimal for promoting success. However, calling additional personnel into the birth room may frighten the birthing person and their family and distract attention from important instructions given by the caregiver. Therefore, the caregiver should try to maintain a calm but firm tone when she or he requests assistance and gives instructions. Clinical staff should be ready to assist with maneuvers as instructed by the midwife or physician.

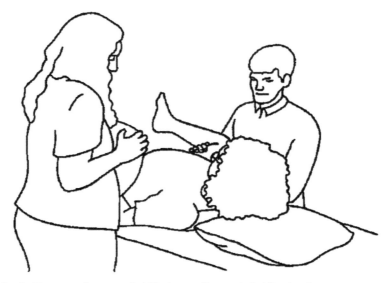

Fig. 8.44. McRobert's Maneuver (exaggerated lithotomy with people holding legs).

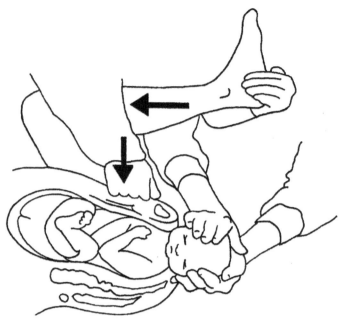

Fig. 8.45.   Suprapubic pressure. Assistant presses down while birth attendant uses gentle pressure.

The doula's role is to help the birthing person stay calm, to cooperate with the caregiver, and, if the caregiver requests, to help facilitate rapid positions changes.

Suprapubic pressure

Suprapubic pressure (Fig. 8.45) is an essential adjunct to the McRoberts' maneuver. To provide suprapubic pressure, an assistant presses down above the symphysis pubis to help deliver the anterior shoulder of the fetus. In providing suprapubic pressure, the attendant is essentially dislodging the trapped shoulder from above the pubic bone using gentle pressure. The caregiver guides the assistant's use of suprapubic pressure.

Fundal pressure is not the same as suprapubic pressure and is never appropriate in cases of shoulder dystocia. Fundal pressure is defined as mechanical pressure on the fundus (top) of the uterus and has been used to hasten the birth process. It is not recommended for use during management of shoulder dystocia, nor routinely at any time in the care of people in labor. In fact, the practice is considered obsolete and potentially hazardous in most developed countries.[91] In one study it was found that fundal pressure increased the force of expulsion by as much as 28%[89] however there is no evidence that it hastens birth.[91] Risks of fundal pressure to the birthing person include uterine rupture and an increased incidence of severe perineal damage. Newborn risks include bone fracture and braindamage.[91]

Hands and knees position, or the Gaskin maneuver

Moving a birthing person to the hands-and-knees position when delivery of the shoulder appears to be obstructed, sometimes referred to as the "Gaskin maneuver," has been found useful in cases of shoulder dystocia.[92]

The hands-and-knees position appears to work by several mechanisms. First, the position allows the sacrum to move freely, which can increase the pelvic outlet sagittal diameter by 1–2 cm.[92] Further, the movement to this position appears to dislodge the impacted shoulders. Additionally, when there is bilateral impaction of the shoulders, the position may allow gravity to move the posterior shoulder forward over the sacral promontory. In this situation, it may be possible to attempt to deliver the posterior shoulder first, using gentle downward pressure.

Shrug maneuver

The Shrug maneuver (Fig. 8.46) is described by Sancetta et al.,[93] as a modification of earlier techniques to deliver the posterior arm and shoulder. The steps are described as follows: first, use one hand to flex the neck toward the anterior shoulder; second, slide the other hand behind the posterior shoulder; third use the thumb and index finger to grasp through the axilla, making an "OK" sign; fourth move the posterior shoulder in the shrug position (move the shoulder toward the ears); fifth release the flexion on the head so the head is returned to a neutral position and use the "OK" hand on the posterior shoulder to rotate the fetus 180 degrees in the direction of the fetal chest.[93] This means the posterior shoulder is now the anterior shoulder, and the anterior shoulder is now the posterior shoulder. Proceed with usual normal delivery.

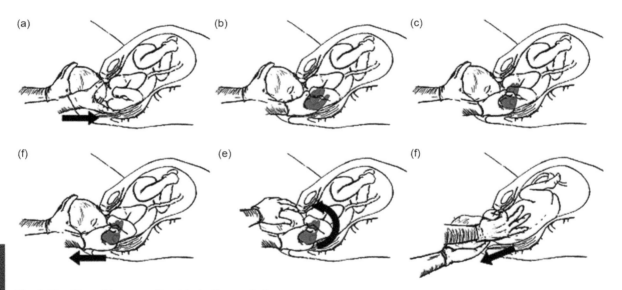

Fig. 8.46.   Shrug Maneuver. Reprinted with permission.

Posterior axilla sling traction (PAST)

The posterior axilla sling traction (PAST) technique for shoulder dystocia involves the use of urinary or suction catheter looped underneath the neonatal posterior shoulder.[94] First, the catheter is folded in half to create a loop (Image 8.47). Next the loop is threaded behind the posterior shoulder and pulled through using the index finger, to create a sling. The sling is then used to apply traction to either deliver the posterior shoulder or posterior arm. If delivery of the posterior arm and shoulder fail, the sling can be used to attempt to rotate the posterior shoulder.[94,95]

Tully's FlipFLOP pneumonic

The FlipFLOP mnemonic (Fig. 8.48) was developed by Gail Tully,[96] and may be used as a low intervention option to alleviate shoulder dystocia for pregnant people with good mobility, usually those without an epidural although it is also possible in some cases where the person exhibits more motor control.[96] This mnemonic may be used as an alternative to the HELPERR mnemonic.

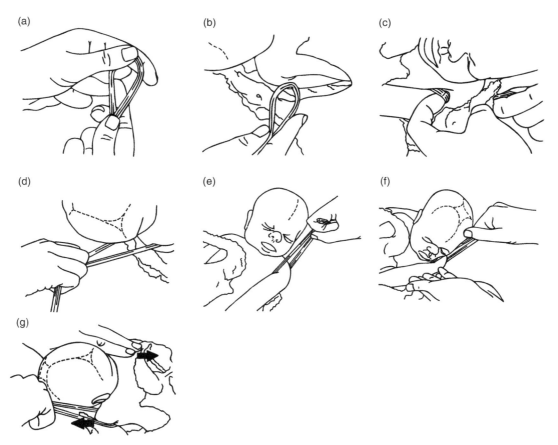

Fig. 8.47. (**a**) Neonatal suction tube is folded and held with thumb and index finger. (**b**) The loop is then fed behind the posterior shoulder with the index finger of one hand. (**c**) With the fingers of the other hand, the suction tube is caught on the other side of the armpit and pulled underneath. (**d**) The suction tube is positioned under the posterior axilla of the fetus. (**e**) The sling is gently pulled to deliver the posterior shoulder. (**f**) Sweeping out the posterior arm with the sling in place. (**g**) Shoulder rotation using sling. Source: Schom and Blanco.

F: Flip the pregnant person to Gaskin's position (hands and knees)
L: Lift the leg into a lunge, if possible, the leg that lunges forward should be on the same side as the fetal back
O: Oblique, use the hand or two fingers to rotate the anterior shoulder to an oblique position
P: Posterior arm, deliver the posterior arm

Somersault maneuver

Twenty-five percent of neonates are born with the umbilical cord wrapped around the neck, which is referred to as a "nuchal cord."[97] Common practice is for the caregiver to slip the nuchal cord over the fetal head, prior to delivery of the shoulders if it is loose enough to allow for this simple maneuver. However, a small percentage of nuchal cords are too tight to allow for this action. A tight nuchal cord can delay progress during birth and may also limit circulation to the fetus during contractions, resulting in variable type fetal heart rate decelerations. In very

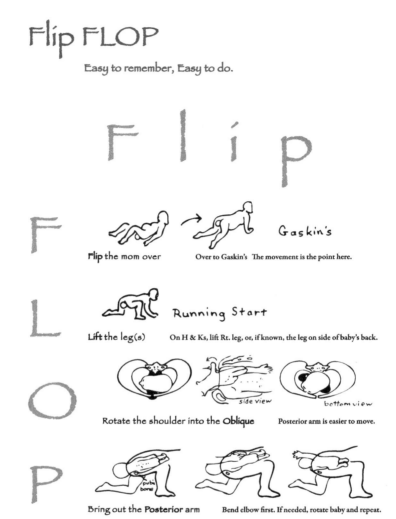

Flip FLOP

Easy to remember, Easy to do.

Flip

Flip the mom over   Over to Gaskin's The movement is the point here.   **Gaskin's**

Lift the leg(s)   On H & Ks, lift Rt. leg, or, if known, the leg on side of baby's back.   **Running Start**

Rotate the shoulder into the Oblique   side view   bottom view   Posterior arm is easier to move.

Bring out the Posterior arm   pubic bone   Bend elbow first. If needed, rotate baby and repeat.

©2005 **Maternity House Publishing** Gail Tully, CPM www.spinningbabies.com Permission to copy as whole.

Fig. 8.48. Flip Flop Pneumonic.

rare cases, on strategy to manage a tight nuchal cord at birth is to double clamp the cord and cut it, freeing the baby from this impediment. This strategy is effective but prevents the neonate from benefiting from both the oxygenated blood flow to the fetus prior to delivery and the placental blood transfusion following birth when cord clamping is delayed as is widely recommended.

In order to avoid clamping and cutting a tight nuchal cord prior to the birth, the caregiver can deliver the fetus using a somersault maneuver. This maneuver was first described by Schom and Blanco.[98] The four steps in the process (Fig. 8.49) include unhurried shoulder delivery, flexion of the baby's head toward the mother's thigh, maintaining the neonate's head near the perineum while allowing the body to deliver in a somersault manner, and finally unwrapping the baby from the cord. The use of the somersault maneuver allows caregivers to safely manage tight nuchal cords while maintaining the benefits of the intact cord for the newborn.[97–99] Following the somersault

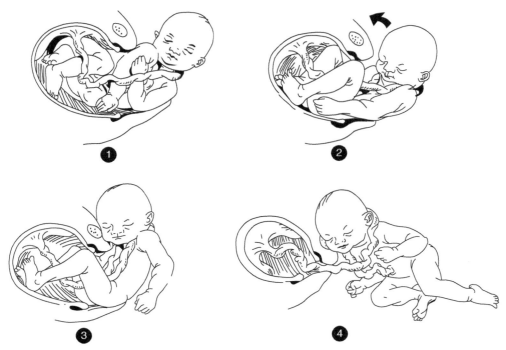

Fig. 8.49. Somersault maneuver. The somersault maneuver involves holding the infant's head flexed and guiding it upward or sideways toward the pubic bone or thigh, so the baby does a "somersault," ending with the infant's feet towards the laboring person's knees and the head still at the perineum. (**1**) Once the nuchal cord is discovered, the anterior and posterior shoulders are slowly delivered under control without manipulating the cord. (**2**) As the shoulders are delivered, the head is flexed so that the face of the baby is pushed toward the maternal thigh. (**3**) The baby's head is kept next to the then unwrapped, and the usual management ensues.[97]

maneuver, the caregiver can delay cord clamping and watch for improvements in the color and tone of the fetus, who might be somewhat compromised due to the tight cord, thereby providing the benefits of placental transfusion.

Decreased contraction frequency and intensity

If contraction intensity and/or frequency decrease during the second stage, the possible causes should be considered. Immobility, medications, dehydration, and exhaustion are all possible causes. Contractions might be improved by such measures as changing positions, allowing the medications or epidural to wear off (if the birth giver can tolerate it), breast stimulation, acupressure, hydration, encouraging the birth giver to avoid voluntary pushing for a number of contractions, or immersion in water. These are almost the same measures as those suggested for inadequate contractions during the active phase of first stage.

The essence of coping during the second stage of labor

When the second stage begins, the birth giver, if undisturbed and unrestricted, often becomes more aware of their surroundings, alert, and energetic.[43] Then, as the reflexive urge to push intensifies, it guides them to bear down and find a position that feels right. As the fetus moves down the vaginal canal, the birth giver may temporarily "hold back" (i.e., tense her perineum, fearing the stretching feeling). Then the body's strong urges take over and they let go, releasing the pelvic floor and their attempts to control the process. The birth giver may grunt, moan, or even bellow with contractions as she instinctively moves into different positions. The 3 Rs—relaxation, rhythm, and ritual—no longer apply.

The caregiver's role when a birth giver is coping in this way is to monitor the wellbeing of the fetus and birth giver as unobtrusively as possible, provide encouragement and reassurance as needed, and accommodate and support instinctive behaviors as much as possible. There are many safe and effective positions and ways of bearing down. As long as birth giver and baby are tolerating the second stage and some progress is being made, there is no reason to intervene. When it is clear that the baby will be born soon, it may be necessary to ask the birth giver to adopt a position which provides the clinical caregiver with adequate access to the perineum and baby.

In summary, "coping well" during the second stage includes grunting and bearing down reflexively with the urge to push (even bellowing at times), breathing as desired between bearing down efforts, and moving into positions that feel right. These behaviors are signs of normal coping, not signs of distress.

IF EMOTIONAL DYSTOCIA IS SUSPECTED

Emotional distress sometimes underlies a lack of progress in the second stage.

Signs of emotional stress during second stage can include:

- verbal or facial expressions of fear;
- crying or panic;
- inability to get beyond holding back to releasing the pelvic floor;
- holding their legs together;
- diffuse bearing down (see "Diffuse pushing" earlier in this chapter);
- begging the caregiver to take the baby out or to "knock" them out with drugs;
- desperation, inability to follow caregiver's suggestions.

Triggers of emotional distress unique to the second stage

These factors might trigger emotional distress and interfere with the birth giver's ability to cope during the second stage:

- Fatigue or exhaustion, which can lead to hopelessness or anxiety.
- The intense sensations of second stage or of manual stretching of the vagina. These sensations may be especially frightening if the birth giver has been sexually abused or otherwise traumatized in the genital region in the past, as they may trigger flashbacks.
- Fear of behaving inappropriately or offensively (making noise, passing stool while pushing).
- The immediacy of the birth and the responsibility of parenting the child, especially if their own parents were dysfunctional or they have relinquished a child for adoption or had a child removed from their care.
- Fear for the baby's wellbeing, especially if a sibling or a previous child died around birth or had another adverse outcome.
- The loss of privacy, sense of modesty when surrounded by strangers watching their perineum.
- Previous cesarean during second stage.
- Thoughtless or unkind treatment by loved ones or caregiver during labor.

One common response to such fears in the second stage is extreme tension in the pelvic floor as if to deter the fetus's descent, while pushing. The birth giver may be pushing hard but not effectively. Sometimes they unintentionally and unconsciously contract their pelvic floor muscles and buttocks and push with the diaphragm and abdominal muscles. Tension in the perineum and constriction of the anus while pushing indicate that the birth giver is holding back. It is important not to confuse this excessive and prolonged pelvic tension with the normal confusion experienced by many individuals when they first begin to push. As second stage begins it is normal for people in labor to experiment for several contractions in order to discover how to push effectively. This is particularly true in the absence of a strong urge to push. In such cases, it may be best for them to rest and await a stronger urge to push.

If a birth giver exhibits "diffuse pushing" and does not benefit from the suggestions to improve bearing-down efforts consider the possibility of emotional dystocia. Whatever fears or anxieties cause the birth giver to hold back may be difficult to set aside and move beyond; it is unlikely that they will simply be able to "snap out of it." However, those around them may be able to address and alleviate fears. The following measures may be helpful:

- Encourage the birth giver to express their feelings. Ask them, "What was going through your mind during that last contraction?" Listen to them, acknowledge and validate their concerns, and try to give appropriate reassurance, encouragement, or information and suggestions. Often, all the birth giver needs is a chance to express their concerns. They need to know they are being heard, that their fears are normal, and that they will get through this event.
- Sometimes, when it is clear to everyone including the birth giver, that there is a delay, asking them why they think labor has slowed down, reveals useful information. Answers such as, "I can't push right" or "The baby doesn't want to come out" or "It hurts too much!" might indicate emotional dystocia.
- Provide appropriate information. For example, if the birth giver is afraid of having a bowel movement as they push (and it is too late for them to go to the bathroom), they can be reassured that passing stool indicates effective pushing, that this is a common event, that any fecal material will be quickly wiped away and disposed of. In fact, this is one of many good reasons to apply warm compresses to the perineum—to be able to unobtrusively remove any stool. This may also be a good time to allow the birth giver to push on the toilet if they and the clinicians are comfortable with that option.
- If the birth giver is afraid they will "tear" while pushing, reassure them that, by relaxing their perineum or letting the baby come, the perineum will actually stretch more and be less likely to tear. Also, unless there is a good reason not to do so, let them try a few contractions without pushing. "Let's try breathing through this next one," so that they feel they have some options during what might feel like a frightening time. Allowing the birth giver to hold a warm compress on their own perineum or to simply provide support to the perineum with their own hand may also be reassuring and allow them to push more effectively.
- Give the birth giver time to adjust to the intense sensations and emotions of second stage. Avoid creating a sense of rushing. Speak in a calm and quiet voice. There is usually no need for the caregiver to raise their voice.
- Encourage the birth giver to relax their perineum between contractions and let it bulge during contractions. The application of hot compresses (washcloths soaked in warm water, wrung out) to the perineum often feels good and promotes relaxation. The compresses should not be too hot for the person applying them to hold comfortably in their hand. If they are reluctant to push because of an intense burning sensation a cool compress may provide more comfort. Encourage the birth giver to push as though they were blowing up an imaginary balloon, or trying to urinate rapidly. Give them positive reinforcement whenever they bear down effectively. Pushing in this manner sometimes causes the pelvic floor to bulge, which the caregiver can see. If they seem reluctant to sustain a bearing-down effort and are not making progress, advise them to "push to the pain, and right through it. It will feel better when you push through it." Allowing them to place their hand on their perineum will also provide good feedback about the progress they've made and the reason for the burning.
- Have the birth giver try pushing while sitting on the toilet. This may be especially helpful when there is concern about passing stool. Toilet-sitting also elicits the conditioned response of releasing the pelvic floor. Whoever is responsible for the birth giver's care can monitor what the birth giver is feeling and ensure that they move to an appropriate place for the birth to occur.

CONCLUSION

Some birth givers experience a latent phase of the second stage, and have no immediate urge to bear down once the cervix is completely dilated. The redefined second stage of labor begins when birth givers experience an urge to bear down. The duration of the second stage is best determined by the condition of the laboring person and fetus, rather than a strict time limit. Non-supine positions offer numerous advantages and are prefered by birth givers. Spontaneous bearing down can be supported by words of encouragement. During crowning of the fetal head a variety of approaches can be used for comfort and to promote an intact perineum. Various maneuvers are used by birth attendants to manage a nuchal cord and to relieve shoulder dystocia. Emotional support of the birth giver during second stage labor will help promote comfort and coping.

REFERENCES

1. Hanson L. (2009) Second stage labor care: Challenges in spontaneous bearing down. *Journal of Perinatal and Neonatal Nursing* 23, 31–39.
2. Aderhold KJ, Roberts JE. (1991) Phases of second stage labor. Four descriptive case studies. *Journal of Nurse-midwifery* 36(5), 267–275. doi: 10.1016/0091-2182(91)90041-m
3. Simkin P. (1984). Active and physiologic management of second stage: A review and hypothesis. In: S Kitzinger, P Simkin (eds), *Episiotomy and the Second Stage of Labor*. Seattle: Penny Press, pp. 7–21.
4. Simkin P. (2013) *The Birth Partner*, 4th edn. Boston: Harvard Common Press, pp. 57–109.
5. Cohen W, Friedman E. (1983) Normal labor. In: *Labor: Clinical Evaluation and Management* (2nd ed.). pp. 11–23. c08. indd 213 13-09-2023 18:25:20
6. Vasicka A, Kumaresan P, Han G, Kumaresan M. (1978) Plasma oxytocin in initiation of labor. *American Journal of Obstetrics and Gynecology* 130(3), 263–273.
7. Fuchs A, Romero R, Keefe D, Parra M, Oyarzun E, Behnke E. (1991) Oxytocin secretion and human parturition: Pulse frequency and duration increase during spontaneous labor in women. *American Journal of Obstetrics and Gynecology* 165(4), 1515–1523.
8. Rahm VA, Hallgren A, Högberg H, Hurtig I, Odlind V. (2002) Plasma oxytocin levels in women during labor with or without epidural analgesia: A prospective study. *Acta Obstetricia Et Gynecologica Scandinavica* 81(11), 1033–1039.
9. Beynon C. (1957) The normal second stage of labour: A plea for reform in its conduct. *Journal of Obstetrics and Gynaecology of the British Commonwealth* 64(6), 815–820.
10. Roberts J. (2002) The "push" for evidence: Management of the second stage. *Journal of Midwifery & Women's Health* 47(1), 2–15.
11. Friedman E. (1978) *Labor: Clinical Evaluation and Management*, 2nd ed. New York: Appleton-Century-Crofts, pp. 45–58.
12. Kopas ML. (2014) A review of evidence-based practices for management of the second stage of labor. *Journal of Midwifery & Women's Health* 59(3), 264–276.
13. Clark SL, Simpson KR, Knox GE, Garite TJ. (2009) Oxytocin: New perspectives on an old drug. *American Journal of Obstetrics and Gynecology* 200(1), 35–e1.
14. Rooks JP. (2009) Oxytocin as a "high alert medication": A multilayered challenge to the status quo. *Birth* 36(4), 345–348.
15. Fraser DM, Cooper MA. (2009) *Myles Textbook for Midwives*, 15th edn. Churchill Livingstone.
16. Rosevear S, Stirrat G. (1996) *The Handbook of Obstetric Management*. Oxford: Blackwell Scientific.
17. Osborne K, Hanson L. (2012) Directive versus supportive approaches used by midwives when providing care during second stage labor. *Journal of Midwifery and Women's Health* 57(1), 3–11.
18. Roberts J, Hanson L. (2007) Best practices in second stage labor care: Maternal bearing down and positioning. *Journal of Midwifery and Women's Health* 52, 238–245. doi: 10.1016/j.jmwh.2006.12.011
19. Szu LT, Chou PY, Lin PH, Chen C, Lin WL, Chen KH. (2021) Comparison of maternal and fetal outcomes between delayed and immediate pushing in the second stage of vaginal delivery: Systematic review and meta-analysis of randomized controlled trials. *Archives of Gynecology and Obstetrics* 303(2), 481–499. doi: 10.1007/s00404-020-05814-w

20. Isaac Ashford J. (1988) *Mothers and Midwives: A history of traditional childbirth.* Self published. ISBN: 0961996811, 9780961996819.

21. Leavitt JW. (1983) "Science" enters the birthing room: Obstetrics in America since the eighteenth century. *The Journal of American History* 70(2), 281–304. doi: 10.2307/1900205

22. Caldeyro-Barcia R. (1979) The influence of maternal bearing-down efforts during second stage on fetal well-being. *Birth* 6(1), 17–21.

23. Bloom SL, Casey BM, Schaffer JI, McIntire DD, Leveno KJ. (2006) A randomized trial of coached versus uncoached maternal pushing during the second stage of labor. *American Journal of Obstetrics and Gynecology* 194(1), 10–13.

24. Aldrich CJ, d'Antona D, Spencer JAD, Wyatt JS, Peebles DM, Delpy DT, Reynolds EOR. (1995) The effect of maternal pushing on fetal cerebral oxygenation and blood volume during the second stage of labour. *BJOG: An International Journal of Obstetrics & Gynaecology* 102(6), 448–453.

25. Simpson KR, James DC. (2005) Effects of immediate versus delayed pushing during second-stage labor on fetal well-being: A randomized clinical trial. *Nursing Research* 54(3), 149–157.

26. Roberts J. (2003) A new understanding of the second stage of labor: Implications for nursing care. *JOGNN* 32(6), 794–801.

27. Le Goueff F, Garite TJ. (2003). 14. *American College of Obstetricians and Gynecologists.* Dystocia and augmentation of labor. Washington (DC): The College. ACOG Practice Bulletin no.: 49. 15. Goffinet F, Langer B, Carbonne B, Berkane N, Tardif D.

28. Oppenheimer L, Black A. (2013) The second stage of labor. In: GD Posner, J Dy, AY Black, GD Jones (eds), *Oxorn-Foot Human Labor & Birth*, 6th edn. McGraw Hill, pp. 266–281.

29. Zhang J, Landy HJ, Branch DW, Burkman R, Haberman S, Gregory KD, … Reddy UM. (2010) Contemporary patterns of spontaneous labor with normal neonatal outcomes. *Obstetrics and Gynecology* 116(6), 1281–1287.

30. Spong CY, Berghella V, Wenstrom KD, Mercer BM, Saade GR. (2012) Preventing the first cesarean delivery: Summary of a joint Eunice Kennedy Shriver national institute of child health and human development, society for maternal-fetal medicine, and American college of obstetricians and gynecologists workshop. *Obstetrics and Gynecology* 120(5), 1181–1193.

31. (ACOG) American College of Obstetricians and Gynecologists & (SMFM) Society for Maternal-Fetal Medicine. (2014) Obstetric care consensus No. 1: Safe prevention of the primary cesarean delivery. *Obstetrics & Gynecology* 123, 693–711.

32. ACOG. (2019) ACOG Committee Opinion: Approaches to Limit Interventions during labor and birth. *Obstetrics & Gynecology* e164–e173.

33. Osborne K, Hanson L. (2014) Labor down or bear down: A strategy to translate second-stage labor evidence to perinatal practice. *The Journal of Perinatal & Neonatal Nursing* 28(2), 117–126.

34. Thies-Lagergren L, Hildingsson I, Christensson K, Kvist LJ. (2013) Who decides the position for birth? A follow-up study of a randomised controlled trial. *Women and Birth* 26(4), e99–e104.

35. Fenwick L, Simkin P. (1987) Maternal positioning to prevent or alleviate dystocia in labor. *Clinical Obstetrics and Gynecology* 30(1), 83–89.

36. Michel SC, Rake A, Treiber K, Seifert B, Chaoui R, Huch R, … Kubik-Huch RA. (2002) MR obstetric pelvimetry: Effect of birthing position on pelvic bony dimensions. *American Journal of Roentgenology* 179(4), 1063–1067.

37. Elvander C, Ahlberg M, Thies-Lagergren L, Cnattingius S, Stephansson O. (2015) Birth position and obstetric anal sphincter injury: A population-based study of 113 000 spontaneous births. *BMC Pregnancy and Childbirth* 15(1), 1–9.

38. Thomson A. (1995) Maternal behavior during spontaneous and directed pushing in the second stage of labour. *Journal of Advanced Nursing* 22, 1027–1034.

39. Schaffer J, Bloom S, Casey B, McIntire D, Nihira M, Leveno K. (2006) A randomized trial of coached versus uncoached maternal pushing during the second stage of labor. *American Journal of Obstetrics and Gynecology* 194(1), 10–13.

40. Hanson L. (1998a) Second-stage positioning in nurse-midwifery practices: Part 1: Position use and preferences. *Journal of Nurse-Midwifery* 43(5), 320–325.

41. Hanson L. (1998b) Second-stage positioning in nurse-midwifery practices: Part 2: Factors affecting use. *Journal of Nurse-Midwifery* 43(5), 326–330.

42. Baxley EG, Gobbo RW. (2004) Shoulder dystocia. *American Family Physician* 69(7), 1707–1714.

43. Odent M. (1999) *The Scientification of Love*. Free Assn Books.

44. Wong CA, Scavone BM, Dugan S, Smith JC, Prather H, Ganchiff JN, McCarthy RJ. (2003) Incidence of postpartum lumbosacral spine and lower extremity nerve injuries. *Obstetrics & Gynecology* 101(2), 279–288.

45. Berta M, Lindgren H, Christensson K, Mekonnen S, Adefris M. (2019 Dec 4) Effect of maternal birth positions on duration of second stage of labor: Systematic review and meta-analysis. *BMC Pregnancy Childbirth* 19(1), 466. doi: 10.1186/s12884-019-2620-0. PMID: 31801479; PMCID: PMC6894325.

46. Graseck A, Tuuli M, Roehl K, Odibo A, Macones G, Cahill A. (2014) Fetal descent in labor. *Obstetrics & Gynecology* 123(3), 521–526.

47. Simkin P. (2003) Maternal positions and pelves revisited. *Birth* 30(2), 130–132.

48. Dudley NJ. (2005) A systematic review of the ultrasound estimation of fetal weight. *Ultrasound in Obstetrics and Gynecology: The Official Journal of the International Society of Ultrasound in Obstetrics and Gynecology* 25(1), 80–89.

49. Stubert J, Peschel A, Bolz M, Glass A, Gerber, B. (2018) Accuracy of immediate antepartum ultrasound estimated fetal weight and its impact on mode of delivery and outcome – a cohort analysis. *BMC Pregnancy and Childbirth* 18(1), 1–8.

50. King TL. (2012, October). Preventing primary cesarean sections: Intrapartum care. In: *Seminars in Perinatology*, Vol. 36, No. 5. WB Saunders, pp. 357–364. c08.indd 215 13-09-2023 18:25:20

51. Sampselle CM, Miller JM, Luecha Y, Fischer K, Rosten L. (2005) Provider support of spontaneous pushing during the second-stage of labor. *Journal of Obstetrics, Gynecology and Neonatal Nursing* 34, 695–702.

52. Huang J, Lu H, Zang Y, Ren L, Li C, Wang J. (2020) The effects of hands on and hands off/poised techniques on maternal outcomes: A systematic review and meta-analysis. *Midwifery* 87, 102712. doi: 10.1016/j.midw.2020.102712

53. Albers LL, Sedler KD, Bedrick EJ, Teaf D, Peralta P. (2005) Midwifery care measures in the second stage of labor and reduction of genital trauma at birth: A randomized controlled trial. *Journal of Midwifery and Women's Health* 50(5), 365–372. doi: 10.1016/j.jmwh.2005.05.012

54. Aasheim V, Nilsen A, Reinar LM, Lukasse M. (2017) Perineal techniques during the second stage of labour for reducing perineal trauma. *The Cochrane Database of Systematic Reviews* 6(6), CD006672. doi: 10.1002/14651858. CD006672.pub3

55. Edqvist M, Hildingsson I, Mollberg M, Lundgren I, Lindgren H. (2017) Midwives' management during the second stage of labor in relation to second-degree tears-an experimental study. *Birth* 44(1), 86–94. doi: 10.1111/birt.12267

56. Jiang H, Qian X, Carroli G, Garner P. (2017) Selective versus routine use of episiotomy for vaginal birth. *Cochrane Database of Systematic Reviews* 2(2).

57. Collins MK, Proter KB, Brook E, Johnson L, Williams M, Jevitt CA. (1994) Vulvar application of lidocaine for pain relief in spontaneous vaginal delivery. *Obstetrics & Gynecology* 84(3), 335–337.

58. Aquino CI, Guida M, Saccone G, Cruz Y, Vitagliano A, Zullo F, Berghella, V. (2020) Perineal massage during labor: A systematic review and meta-analysis of randomized controlled trials. *The journal of maternal-fetal & neonatal medicine: the official journal of the European Association of Perinatal Medicine, the Federation of Asia and Oceania Perinatal Societies, the International Society of Perinatal Obstetricians* 33(6), 1051–1063. doi: 10.1080/14767058.2018.1512574

59. Dekker R, Bertone A. (2018) Evidence based birth signature articles. *The Evidence on: Waterbirth*. Retrieved from: https://evidencebasedbirth.com/waterbirth

60. Duffin C. (2004) Waterbirth findings reveal high levels of satisfaction: Royal College of Midwives annual conference reflects a further move away from medical interventions towards. *Nursing Standard* 18(37), 8–9.

61. Maude RM, Foureur MJ. (2007) It's beyond water: Stories of women's experience of using water for labour and birth. *Women and Birth* 20(1), 17–24.

62. Nutter E, Meyer S, Shaw-Battista J, Marowitz A. (2014) Waterbirth: An integrative analysis of peer-reviewed literature. *Journal of Midwifery & Women's Health* 59(3), 286–319.

63. Cluett ER, Burns E, Cuthbert A. (2018) Immersion in water during labour and birth. *The Cochrane Database of Systematic Reviews* 5(5), CD000111. doi: 10.1002/14651858.CD000111.pub4

64. Torkamani SA, Kangani F, Janani F. (2010) The effects of delivery in water on duration of delivery and pain compared with normal delivery. *Pakistan Journal of Medical Science* 26(3), 551–555.

65. Dahlen HG, Dowling H, Tracy M, Schmied V, Tracy S. (2013) Maternal and perinatal outcomes amongst low risk women giving birth in water compared to six birth positions on land. A descriptive cross sectional study in a birth centre over 12 years. *Midwifery* 29(7), 759–764. doi: 10.1016/j.midw.2012.07.002

66. Pagano E, De Rota B, Ferrando A, Petrinco M, Merletti F, Gregori D. (2010) An economic evaluation of water birth: The cost-effectiveness of mother well-being. *Journal of Evaluation in Clinical Practice* 16(5), 916–919.
67. Harper B. (2020) Waterbirth certification course for providers. Retrieved from: https://birthpedia.net/learn-waterbirth-courses
68. Bovbjerg ML, Cheyney M, Everson C. (2016) Maternal and newborn outcomes following waterbirth: The midwives alliance of North America statistics project, 2004 to 2009 cohort. *Journal of Midwifery & Women's Health* 61(1), 11–20. doi: 10.1111/jmwh.12394
69. Aughey H, Jardine J, Moitt N, Fearon K, Hawdon J, Pasupathy D, Urganci I, Project Team NMPA, Harris T. (2021) Waterbirth: A national retrospective cohort study of factors associated with its use among women in England. *BMC Pregnancy and Childbirth* 21(1), 256. doi: 10.1186/s12884-021-03724-6
70. Bailey JM, Zielinski RE, Emeis CL, Kane Low L. (2020) A retrospective comparison of waterbirth outcomes in two United States hospital settings. *Birth* 47(1), 98–104.
71. Hodgson ZG, Comfort LR, Albert AA. (2020) Water birth and perinatal outcomes in British Columbia: A retrospective cohort study. *Journal of Obstetrics and Gynaecology Canada* 42(2), 150–155. doi: 10.1016/j.jogc.2019.07.007
72. Jacoby S, Becker G, Crawford S, Wilson RD. (2019) Water birth maternal and neonatal outcomes among midwifery clients in Alberta, Canada, from 2014 to 2017: A retrospective study. *Journal of Obstetrics and Gynaecology Canada* 41(6), 805–812. c08.indd 216 13-09-2023 18:25:20.
73. Neiman E, Austin E, Tan A, Anderson CM, Chipps E. (2020) Outcomes of waterbirth in a US hospital-based midwifery practice: A retrospective cohort study of water immersion during labor and birth. *Journal of Midwifery & Women's Health* 65(2), 216–223.
74. Sidebottom AC, Vacquier M, Simon K, Fontaine P, Dahlgren-Roemmich D, Hyer B, … Saul L. (2019) Who gives birth in the water? A retrospective cohort study of intended versus completed Waterbirths. *Journal of Midwifery & Women's Health* 64(4), 403–409.
75. Ulfsdottir H, Saltvedt S, Georgsson S. (2018) Waterbirth in Sweden – a comparative study. *Acta Obstetricia Et Gynecologica Scandinavica* 97(3), 341–348. doi: 10.1111/aogs.13286
76. Vanderlaan J, Hall P, Lewitt M. (2018 April) Neonatal outcomes with water birth: A systematic review and meta-analysis. *Midwifery* 59, 27–38.
77. ACOG: American College of Obstetricians and Gynecologists. (2017a) ACOG practice bulletin No 178: Shoulder dystocia. *Obstetrics and Gynecology* 129(5), e123–e133. doi: 10.1097/AOG.0000000000002043
78. Beta J, Khan N, Khalil A, Fiolna M, Ramadan G, Akolekar R. (2019) Maternal and neonatal complications of fetal macrosomia: Systematic review and meta-analysis. *Ultrasound in Obstetrics & Gynecology* 54(3), 308–318. doi: 10.1002/uog.20279
79. Mehta SH, Sokol RJ. (2014) Shoulder dystocia: Risk factors, predictability, and preventability. *Seminars in Perinatology* 38, 189–193. doi: 10.1053/j.semperi.2014.04.003
80. Hansen A, Chauhan SP. (2014) Shoulder dystocia: Definitions and incidence. *Seminars in Perinatology* 38, 184–188.
81. Gherman RB. (2002) Shoulder dystocia: An evidence-based evaluation of the obstetric nightmare. *Clinical Obstetrics and Gynecology* 45(2), 345–362. doi: 10.1097/00003081-200206000-00006
82. Dajani NK, Magann EF. (2014) Complications of shoulder dystocia. *Seminars in Perinatology* 38(4), 201–204. doi: 10.1053/j.semperi.2014.04.005
83. Locatelli A, Incerti M, Ghidini A, Longoni A, Casarico G, Ferrini S, Strobelt N. (2011) Head-to-body delivery interval using 'two-step' approach in vaginal deliveries: Effect on umbilical artery pH. *The Journal of Maternal-Fetal & Neonatal Medicine* 24(6), 799–803.
84. Hishikawa K, Kusaka T, Fukuda T, Kohata Y, Inoue H. (2020) Neonatal outcomes of two-step delivery in low-risk pregnancy: A prospective observational study. *The Journal of Obstetrics and Gynaecology Research* 46(7), 1090–1097. doi: 10.1111/jog.14272
85. Grobman WA. (2014) Shoulder dystocia: Simulation and a team-centered protocol. *Seminars in Perinatology* 38, 205–209.
86. Hoffman MK, Bailit JL, Branch DW, Burkman RT, Van Veldhusien P, Lu L, … Zhang J. (2011) A comparison of obstetric maneuvers for the acute management of shoulder dystocia. *Obstetrics and Gynecology* 117(6), 1272.
87. Sagi-Dain L, Sagi S. (2015) The role of episiotomy in prevention and management of shoulder dystocia: A systematic review. *Obstetrical and Gynecological Survey* 70(5), 354–362.

8

88. Mahlmeister LR. (2008) Best practices in perinatal nursing: Risk identification and management of shoulder dystocia. *Journal of Perinatal and Neonatal Nursing* 22(2), 91–94.

89. Buhimschi CS, Buhimschi IA, Malinow A, Weiner CP. (2001) Use of McRoberts' position during delivery and increase in pushing efficiency. *Lancet (London, England)* 358(9280), 470–471. doi: 10.1016/S0140-6736(01)05632-X

90. Gherman RB, Tramont J, Muffley P, Goodwin TM. (2000) Analysis of McRoberts' maneuver by x-ray pelvimetry. *Obstetrics and Gynecology* 95(1), 43–47. doi: 10.1016/s0029-7844(99)00445-7

91. Verheijen EC, Raven JH, Hofmeyr GJ. (2009) Fundal pressure during the second stage of labor. *Cochrane Database of Systematic Reviews* 4, Art. No.: CD006067. doi: 10.1002/14651858.CD006067.pub2

92. Bruner JP, Drummond SB, Meenan AL, Gaskin IM. (1998) All-fours maneuver for reducing shoulder dystocia during labor. *The Journal of Reproductive Medicine* 43(5), 439–443.

93. Sancetta R, Khanzada H, Leante R. (2019) Shoulder shrug maneuver to facilitate delivery during shoulder dystocia. *Obstetrics and Gynecology* 133(6), 1178–1181. doi: 10.1097/AOG.0000000000003278

94. Taddei E, Marti C, Capoccia-Brugger R, Brunisholz Y. (2017) Posterior axilla sling traction and rotation: A case report of an alternative for intractable shoulder dystocia. *Journal of the Institute of Obstetrics and Gynaecology* 37(3), 387–389. doi: 10.1080/01443615.2016.1264070

95. Cluver CA, Hofmeyr GJ. (2015) Posterior axilla sling traction for shoulder dystocia: Case review and a new method of shoulder rotation with the sling. *American Journal of Obstetrics and Gynecology* 212(6), 784–e1. c08.indd 217 13-09-2023 18:25:20

96. Tully G. (2012) FlipFLOP: Four steps to remember. *Midwifery Today with International Midwife* (103), 9–11.

97. Mercer JS, Skovgaard RL, Peareara-Eaves J, Bowman TA. (2005) Nuchal cord management and nurse-midwifery practice. *Journal of Midwifery & Women's Health* 50(5), 373–379. doi: 10.1016/j.jmwh.2005.04.023

98. Schorn MN, Blanco JD. (1991) Management of the nuchal cord. *Journal of Nurse-midwifery* 36(2), 131–132. doi: 10.1016/0091-2182(91)90063-u

99. Mercer JS, Erickson-Owens, DA. (2014) Is it time to rethink cord management when resuscitation is needed? *Journal of Midwifery & Women's Health* 59(6), 635–644. doi: 10.1111/jmwh.12206

8

Chapter 9

Optimal Newborn Transition and Third and Fourth Stage Labor Management

Emily Malloy, PhD, CNM, Lisa Hanson, PhD, CNM, FACNM, and Karen Robinson, PhD, CNM, FACNM

OVERVIEW OF THE NORMAL THIRD AND FOURTH STAGES OF LABOR FOR UNMEDICATED MOTHER AND BABY

The third stage of labor encompasses both the delivery of the placenta and an enormous physiologic shift for the birthing person and newborn. The newborn transitions from complete in utero dependence on the placenta for life-sustaining nutrients and oxygen to the independent transition to breathing and eating. The newborn now takes in and uses oxygen and food. Simultaneously, the newborn adapts to the new surroundings, and regulates body temperature and conducts all life functions. A compelling drama that began with the stimulation and beneficial stress caused by labor contractions continues to unfold with the first breath and first cry, a joyous sound for the birthing person and family. The transition from fetus to neonate is underway and completed in a few minutes. During those first minutes after birth, the newborn's lungs are inflated, and take over as the organs of respiration, circulation is rerouted and the heart is restructured so that soon all blood will circulate through the lungs to transfer the oxygen needed throughout the body. The skin tones become ruddy due to the increased oxygenation in the blood. Initially, the newborn is wet and streaked with blood, mucus, amniotic fluid, and vernix. However, the neonate begins to lose heat, which stimulates the temperature-regulating system and is additionally stabilized by placing the newborn skin to skin on the birthing person's abdomen or chest, depending on the length of the umbilical cord. A nurse may gently dry and rub the newborn and places a warm blanket over the dyad.

Although the newborn's senses develop in utero, they are not used until after the birth during the transition to extra uterine life. The neonate calms down, and stares alertly and intently at the parent. Throughout the time that the baby passes through the vaginal canal and is placed skin to skin, the baby is becoming "seeded" by the birthing person's vaginal and skin microbes, which, along with microbes from other parts of the body, will play a vital role in establishing the lifelong health and wellbeing of the baby. Heavily colonized places on the human microbiome—the vaginal and rectum and the underarms—are the sites where the neonate is exposed to additional adult microbes, first during the birth and next being cradled in their parent's arms during feedings.

After 15–30 minutes of life the neonate initiates the breast crawl (TBC), becoming active, crawling in a rudimentary way, bringing hands to mouth, bobbing the head, indicating interest in finding the breast.[1] Guided by the scent of breastmilk and other mysterious knowledge the newborn travels toward the breast. Once there, the newborn opens their mouth and bobs her way onto the nipple, adjusting as necessary, latches on and impresses the mother with their strength, power, and innate knowledge.[2] The first 1.5–2 hours after the birth have been referred to as the "golden hour" or the "magical hour" during which the newborn cries, relaxes, awakens, and begins the breast crawl.[3] For the birthing person, the third stage of labor represents the final act of pregnancy—giving birth to the placenta—and an enormous shift within the body and psyche from the task of maintaining the pregnancy to taking on the complex new role of motherhood/parenthood. As the uterus contracts to expel the placenta, a cocktail of hormones floods the body to give their what she needs to make the shift.[4] The fourth stage, beginning after the birth of the placenta, and lasting for 1–2 hours, is sometimes referred to as the "recovery" or "stabilization" stage for the mother. It is inappropriate to discuss the fourth stage in terms of only the birthing person or the baby, because as with all other mammals, the two are thoroughly or other family members entwined and mutually dependent. With today's customary involvement in birth by the father, partner, or significant or other family members, the fourth stage also includes other family members.

Oxytocin, which began to surge during the baby's journey down the birth canal, is at high levels, endorphins are flowing, and these combine to give "high" spirits and feelings of love and gratefulness.[4] These hormones also help override the fatigue, pain, and discouragement felt earlier during the labor.

With baby in the mother/parent's arms, a mutually beneficial relationship occurs. Not only does the mother/birthing person provide everything the baby needs at this time, but the baby reciprocates by enhancing involution, successful breastfeeding, and attachment. The baby squirming on the mother/parent's abdomen stimulates the uterus to contract and expel the placenta. Once the baby begins nuzzling and suckling at the breast, oxytocin flows, contracting the uterus, increasing feelings of joy and love, and stimulating the pituitary gland to secrete prolactin, the key to the production of breastmilk.[4]

This ideal scenario for third and fourth stages, however, presents a challenge for the nurse, midwife, or doctor—to preserve a calm, peaceful, private environment, while remaining watchful and cautious. The caregiver and nurse assess and monitor the dyad calmly and unobtrusively, and cannot be swept up in the emotions of joy and relief. The caregivers know the importance of the third and fourth stages to the wellbeing of mother and baby and remain vigilant for problems that may require quick action. These concerns sometimes dominate and lead to practices that interrupt the normal maternal–infant tasks of third and fourth stages. If the delicate hormonal interaction and mutual regulation between baby and mother/birthing person are postponed, rushed, disturbed, altered with medications, or interrupted by surgery, they may not resume as smoothly later, when the delay is over. A difficult childbirth may put the birthing person at risk of postpartum PTSD.[5] Disruptions in the early postpartum time increase the chance of emotional stress for mother/parent and baby, may lead to more crying by the baby, temperature drops in the baby, less uterine muscle tone, challenges in the initiation of breastfeeding, and increased need for medical interventions. Further, there is a relationship between breastfeeding and postpartum depression, and difficulty initiating breastfeeding may increase the birthing person's chance of postpartum depression.[6,7]

In this chapter, we describe common third and fourth stage labor care practices, with a critical examination of common practices and suggestions for alternative approaches that help to foster the mother–infant dyad and family interactions described above. Topics to be discussed include routine intrapartum oral and nasal suctioning, management of the umbilical cord, evidence-based third stage management approaches, microbial health of the infant, and fostering uninterrupted maternal–newborn contact and breastfeeding.

THIRD STAGE MANAGEMENT: CARE OF THE BABY

Oral and nasopharynx suctioning

Over millennia, during the birth process, the fetal chest has been compressed tightly as it passes through the vagina, providing pressure that helps to clear amniotic fluid and mucus from the respiratory passages. For decades, babies have had their noses and mouths suctioned during the birth process in order to clear them of amniotic fluid and secretions. However, there is no evidence that routine suctioning of the oral cavity and nasopharynx of the neonate prior to delivery of the shoulders is necessary, nor does it improve neonatal outcomes.[8,9] In fact, routine intrapartum suctioning may lead to instability in neonatal breathing, heart rate, and oxygen saturation.[8,9] Just as suctioning prior to birth is unnecessary and potentially harmful, the routine of bulb suctioning a vigorous newborn's nose and mouth immediately following birth has no known benefits, since healthy newborns can usually clear their own airways. Kelleher and colleagues[10] conducted a randomized trial of 503 infants to compare the outcomes of bulb suctioning with gentle wiping of the face, nose, and mouth. The researchers found that the practice of face wiping led to equivalent outcomes in normal newborns.

Historically, birth attendants have used various strategies to deeply suction babies born with meconium stained amniotic fluid, but this is no longer recommended as a routine.[11] Randomized controlled trials have shown that suctioning term newborns with meconium stained amniotic fluid does not prevent meconium aspiration syndrome nor does it improve neonatal outcomes.[12] Vigorous newborns should receive routine care and observation. Depressed infants are immediately placed in the radiant warmer, and carefully evaluated for resuscitation needs.[11] When thick meconium fluid is present, a professional trained in endotracheal intubation should be in attendance at birth. However, routine endotracheal intubation to assess for meconium is not recommended for vigorous infants.[11] Instead oral and nasopharynx bulb suctioning to clear meconium fluid prior to the initiation of resuscitation measures is recommended.[11]

Delayed clamping and cutting of the umbilical cord

In the past, clamping and cutting the umbilical cord happened routinely within 10–15 seconds after the birth. Scientific evidence now shows that delayed clamping and cutting of the umbilical cord is beneficial and standard practice. What is unknown is optimal time when the cord should be cut and clamped, with recommendations varying from delaying for 60 seconds, 2–3 minutes, five minutes, and up to the time when the umbilical stops pulsing and appears white and blanched. The World Health Organization[13] recommends clamping the cord any time after 60 seconds up to the point at which the umbilical cord stops pulsing. Both term and preterm neonates benefit significantly from delayed cord clamping and it is not associated with adverse outcomes.[14–16] Further, compared with immediate cord clamping, DC lowered the odds of neonatal morality for preterm newborns.[17]

After the birth of a full-term infant, approximately 30% of the fetal-placental blood remains in the placenta. Immediate cord clamping robs the baby of this iron-rich blood supply.[14] Delaying clamping (DC) of the umbilical cord allows the placental blood to transfer to the infant. For a 3-kg newborn, this amounts to 50–85 mL of whole blood[15] that contains red blood cells (RBCs), iron, and stem cells.[14] With DC the infant receives 15 mL/kg of RBCs; with iron sufficient to be protective against the development of anemia during the first 6 months of life.[15,18] DC facilitates physiologic transitioning to extrauterine life through optimal perfusion of vital organs and appears to reduce inflammation and risk for infection in vulnerable infants.[14,15] Furthermore, one randomized controlled trial showed continued benefit of delayed cord clamping at four months of life, with newborns in the delayed cord clamping groups showing higher levels of ferritin and increased brain myelination.[19]

A healthy term infant can be placed immediately on the mother/parents' abdomen, cared for, and assessed while maintaining skin-to-skin contact.[11] The birth attendant can easily assess the neonatal heart rate by palpating the pulse off the cord, and can evaluate when it stops pulsating. While the neonate is skin-to-skin (>10 cm above the level of the placenta), it takes approximately 5 minutes for the neonate to receive all the placental blood.[14]

Researchers systematically reviewed 15 randomized clinical trials of early versus late cord clamping in term infants to study maternal and neonatal outcomes.[18] Delayed cord clamping did not significantly impact the incidence of postpartum hemorrhage or amount of blood loss in the birthing person.[18] The analysis of neonatal outcomes revealed that there were no significant differences in neonatal mortality, Apgar scores, or admissions to neonatal intensive care units between groups. Infants born to mothers in the DC group were significantly heavier than those whose cords were clamped immediately (101 g increase; 95% CI 45–157; random-effects model; 12 trials; 3139 infants; I2 62%). Seven clinical trials (including a total of 2324 infants) assessed phototherapy as an outcome. Although the diagnosis of clinical jaundice was not significantly different between groups (2098 infants; RR 0.84; 95% CI 0.66–1.07), more infants in the DC group required phototherapy than those in the immediate cord clamping group (RR 0.62; 95% C0.41 to 0.96).[18] In the five trials that studied polycythemia as an outcome, there was no difference between groups (RR 0.39; 95% CI 0.12–1.27; 1025 infants). However, hemoglobin concentrations at 24 and 48 hours were significantly lower in the early cord clamping group infants (MD−1.49 g/dL; 95% CI−1.78 to−1.21). Five studies could be analyzed for the outcome of infant anemia. Late clamping resulted in improved infant iron stores as it significantly reduced the likelihood of iron deficiency (average RR 2.65; 95% CI 1.04–6.73). The authors recommended more use of delayed cord clamping as long as phototherapy is available.[18] This recommendation remains controversial. Experts in delayed cord clamping criticized that the relationship in the systematic review between delayed cord clamping and hyperbilirubinemia was based on the inclusion of a trial that was not peer reviewed or blinded and was therefore unsubstantiated.

The American College of Obstetrics and Gynecology (ACOG) committee opinion[20] endorsed by the American Academy of Pediatrics supports the practice of delayed cord clamping in both term and preterm infants for 30–60 seconds because of the documented benefit, including improved transitional circulation and red blood cell volume, less need for blood transfusion, and less incidence of both necrotizing enterocolitis and intravascular hemorrhage.[20]

The 7th edition of the Neonatal Resuscitation Guidelines and the 2020 update includes delayed cord clamping for at least 30–60 seconds in vigorous term and preterm newborns,[11] AAP 2020 https://www.aappublications.org/news/2020/10/21/nrp102120. Further, the authors of the WHO guidelines consider that the benefits of delayed cord clamping outweigh the risks (bilirubin level requiring phototherapy).[21,22]

When a newborn is pale or slightly cyanotic following a tight nuchal cord, the baby can be held at a level lower than the perineum for 30 seconds to 1 minute (in order to maximize the blood that is transfused), then placed on the mother's abdomen while cord clamping is delayed for at least a total of 3 minutes.[23] This strategy promotes optimal transition to extrauterine life and can improve the color and the tone of neonates who are otherwise healthy at birth. Although the WHO guidelines[21] did not specify, initial newborn resuscitation with an intact cord can be done on a flat surface near the mother/parent, for example, on the bed between the mother/parent legs.[24] A mobile trolley (cart) has been developed to allow newborn resuscitation to occur at the mother's bedside (within 50 cm of her perineum) while maintaining an intact cord.[25] An assessment of the use of the resuscitation trolley during 78 births of neonates born at 24–41 weeks gestation found that the trolley allowed the use of the full range of resuscitation procedures while maintaining neonatal temperature.[26] The trolley was not useful in 18 cases where the umbilical cord was too short for the infant to reach the trolley. One trial of 60 neonates who received resuscitation with the cord intact found that while parents were comfortable with it, although some providers expressed concerns about access to the infant.[27] Research continues to be ongoing, and one recent trial successfully implemented a mobile resuscitation cart for use during operative vaginal deliveries, eliminating all cases of early cord clamping in their setting.[28] Additional studies optimizing the practice of neonatal resuscitation with the umbilical cord intact are ongoing.[29]

Umbilical cord milking is a strategy that has been suggested for both term and preterm infants in the event that delayed cording clamping is not possible. The midwife or physician gently "milks" the umbilical cord toward the baby 3–4 times before it is clamped.[30] Cord milking achieves transfer of placental blood similar to that of DC, but the transfer occurs in 30 seconds or less.[14] Umbilical cord milking can be safely done in term and late preterm neonates.[31] However, for very preterm infants one systematic review and meta-analysis found that umbilical cord milking increased the risk of intraventricular hemorrhage.[32] No adverse outcomes have been reported with umbilical cord milking for term infants. Therefore, cord milking can be used during cesarean birth or rapidly before the cord is cut for a term or late preterm infant who needs to be passed to care providers for resuscitation but should not be used for very preterm infants.[14,15]

THIRD STAGE MANAGEMENT: THE PLACENTA

The third stage of labor begins following the birth of the baby and ends with delivery of the placenta. Placental separation follows a predictable pattern. Initially strong contractions lead to thickening of the uterus, which results in shearing off, eventual separation from the uterine wall, and finally, expulsion of the placenta.[33] The signs of placental separation include: (a) the uterus rising in the maternal abdomen; (b) the uterus changing shape from discoid to globular; (c) the umbilical cord lengthening; and (d) a small gush of blood flowing from the mother's vagina. Recognition of placental separation is important to appropriate management. The average duration of the third stage of labor is 10 minutes, with only 3% of births having a third stage longer than 30 minutes.[34] The risk of postpartum hemorrhage increases when the third stage of labor duration is longer than 30 minutes.[34]

During the third stage of labor, most birth attendants use one of two approaches to provide care—active management or expectant management. However, some practitioners use a combination of both approaches.[34,35]

Physiologic (expectant) management of the third stage of labor

Physiologic management (also called expectant management) of the third stage of labor allows the placenta to deliver spontaneously without the routine administration of oxytocic medications. However, there are variations in definitions between sources.[35] Birth attendants who use expectant management await the signs of placental separation. Once these signs have occurred, however, some birth attendants guard the uterus (Fig. 9.1) and use gentle traction to deliver the placenta; others await completely spontaneous placental delivery aided by gravity. Although physiologic management is congruent with the non-interference philosophy held by most midwives and some low-intervention doctors,[36] it has not been adequately studied with a population of women at low risk for postpartum hemorrhage, using the criteria for low risk that have been defined by midwives.[35] The following are criteria for the midwifery designation of low risk; all criteria must be present:

1. Good maternal health and nutrition.
2. Single baby at term.
3. Maternal/birthing person desire for spontaneous placental birth, active participation in the process, prolonged skin-to-skin contact, and early breastfeeding.
4. A trusting relationship with the birth attendant.
5. An informed and supportive birth team.
6. An environment where the birthing person feels safe.
7. A midwife who is skilled in physiologic management.
8. Normal pregnancy, first and second stages.
9. A healthy infant.
10. Birthgiver's willingness to accept uterotonic medications if indicated.[35]

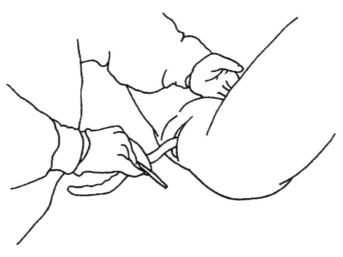

Fig. 9.1.   Guarding the uterus.

The midwifery criteria (coined as "psycho-physiologic management"[37]) that define birthing people as low risk for postpartum hemorrhage are more stringent than the obstetric criteria used to define low risk; midwifery criteria include additional psychological and environmental factors. The trials that compared expectant management with active management of third stage included birthing who met the obstetric criteria for low risk. However, if the midwifery criteria listed above had been used instead, many of these birthing people would have been identified as high risk. Most existing randomized trials have found that expectant management is associated with greater blood loss and a higher incidence of immediate postpartum hemorrhage compared to an active management approach to third stage care.[35] Because scientific evidence supporting expectant management for low-risk laboring people is limited,[35,38] all birth attendants have been encouraged to adopt active third stage management.[21,39] This topic has remained controversial among midwives and low-intervention physicians. Clearly, randomized controlled trials comparing "psycho-physiologic" management with active management of third stage are sorely needed.

Active management of the third stage of labor

Active management of the third stage has been promoted worldwide for decades to shorten the third stage and prevent maternal hemorrhage, a leading cause of maternal death especially in low-resource areas.[40] Numerous organizations have published guidelines that include Active Management of Third Stage (AMTS) labor to prevent postpartum hemorrhage.[21,41,43] Current evidence-based recommendations for active management of the third stage include three components: 1) Prophylactic oxytocin (or uterotonic agent) 2) Delayed cord clamping, and 3) Controlled cord traction (CCT).[44] Prophylactic oxytocin and controlled cord traction are associated with decreased postpartum blood loss.[44]

A Cochrane review by Begley and colleagues[40] concludes that while studies favor active management of the third stage over physiologic management for the prevention of postpartum hemorrhage, the evidence is low quality, and more studies are needed. Numerous organizations have published guidelines that include Active Management of Third Stage (AMTS) labor to prevent postpartum hemorrhage.[23,41–43]

CCT reduces the risk of manual removal of the placenta and may be offered routinely by skilled birth attendants.[45] CCT is appropriate once the signs of placental separation have occurred. Overly vigorous CCT may lead to cord evulsion or life-threatening uterine inversion.[34] CCT is not necessary if the birthing person is upright or in a squatting position.[34] Guarding of the uterus (Fig. 9.1) is a technique that can be used to safely perform CCT. Birthing people who hope to avoid CCT may safely do so if a uterotonic agent is used; however, they may be at higher risk for manual removal of the placenta.[45]

Although routinely done during the third stage of labor, the evidence on uterine massage to prevent postpartum hemorrhage is limited.[44] Uterine massage is recommended only after placental delivery[43] and especially if uterotonic medications are not used. There appears to be no or limited benefit to uterine massage when oxytocin is used (Abdel-Aleem et al., 2010). The authors of a Cochrane review reported inconclusive findings concerning the independent value of uterine massage, because the women in the two trials included all received uterotonic medications as part of third stage management.[46] The authors did not recommend a change in practice based on their findings but described the need for more research. Uterine massage before separation of the placenta is a dangerous practice that can lead to partial separation of the placenta and an increased risk of postpartum hemorrhage.[34]

One critical AMTS feature that has consistently been promoted in all birth settings is the prophylactic administration of a uterotonic medication.[21,42,43] Drugs commonly used in active management of the third stage include synthetic oxytocin (e.g., Pitocin), Ergot alkaloids such as methylergonovine maleate (Methergine), misoprostol (Cytotec), Carbetocin, and tranexamic acid. Each of these agents plays a role in preventing postpartum hemorrhage by stimulating uterine contractions.

Synthetic oxytocin is recommended as first-line postpartum hemorrhage prophylaxis in a number of international postpartum hemorrhage prevention guidelines and is associated with less postpartum blood loss.[21,41–47] Synthetic oxytocin can be administered intramuscularly or diluted in an intravenous solution. Synthetic oxytocin may not be as effective for birthing people who have undergone a long induction of labor using oxytocin, and a different uterotonic agent may be considered.[34] Intravenous administration of oxytocin is more effective than intramuscular administration at preventing postpartum hemorrhage.[48] Recently evidence has suggested that the use of two uterotonic agents, such as oxytocin plus misoprostol or oxytocin plus tranexamic acid, may be more effective than oxytocin alone but also may increase side effects.[49] All of the uterotonic agents above have been found to be superior to no treatment for the prevention of postpartum hemorrhage.[49] Additionally, the antifibrinolytic age tranexamic acid has been given prophylactically and found to reduce the risk of postpartum hemorrhage.[50]

If synthetic oxytocin is unavailable, birth attendants in low-resource areas are encouraged to use misoprostol.[51] Several studies indicate that misoprostol is equally effective as synthetic oxytocin[52] and methergine[53] with the added benefits of low cost and administration that requires no needles and no refrigeration. However, misoprostol has side effects, including shivering and the development of a transient fever, found to be unacceptable to women who had received it.[54] While misoprostol has potential to reduce postpartum hemorrhage in developing countries,[53] the World Health Organization[21] guideline for hemorrhage prevention contains a recommendation that oxytocin be administered by skilled birth attendants prophylactically and in preference to misoprostol. Therefore, careful selection of appropriate uterotonics requires continuing critical evaluation of the current literature as well as weighing the risks and benefits of the available options.

The exact optimal timing of the administration of uterotonics as a part of active management is unclear.[42] However, birth attendants who delay cord clamping also delay the administration of medication until the cord is clamped and cut. A Cochrane review was conducted to address the issue of optimal timing of prophylactic uterotonics.[55] Findings from three clinical trials that included 1671 birthing people were included in the systematic review. The main uterotonic used in the trials was intravenous oxytocin. Although more research is needed, the authors concluded that the timing of the prophylactic uterotonic administration (after the birth of the anterior shoulder, after the birth of the neonate, or after the delivery of the placenta) did not have a significant impact on third stage labor outcomes such as incidence of postpartum hemorrhage, retained placenta, or length of third stage labor. Since the newer guidelines on the prevention of postpartum hemorrhage include a provision for delayed cord clamping, and evidence supports this practice, a delay in the administration of uterotonics until after the cord is clamped and cut does not appear to increase the risk of postpartum hemorrhage.

All skilled birth attendants should be well prepared to manage postpartum hemorrhage. The reported incidence of postpartum hemorrhage is 5–15%, with variation between sources and populations.[41] Birthing people who have large babies, long labors, a history of postpartum hemorrhage, multiple gestation, or a history of five or more births are at higher risk.[56] However, risk factors do not adequately predict those birthing people who will actually experience postpartum hemorrhages (Anderson and Etches, 2007).[56] Therefore, the international focus on postpartum hemorrhage prevention as previously described is an essential public health initiative to reduce maternal morbidity. Uterine atony accounts for approximately 80% of postpartum hemorrhages, followed by lacerations, infection, retained placental tissue, subinvolution, and coagulopathies.[34]

While synthetic oxytocin is the typical first-line prophylactic uterotonic, during a postpartum hemorrhage the birth attendant may ask for the following depending on the setting: help; a large-bore intravenous line if one is not in place; additional uterotonic agent plus tranexamic acid and use of vigorous uterine massage. If these strategies do not succeed in contracting the uterus, the birth attendant will compress the uterus between both hands (bimanual compression; Fig. 9.2). A combination of the administration of uterotonic medications and bimanual compresses is successful in most cases of postpartum hemorrhage management.[34,43] Careful examination of the placenta for completeness and of the cervix, vagina, and perineum for lacerations and/or hematomas is essential in the management of postpartum hemorrhage. The "Four Ts" mnemonic (Tone, Trauma, Tissue, and Thrombin) is used to assist birth attendants to find the cause of the hemorrhage in order to direct appropriate management.[34,43] Some or all of the uterotonic medications previously described may be used in sequence, including the final addition of another prostaglandin agent (carboprost tromethamine [Hemabate]) to stop the bleeding.[34,43] While this agent has unpleasant side effects for the birthing person, such as nausea, vomiting, and diarrhea, administration can be a lifesaving measure. Aortic compression is a life-saving skill when hemorrhage is unrelenting.[43] Skilled birth attendants are encouraged to review this technique. In low-resource settings the use of non-pneumatic

9

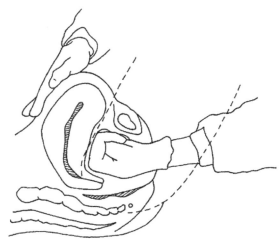

Fig. 9.2.   Bimanual compression.

anti-shock (when available) can save the lives of birthing people who experience severe hypovolemic shock during or following a postpartum hemorrhage.[43]

The management of a hemorrhage can be frightening for the person and their family. The doula can support the birthing person and their family during the sometimes painful procedures required to achieve resolution.

THE FOURTH STAGE OF LABOR

The "fourth stage of labor" refers to the time from birth of the placenta through the first one or two postpartum hours. Most definitions focus on the birthing person—stabilization of vital signs, control of bleeding, repair of any lacerations, and evidence of the beginnings of involution. However, in keeping with the description of the fourth stage that introduces this chapter, our definition includes family integration. The fourth stage is not complete until birthing parent and baby are together, preferably skin to skin and breastfeeding or chest feeding, and "ready to adjust together to their new roles in continuing the lifecycle of the [person] and the family."[57] In other words, rather than stating a specific time frame for fourth stage, we suggest specific processes of the dyad—both birthing parent and baby—as defining criteria.

Keeping the mother and baby together Klaus, Kennell, and colleagues[58] first suggested that birthing people and their infants benefit from being together during the first hour after birth, in terms of parent– infant attachment. Over several decades, they further developed their concept of the "sensitive period" lasting about 1 hour after birth.[59] Their work was pivotal in highlighting the third and fourth stages as times when feelings of love and attachment develop. Furthermore, parent–baby contact fosters other outcomes such as neonatal adaptation, breastfeeding, and maternal recovery. A Cochrane systematic review of 46 randomized controlled trials from 21 different countries (38 trials contributed data) of early skin-to-skin contact (SSC) has confirmed numerous benefits on both mother and baby.[60] Yet, even though many hospitals have established protocols that allow or encourage early maternal–infant contact immediately and for hours afterward, a large American survey of birthing people's experiences during birth found that only 58% reported having their babies in their arms during the first hour after birth and 60% said the baby "roomed in" with them during the hospital stay.[61] Although clear guidance from the World Health Organization recommends immediate SSC, one systematic review evaluation practices in 28 countries found the practice varied greatly, from 1 to 98% of the time, depending on location.[62]

Currently, in hospitals that are committed to keeping the parent–newborn dyad together, initial third and fourth stage management practices include drying the baby and placing the baby directly on the birthing person's bare abdomen or chest, with the umbilical cord still attached and pulsating. Both the birthing person and baby are covered with a prewarmed blanket. This SSC is considered an important component of the initiation of breast-feeding. The specific benefits of early SSC include the following: more successful first feeding, and longer duration (in months) of breastfeeding; and improved neonatal stability.[60] SSC was not associated with any negative outcomes.

The baby's temperature is stabilized by SSC with the birthing parent in a manner that is superior to that of the electronic radiant warmers.[8] Based on the evidence, there appears to be no rationale for using the radiant warmer instead of SSC. The 7th edition NRP Guidelines include SSC.[11]

The term "kangaroo care" (KC) refers to a practice where low-birth-weight neonates are given early and prolonged SSC between the breasts of their birthing parent/mother. When compared with conventional neo-natal care, a Cochrane Systematic Review found that KC is associated with improved outcomes, such as lower mortality and reduced risk of infections, hypothermia, severe illness, and length of hospital stay.[63] In addition, KC increased growth, breastfeeding, and parent satisfaction with their care.[63] For infant who are premature and low-birth weight, one randomized control trial conducted in five countries—Ghana, India, Malawi, Nigeria, and Tanzania—found an increase in survival for those who received KC.[64] Furthermore, KC has great appeal to worried parents of premature babies who feel helpless.[63] Holding their babies skin to skin may be important for attachment and a sense of being capable of nurturing their babies. The involvement they feel and the opportunity to know their babies well are worth making the practice commonplace, even if there were no other benefits. In fact, many believe that KC should be the standard method of care for all newborn babies, both low birth weight and full term.[65]

BABY-FRIENDLY (BREASTFEEDING) PRACTICES

Globally, the World Health Organization estimates that 3 out of 5 babies are not breastfed in the first hour of life.[66] The World Health Organization's Baby-Friendly Initiative, revised in 2018, encourages all birthing people to be offered assistance breast/chest-feeding within the first 30 minutes of birth.[67] Instinctual infant suckling behaviors manifest in a predictable pattern within the first hour of life.[67] The initiation of breastfeeding promotes uterine contractility and therefore placental separation and expulsion. Breastfeeding stimulates the release of oxytocin from the posterior pituitary gland in the birthing person's brain. This hormone is also strongly associated with maternal/parental love.[4,59,68] Breastfeeding is a synergy between mother/parent and baby where both benefit physically and emotionally.

Table 9.1 contains the 10 steps to successful breastfeeding that are a part of the Baby-Friendly Initiative. These principles can guide healthcare providers and doulas while they support breastfeeding.

Newborns, placed in the middle of their mother/birthing parent's abdomen (nose at the level of the nipples), have the ability to move to find the nipple and initiate breastfeeding/chestfeeding rather independently.[69] This has been called the "breast crawl" and is being promoted internationally as a strategy to initiate and to encourage breastfeeding/chestfeeding.[65]. Infants born following unmedicated births have more coordinated suckling activity during the breast crawl than those born to mothers who have received analgesics.[70] The breast crawl benefits the mother by enhancing placental expulsion and reducing postpartum blood loss.[71] This occurs mechanically, as the newborn kicks their legs and stimulates uterine contractions, and also hormonally, as the stimulation to the nipples releases oxytocin into the maternal/birthing parent's circulation. Therefore, this instinctual breastfeeding behavior benefits both the birthing person and the newborn and sets the stage for successful breastfeeding or chestfeeding.

Immediate newborn bathing disrupts skin-to-skin time, the initiation of breastfeeding, and removes the protective vernix and healthy microbes on the neonate's skin. The World Health Organization recommends delaying bathing for 24 hours.[21] If this is not possible for cultural reasons, WHO recommends a delay of at least 6 hours. A policy of "wait for 8" has been initiated in some settings.[73] Preer et al. studied the impact of a policy of a 12-hour delay in newborn bathing and breastfeeding initiation using a retrospective chart review that included 702 newborns.[74] Prior to the policy change, newborns were bathed at an average of 2.4 hours after birth; after the policy change, the time of the first bath averaged 13.5 hours after birth. Delayed bathing was associated with a significant increase in breastfeeding initiation and increased in-hospital breastfeeding rates.

Table 9.1.   Ten steps to successful breast/chest feeding.

Every facility providing maternity services and care for newborn infants should enact the following:

Critical management procedures:

1a. Comply fully with the *International Code of Marketing of Breast-milk Substitutes* and relevant World Health Assembly resolutions.

1b. Have a written infant feeding policy that is routinely communicated to staff and parents.

1c. Establish ongoing monitoring and data-management systems.

2. Ensure that staff have sufficient knowledge, competence and skills to support breastfeeding.

Key clinical practices:

3. Discuss the importance and management of breastfeeding with pregnant women and their families.

4. Facilitate immediate and uninterrupted skin-to-skin contact and support mothers to initiate breastfeeding as soon as possible after birth.

5. Support mothers to initiate and maintain breastfeeding and manage common difficulties.

6. Do not provide breastfed newborns any food or fluids other than breast milk, unless medically indicated.

7. Enable mothers and their infants to remain together and to practise rooming-in 24 hours a day.

8. Support mothers to recognize and respond to their infants' cues for feeding.

9. Counsel mothers on the use and risks of feeding bottles, teats and pacifiers.

10. Coordinate discharge so that parents and their infants have timely access to ongoing support and care.

According to the WHO, "There is substantial evidence that implementing the Ten Steps significantly improves breastfeeding rates."[67] The practice is supported by a systematic review of 58 studies.[72]

Ten Steps to Successful Breastfeeding is a summary of the guidelines for maternity care facilities presented in the joint WHO/UNICEF statement "Protecting, promoting and supporting breastfeeding in facilities providing maternity and newborn services: the revised Baby-friendly Hospital initiative[67] which have been accepted as the minimum global criteria for attaining the status of a Baby-Friendly Hospital."
Source: WHO/https://www.who.int/publications/i/item/9789241513807/last accessed February 22, 2023. Reproduced with permission of WHO.

SUPPORTING MICROBIAL HEALTH OF THE INFANT

For decades hospital staff have made various attempts to keep the birth process as clean as possible, using enemas, perineal shaves, various soap scrubs, and sterile drapes. Following birth, the baby was quickly bathed to remove vernix and blood. These strategies are not evidence-based, and in places where they are still used, they should be abandoned. It is now understood that these practices are harmful.

Bacteria and other microbes form a large proportion of the cells in the human body.[75] There has been increasing interest in the microbial health of neonates, and scientific knowledge of the human microbiome is developing rapidly.

During pregnancy and through the process of normal vaginal birth, the baby is exposed to the bacterial communities of the birthing person.[76] Table 9.2 contains a glossary of microbiome terminology. The vaginal canal of healthy pregnant people is colonized with lactobacilli while the gastrointestinal tract is colonized with bifidobacteria.[76,77] Infants born vaginally to healthy pregnant people are colonized with these and other "commensal" or healthy microbes. Vaginal birth and breastfeeding/chestfeeding allow the infant maximal exposures to pioneer microbiota

Table 9.2.   Microbiome glossary.

Term	Definition
Probiotic	Live microorganisms
	Can be ingested in amounts sufficient to produce a health effect[79]
	Lactobacillus and *Bifidobacterium* are two common types of probiotic bacteria
Prebiotic	Not living organisms; food for the probiotic bacteria
Symbiotic	Probiotic and prebiotic microorganisms that live together and are interdependent
Pioneer microbiota	Bacteria that initially colonize the newborn

Source: Sousa E Silva and Freitas.[75] Reproduced with permission of Taylor & Francis.

Table 9.3. Microbe-challenging and microbe-friendly practices.

Practice/event	Microbe-challenging practices and event	Microbe-friendly practices and event
Gestational age	Premature birth	Full term
Labor practices	Multiple vaginal examinations	Limited vaginal exams
Mode of birth	Cesarean birth	Spontaneous labor resulting in vaginal birth
Medications	Antibiotics during labor or given to the neonate	No antibiotics
Care practices immediately after birth	Wrapped in hospital blanket Separated from parents (e.g., in nursery)	Immediate skin-to-skin contact with one or both parents; blankets from family's home used to cover baby
Bathing	Early (first few hours of life)	Delayed bathing for 24 hours and then only water, no soap
Feeding	Formula or glucose water	Breastmilk exclusively

that serve to activate the infant's immune system in preparation for the extrauterine environment[76]. Breastmilk is a symbiotic food, and has a microbiome that is uniquely beneficial to babies.[78] Breastfeeding/chestfeeding allows the baby to remain in physical contact with the mother/parent's skin and receives symbiotic breastmilk, which contains prebiotic sugars that nourish the microbes that are vital to the infant's developing immune system.

Intrapartum caregivers can make an impact on the microbial health of the newborn. Table 9.3 contains a summary of microbe-challenging and microbe-friendly practices.

The bacterial communities on the skin of infants born by cesarean reflect the hospital's microbiome rather than the mother's.[80] Unplanned cesareans have a slight microbiologic advantage over planned cesarean birth. Both cesarean- born and formula-fed infants experience a delay in the development of a mature microbiome. Studies have shown that infants born by cesarean have significantly more immune-related diseases such as type 1 diabetes, asthma, and allergic disorders.[76]

One innovative strategy known as "vaginal seeding" aimed at microbial restoration for cesarean-born neonates is currently hotly debated.[81,82]

One small study by Dominguez-Bello and colleagues[83] of 18 maternal infant dyads included 11 delivered by planned cesarean and 7 born vaginally showed that the microbial restoration was successful in the four cesarean-born infants who received the vaginal microbial transfer. The microbial composition of the intervention infants resembled that of vaginally born infants, particularly the predominance of Lactobacillus and Bacteroides at 1 and 2 weeks of life respectively. The benefits of microbial transfer persisted for 30 days, the duration of the study. The researchers confirmed that the mode of birth shapes the infant's microbiome.[83] However, another small randomized control trial found limited colonization and that the neonatal gut was not altered, and questioned the practice.[84] The ACOG recommends that vaginal seeding only be performed as a part of an approved research protocol.[20,85] The practice guideline further states that after informed consent, if a pregnant person decides to perform vaginal seeding themselves, they should be screened for Gonorrhea, Chlamydia, and Group B Streptococcus.

ROUTINE NEWBORN ASSESSMENTS

In many hospitals, a high priority is placed on efficiently completing a checklist of routine newborn assessments and procedures before uniting the birthing person and baby for extended time together. However, the WHO recommends a series of newborn care practices based on scientific evidence.[20] These guidelines include that breastfeeding should be initiated as soon as possible following birth, and that skin-to-skin contact be promoted during the first hour after birth for thermoregulation and to promote breastfeeding. WHO also recommends the administration of vitamin K after the first hour of life.

It is not necessary or advisable to separate the parent/mother and baby to provide adequate assessment and care. The midwife or nurse can observe the baby's initial transition with assessments of the baby's color, respirations, muscle tone, and pulse while the baby is in the birthing parent's arms and without the need for equipment. For example, the pulse of the baby is readily palpable on the umbilical cord or the stump of the cord if it was already clamped and cut. It is optimal if the immediate postpartum care of the newborn is discussed with the birth person and family prior to the birth to help them prepare to actively participate in optimal newborn transitioning.

Following this initial transition period and the initiation of breastfeeding or chestfeeding, numerous routine assessments and required procedures are performed and, when they take place in the radiant warmer can interfere with parent–infant interactions. In some countries, such as the United States, erythromycin ophthalmic ointment is administered to the infant to prevent neonatal conjunctivitis, and vitamin K injections are given to prevent hemorrhagic disease of the newborn. Last, the careful documentation of the baby's identification through the use of matching bands on both the parent and the infant requires significant nursing time.

For healthy newborns, all of these tasks can occur with the baby in the parent's arms and with minimal interference with parental interaction. Alternatively, another option is to postpone whatever tasks can be delayed to allow for SSC and the initiation of breastfeeding. Parents who wish to remain in constant contact with their newborn need to clearly communicate this to the staff. If there is no other option, the radiant warmers have wheels that allow them to be rolled next to the birthing bed. A doula can help parents with their desires regarding SSC and minimal separation from their babies by learning their preferences in advance and encouraging them to voice them early in a birth plan, during labor and again after the birth.

CONCLUSION

The third and fourth stages of labor are busy times in terms of care and observation of mother or birthparent and baby, yet they are also times of mutual regulation by the newborn and parent. The underlying basis of optimal care of the mother/birthing parent and newborn is continuous skin-to-skin contact (SSC), which fosters newborn adaptation, maternal recovery, and deep emotional connections within the family. Sensitive care at this time includes respect for the benefits of SSC and a belief by the staff in the importance of minimal disturbance combined with vigilant oversight.

REFERENCES

1. Henderson A. (2011) Understanding the breast crawl: Implications for nursing practice. *Nursing for Women's Health* 15(4), 296–307. doi: 10.1111/j.1751-486X.2011.01650.x

2. Widström AM, Lilja G, Aaltomaa-Michalias P, Dahllöf A, Lintula M, Nissen E. (2011) Newborn behaviour to locate the breast when skin-to-skin: A possible method for enabling early self-regulation. *Acta Paediatrica (Oslo, Norway 1992)* 100(1), 79–85. doi: 10.1111/j.1651-2227.2010.01983.x

3. Sharma D, Sharma P, Shastri S. (2017) Golden 60 minutes of newborn's life: Part 2: Term neonate. *The Journal of Maternal-fetal & Neonatal Medicine: The Official Journal of the European Association of Perinatal Medicine, the Federation of Asia and Oceania Perinatal Societies, the International Society of Perinatal Obstetricians* 30(22), 2728–2733. doi: 10.1080/14767058.2016.1261399

4. Buckley SJ. (2015) *Hormonal Physiology of Childbearing: Evidence and Implications for Women, Babies, and Maternity Care.* Washington, DC: Childbirth Connection Programs, National Partnership for Women and Families.

5. Grekin R, O'Hara MW. (2014) Prevalence and risk factors of postpartum posttraumatic stress disorder: A meta-analysis. *Clinical Psychology Review* 34(5), 389–401. doi: 10.1016/j.cpr.2014.05.003

6. Dennis CL, McQueen K. (2009) The relationship between infant-feeding outcomes and postpartum depression: A qualitative systematic review. *Pediatrics* 123(4), e736–e751. doi: 10.1542/peds.2008-1629

7. de Graaff LF, Honig A, van Pampus MG, Stramrood C. (2018) Preventing post-traumatic stress disorder following childbirth and traumatic birth experiences: a systematic review. *Acta Obstetricia et Gynecologica Scandinavica* 97(6), 648–656. doi: 10.1111/aogs.13291

8. Mercer JS, Erickson-Owens DA, Graves B, Haley MM. (2007) Evidence-based practices for the fetal to newborn transition. *Journal of Midwifery & Women's Health* 52(3), 262–272. doi: 10.1016/j.jmwh.2007.01.005

9. Velaphi S, Vidyasagar D. (2008) The pros and cons of suctioning at the perineum (intrapartum) and post-delivery with and without meconium. *Seminars in Fetal & Neonatal Medicine* 13(6), 375–382. doi: 10.1016/j.siny.2008.04.001

10. Kelleher J, Bhat R, Salas AA, Addis D, Mills EC, Mallick H, Tripathis A, Pruitt EP, Roane C, McNair T, Owen J, Ambalavanan N, Carlo WA. (2013) Oronasopharyngeal suction versus wiping of the mouth and nose at birth: A randomized equivalency trial. *Lancet (London, England)* 382(9889), 326–330. doi: 10.1016/S0140-6736(13)60775-8

11. Weiner GM, Zaichkin, J. (eds) (2016) *Textbook of Neonatal Resuscitation (NRP)*, 7th edn. Elk Grove Park: American Academy of Pediatrics and American Heart Association.

12. Vain NE, Szyld EG, Prudent LM, Wiswell TE, Aguilar AM, Vivas NI. (2004) Oropharyngeal and nasopharyngeal suctioning of meconium-stained neonates before delivery of their shoulders: Multicentre, randomised controlled trial. *Lancet (London, England)* 364(9434), 597–602. doi: 10.1016/S0140-6736(04)16852-9

13. World Health Organization. (2019) Optimal timing of cord clamping for the prevention of iron deficiency anaemia in infants. Retrieved from https://www.who.int/elena/titles/cord_clamping/en.

14. Mercer JS, Erickson-Owens DA. (2012) Rethinking placental transfusion and cord clamping issues. *The Journal of Perinatal & Neonatal Nursing* 26(3), 202–219. doi: 10.1097/JPN.0b013e31825d2d9a

15. Mercer JS, Erickson-Owens DA. (2014) Is it time to rethink cord management when resuscitation is needed? *Journal of Midwifery & Women's Health* 59(6), 635–644. doi: 10.1111/jmwh.12206

16. Rabe H, Gyte GM, Díaz-Rossello JL, Duley L. (2019) Effect of timing of umbilical cord clamping and other strategies to influence placental transfusion at preterm birth on maternal and infant outcomes. *The Cochrane Database of Systematic Reviews* 9(9), CD003248. doi: 10.1002/14651858.CD003248.pub4

17. Jasani B, Torgalkar R, Ye XY, Syed S, Shah PS. (2021) Association of umbilical cord management strategies with outcomes of preterm infants: A systematic review and network meta-analysis. *JAMA Pediatrics* 175(4), e210102. doi: 10.1001/jamapediatrics.2021.0102

18. McDonald SJ, Middleton P, Dowswell T, Morris PS. (2013) Effect of timing of umbilical cord clamping of term infants on maternal and neonatal outcomes. *The Cochrane Database of Systematic Reviews* 2013(7), CD004074. doi: 10.1002/14651858.CD004074.pub3

19. Mercer JS, Erickson-Owens DA, Deoni S, Dean DC, 3rd, Collins J, Parker AB, Wang M, Joelson S, Mercer EN, Padbury JF. (2018) Effects of delayed cord clamping on 4-Month ferritin levels, brain myelin content, and neurodevelopment: A randomized controlled trial. *The Journal of Pediatrics* 203, 266–272.e2. doi: 10.1016/j.jpeds.2018.06.006

20. American College of Obstetricians and Gynecologists, Committee on Obstetric Practice. (2017) Delayed umbilical cord clamping after birth. Committee Opinion No. 684. *Obstetrics & Gynecology* 129, e5–10.

21. World Health Organization. (2012) Guidelines on basic newborn resuscitation. Geneva: WHO. Retrieved from: http://apps.who.int/iris/bitstream/10665/75157/1/9789241503693_eng.pdf?ua=1 (accessed August 20, 2016).

22. WHO. (2014) *Guideline: Delayed Umbilical Cord Clamping for Improved Maternal and Infant Health and Nutrition Outcomes.* Geneva: World Health Organization. https://apps.who.int/iris/bitstream/handle/10665/148793/?sequence=1

23. Coggins M, Mercer J. (2009) Delayed cord clamping: Advantages for infants. *Nursing for Women's Health* 13(2), 132–139. doi: 10.1111/j.1751-486X.2009.01404.x

24. Evans A. (2011) Neonatal resuscitation with intact umbilical cord. *Midwifery Today with International Midwife* (102), 42–43. https://www.midwiferytoday.com/mt-articles/neonatal-resuscitation.

25. Weeks AD, Watt P, Yoxall CW, Gallagher A, Burleigh A, Bewley S, Heuchan AM, Duley L. (2015) Innovation in immediate neonatal care: Development of the Bedside Assessment, Stabilisation and Initial Cardiorespiratory Support (BASICS) trolley. *BMJ Innovations* 1(2), 53–58. doi: 10.1136/bmjinnov-2014-000017

26. Thomas MR, Yoxall CW, Weeks AD, Duley L. (2014) Providing newborn resuscitation at the mother's bedside: Assessing the safety, usability and acceptability of a mobile trolley. *BMC Pediatrics* 14, 135. doi: 10.1186/1471-2431-14-135

27. Katheria AC, Sorkhi SR, Hassen K, Faksh A, Ghorishi Z, Poeltler D. (2018) Acceptability of bedside resuscitation with intact umbilical cord to clinicians and patients' families in the United States. *Frontiers in Pediatrics* 6, 100. doi: 10.3389/fped.2018.00100

28. Sæther E, Gülpen FR, Jensen C, Myklebust TÅ, Eriksen BH. (2020) Neonatal transitional support with intact umbilical cord in assisted vaginal deliveries: A quality-improvement cohort study. *BMC Pregnancy and Childbirth* 20(1), 496. doi: 10.1186/s12884-020-03188-0

29. Katheria AC. (2019) Neonatal resuscitation with an intact cord: Current and ongoing trials. *Children (Basel, Switzerland)* 6(4), 60. doi: 10.3390/children6040060

30. Erickson-Owens DA, Mercer JS, Oh W. (2012) Umbilical cord milking in term infants delivered by cesarean section: A randomized controlled trial. *Journal of Perinatology: Official Journal of the California Perinatal Association* 32(8), 580–584. doi: 10.1038/jp.2011.159

31. Basile S, Pinelli S, Micelli E, Caretto M, Benedetti Panici P. (2019) Milking of the umbilical cord in term and late preterm infants. *BioMed Research International* 2019, 9185059. doi: 10.1155/2019/9185059

32. Balasubramanian H, Ananthan A, Jain V, Rao SC, Kabra N. (2020) Umbilical cord milking in preterm infants: A systematic review and meta-analysis. *Archives of Disease in Childhood. Fetal and Neonatal Edition* 105(6), 572–580. doi: 10.1136/archdischild-2019-318627

33. Herman A, Zimerman A, Arieli S, Tovbin Y, Bezer M, Bukovsky I, Panski M. (2002) Down-up sequential separation of the placenta. *Ultrasound in Obstetrics & Gynecology: The Official Journal of the International Society of Ultrasound in Obstetrics and Gynecology* 19(3), 278–281. doi: 10.1046/j.1469-0705.2002.00557.x

34. Schorn M. (2019) The third stage of labor. In: TL King, MC Brucker, K Osborne, CM Jevitt (eds), *Varney's Midwifery*, 6th edn. Burlington, MA: Jones & Bartlett Learning, pp. 1107–1126.

35. Fahy KM. (2009) Third stage labour care for women at low risk of postpartum hemorrhage. *Journal of Midwifery & Women's Health* 54(5), 380–386. doi: 10.1016/j.jmwh.2008.12.016

36. Tan WM, Klein MC, Saxell L, Shirkoohy SE, Asrat G. (2008) How do physicians and midwives manage the third stage of labor? *Birth (Berkeley, Calif.)* 35(3), 220–229. doi: 10.1111/j.1523-536X.2008.00243.x

37. Fahy K, Hastie C, Bisits A, Marsh C, Smith L, Saxton A. (2010) Holistic physiological care compared with active management of the third stage of labour for women at low risk of postpartum haemorrhage: A cohort study. *Women and Birth: Journal of the Australian College of Midwives* 23(4), 146–152. doi: 10.1016/j.wombi.2010.02003

38. Hastie C, Fahy KM. (2009) Optimising psychophysiology in third stage of labour: Theory applied to practice. *Women and Birth: Journal of the Australian College of Midwives* 22(3), 89–96. doi: 10.1016/j.wombi.2009.02.004

39. Evensen A, Anderson JM, Fontaine P. (2017) Postpartum hemorrhage: Prevention and treatment. *American Family Physician* 95(7), 442–449.

40. Begley CM, Gyte GM, Devane D, McGuire W, Weeks A, Biesty LM. (2019) Active versus expectant management for women in the third stage of labour; *The Cochrane Database of Systematic Reviews* 2(2), CD007412. doi: 10.1002/14651858.CD007412.pub5

41. Dahlke JD, Mendez-Figueroa H, Maggio L, Hauspurg AK, Sperling JD, Chauhan SP, Rouse DJ. (2015) Prevention and management of postpartum hemorrhage: A comparison of 4 national guidelines. *American Journal of Obstetrics and Gynecology* 213(1), 76.e1–76.e10. doi: 10.1016/j.ajog.2015.02.023

42. International Confederation of Midwives, & International Federation of Gynaecologists and Obstetricians. (2004) Joint statement: Management of the third stage of labour to prevent post-partum haemorrhage. *Journal of Midwifery & Women's Health* 49(1), 76–77. doi: 10.1016/j.jmwh.2003.11.005

43. Lalonde AB, Grellier R. (2012) FIGO saving mothers and newborns initiative 2006-2011. *International Journal of Gynaecology and Obstetrics: The Official Organ of the International Federation of Gynaecology and Obstetrics* 119(Suppl 1), S18–S21. doi: 10.1016/j.ijgo.2012.03.010.

44. Saccone G, Caissutti C, Ciardulli A, Abdel-Aleem H, Hofmeyr GJ, Berghella V. (2018) Uterine massage as part of active management of the third stage of labour for preventing postpartum haemorrhage during vaginal delivery: A systematic review and meta-analysis of randomised trials. *BJOG: An International Journal of Obstetrics and Gynaecology* 125(7), 778–781. doi: 10.1111/1471-0528.14923.

45. Hofmeyr GJ, Mshweshwe NT, Gülmezoglu AM. (2015) Controlled cord traction for the third stage of labour. *The Cochrane Database of Systematic Reviews* 1(1), CD008020. doi: 10.1002/14651858.CD008020.pub2.

46. Hofmeyr GJ, Abdel-Aleem H, Abdel-Aleem MA. (2013) Uterine massage for preventing postpartum haemorrhage. *The Cochrane Database of Systematic Reviews* (7), CD006431. doi: 10.1002/14651858.CD006431.pub3.

47. Salati JA, Leathersich SJ, Williams MJ, Cuthbert A, Tolosa JE. (2019) Prophylactic oxytocin for the third stage of labour to prevent postpartum haemorrhage. *The Cochrane Database of Systematic Reviews* 4(4), CD001808. doi: 10.1002/14651858.CD001808.pub3.

48. Oladapo OT, Okusanya BO, Abalos E. (2018) Intramuscular versus intravenous prophylactic oxytocin for the third stage of labour. *The Cochrane Database of Systematic Reviews* 9(9), CD009332. doi: 10.1002/14651858.CD009332.pub3.

49. Gallos ID, Papadopoulou A, Man R, Athanasopoulos N, Tobias A, Price MJ, Williams MJ, Diaz V, Pasquale J, Chamillard M, Widmer M, Tunçalp Ö, Hofmeyr GJ, Althabe F, Gülmezoglu AM, Vogel JP, Oladapo OT, Coomarasamy A. (2018)

9

Uterotonic agents for preventing postpartum haemorrhage: A network meta-analysis. *The Cochrane Database of Systematic Reviews* 7(12), CD011689. doi: 10.1002/14651858.CD011689.pub3

50. Saccone G, Della Corte L, D'Alessandro P, Ardino B, Carbone L, Raffone A, Guida M, Locci M, Zullo F, Berghella V. (2020) Prophylactic use of tranexamic acid after vaginal delivery reduces the risk of primary postpartum hemorrhage. *The Journal of Maternal-fetal & Neonatal Medicine: The Official Journal of the European Association of Perinatal Medicine, the Federation of Asia and Oceania Perinatal Societies, the International Society of Perinatal Obstetricians* 33(19), 3368–3376. doi: 10.1080/14767058.2019.1571576

51. International Federation of Obstetrics and Gynecology (FIGO). (2017) Misoprostol only recommended regimes. Retrieved from: https://www.figo.org/news/misoprostol-dosage-chart-2017

52. Kundodyiwa TW, Majoko F, Rusakaniko S. (2001) Misoprostol versus oxytocin in the third stage of labor. *International Journal of Gynaecology and Obstetrics: The Official Organ of the International Federation of Gynaecology and Obstetrics* 75(3), 235–241. doi: 10.1016/s0020-7292(01)00498-2

53. Garg P, Batra S, Gandhi G. (2005) Oral misoprostol versus injectable methylergometrine in management of the third stage of labor. *International Journal of Gynaecology and Obstetrics: The Official Organ of the International Federation of Gynaecology and Obstetrics* 91(2), 160–161. doi: 10.1016/j.ijgo.2005.07.005

54. McDonald S. (2007) Management of the third stage of labor. *Journal of Midwifery & Women's Health* 52(3), 254–261. doi: 10.1016/j.jmwh.2007.02.012

55. Soltani H, Hutchon DR, Poulose TA. (2010) Timing of prophylactic uterotonics for the third stage of labour after vaginal birth. *The Cochrane Database of Systematic Reviews* (8), 1465–1858. CD006173. doi: 10.1002/14651858.CD006173.pub2

56. Bair ME, Williams J (2007) Management of the third stage of labor. *Journal of Midwifery & Women's Health* 52(4), 412–414. doi: 10.1016/j.jmwh.2007.02.019

57. Gould D. (2000) Normal labour: A concept analysis. *Journal of Advanced Nursing* 31(2), 418–427. doi: 10.1046/j.1365-2648.2000.01281.x

58. Klaus MH, Jerauld R, Kreger NC, McAlpine W, Steffa M, Kennel JH. (1972) Maternal attachment. Importance of the first post-partum days. *The New England Journal of Medicine* 286(9), 460–463. doi: 10.1056/NEJM197203022860904

59. Klaus MH, Kennell JH. (2001) Care of the parents. In: MH Klaus, AA Fanaroff (eds), *Care of the High-Risk Neonate*, 5th edn. Philadelphia: Saunders, pp. 195–222.

60. Moore ER, Bergman N, Anderson GC, Medley N. (2016) Early skin-to-skin contact for mothers and their healthy newborn infants. *The Cochrane Database of Systematic Reviews* 11(11), CD003519. doi: 10.1002/14651858.CD003519.pub4

61. Declercq E, Sakala C, Corry M, Appelbaum S, Herrlich A. (2013) *Listening to 7 Mothers III: Pregnancy and Birth*. New York: Childbirth Connection.

62. Abdulghani N, Edvardsson K, Amir LH. (2018) Worldwide prevalence of mother-infant skin-to-skin contact after vaginal birth: A systematic review. *PloS One* 13(10), e0205696. doi: 10.1371/journal.pone.0205696

63. Conde-Agudelo A, Díaz-Rossello JL. (2014) Kangaroo mother care to reduce morbidity and mortality in low birthweight infants. *The Cochrane Database of Systematic Reviews* 7(4), CD002771. doi: 10.1002/14651858.CD002771.pub3

64. WHO Immediate KMC Study Group, Arya S, Naburi H, Kawaza K, Newton S, Anyabolu CH, Bergman N, Rao S, Mittal P, Assenga E, Gadama L, Larsen-Reindorf R, Kuti O, Linnér A, Yoshida S, Chopra N, Ngarina M, Msusa AT, Boakye-Yiadom A, Kuti BP, Massawe A. (2021) Immediate "Kangaroo Mother Care" and Survival of Infants with Low Birth Weight. *The New England Journal of Medicine* 384(21), 2028–2038. doi: 10.1056/NEJMoa2026486

65. Bergman J. (2011) The importance of skin-to-skin contact for every newborn. *Breastfeeding Today* 6, 4–6.

66. WHO. (2021) Health topics: Breastfeeding. Retrieved from: https://www.who.int/health-topics/breastfeeding#tab=tab_1 (accessed September 2, 2021).

67. WHO. (2018) *Ten steps to.* https://www.who.int/teams/nutrition-and-food-safety/food-and-nutrition-actions-in-health-systems/ten-steps-to-successful-breastfeeding

68. Uvnas-Moberg K. (2003) *The Oxytocin Factor: Tapping the Hormone of Calm, Love and Healing*. Cambridge, MA: Da Capa Press.

69. Varendi H, Porter RH, Winberg J. (1994) Does the newborn baby find the nipple by smell? *Lancet (London, England)* 344(8928), 989–990. doi: 10.1016/s0140-6736(94)91645-4

70. Brimdyr K, Cadwell K, Widström AM, Svensson K, Neumann M, Hart EA, Harrington S, Phillips R. (2015) The association between common labor drugs and suckling when skin-to-skin during the first hour after birth. *Birth (Berkeley, Calif.)* 42(4), 319–328. doi: 10.1111/birt.12186

71. Righard L, Alade MO. (1990) Effect of delivery room routines on success of first breast-feed. *Lancet (London, England)* 336(8723), 1105–1107. doi: 10.1016/0140-6736(90)92579-7

72. Pérez-Escamilla R, Martinez JL, Segura-Pérez S. (2016) Impact of the Baby-friendly Hospital Initiative on breastfeeding and child health outcomes: A systematic review. *Maternal & Child Nutrition* 12(3), 402–417. doi: 10.1111/mcn.12294

73. Lipka D, Schulz M. (2012) Wait for eight: Newborn bath delay. *Journal of Obstetric, Gynecologic & Neonatal Nursing* 41(Suppl.), S46–S47. doi: 10.1111/j.1552-6909.2012.01360.x

74. Preer G, Pisegna JM, Cook JT, Henri AM, Philipp BL. (2013) Delaying the bath and in-hospital breastfeeding rates. *Breastfeeding Medicine: The Official Journal of the Academy of Breastfeeding Medicine* 8(6), 485–490. doi: 10.1089/bfm.2012.0158

75. Sousa E Silva JP, Freitas, AC. (eds) (2014) *Probiotic Bacteria: Fundamentals, Therapy, and Technological Aspects.* Boca Raton, FL: Taylor & Francis Group, CRC Press.

76. Hanson L, Vandevusse L. (2013) The microbiology and immunology of normal physiologic birth: A plea for the nature of mother. *The Journal of Perinatal & Neonatal Nursing* 27(4), 278–280. doi: 10.1097/JPN.0b013e3182a9c996

77. VandeVusse L, Hanson L, Safdar N. (2013) Perinatal outcomes of prenatal probiotic and prebiotic administration: An integrative review. *The Journal of Perinatal & Neonatal Nursing* 27(4), 288–E2. doi: 10.1097/JPN.0b013e3182a1e15d

78. Lyons KE, Ryan CA, Dempsey EM, Ross RP, Stanton C. (2020) Breast milk, a source of beneficial microbes and associated benefits for infant health. *Nutrients* 12(4), 1039. doi: 10.3390/nu12041039

79. Food and Agriculture Organization of the United Nations & World Health Organization (FAO/WHO). (2001) Report on Joint FAO/WHO expert consultation on evaluation of health and nutritional properties of probiotics in food including powder milk with live lactic acid bacteria. Cordoba, Argentina: FAO/WHO. Retrieved from: http://www.fao.org/3/a-a0512e.pdf (accessed September 7, 2016).

80. Dominguez-Bello MG, Costello EK, Contreras M, Magris M, Hidalgo G, Fierer N, Knight R. (2010) Delivery mode shapes the acquisition and structure of the initial microbiota across multiple body habitats in newborns. *Proceedings of the National Academy of Sciences of the United States of America* 107(26), 11971–11975. doi: 10.1073/pnas.1002601107

81. Limaye MA, Ratner AJ. (2020) 'Vaginal seeding' after a caesarean section provides benefits to newborn children: AGAINST: Vaginal microbiome transfer - a medical procedure with clear risks and uncertain benefits. *BJOG : An International Journal of Obstetrics and Gynaecology* 127(2), 302. doi: 10.1111/1471-0528.15977

82. Mueller NT, Dominguez-Bello MG, Appel LJ, Hourigan SK. (2020) 'Vaginal seeding' after a caesarean section provides benefits to newborn children: FOR: Does exposing caesarean-delivered newborns to the vaginal microbiome affect their chronic disease risk? The critical need for trials of 'vaginal seeding' during caesarean section. *BJOG : An International Journal of Obstetrics and Gynaecology* 127(2), 301. doi: 10.1111/1471-0528.15979

83. Dominguez-Bello MG, De Jesus-Laboy KM, Shen N, Cox LM, Amir A, Gonzalez A, Bokulich NA, Song SJ, Hoashi M, Rivera-Vinas JI, Mendez K, Knight R, Clemente JC. (2016) Partial restoration of the microbiota of cesarean-born infants via vaginal microbial transfer. *Nature Medicine* 22(3), 250–253. doi: 10.1038/nm.4039

84. Wilson BC, Butler ÉM, Grigg CP, Derraik J, Chiavaroli V, Walker N, Thampi S, Creagh C, Reynolds AJ, Vatanen T, O'Sullivan JM, Cutfield WS. (2021) Oral administration of maternal vaginal microbes at birth to restore gut microbiome development in infants born by caesarean section: A pilot randomised placebo-controlled trial. *EBioMedicine* 69, 103443. doi: 10.1016/j.ebiom.2021.103443

85. Vaginal seeding. (2017) Committee Opinion No. 725. American College of Obstetricians and Gynecologists. *Obstetrics and Gynecology* 130, e274–8.

Chapter 10

Epidural and Other Forms of Neuraxial Analgesia for Labor: Review of Effects, with Emphasis on Preventing Dystocia

Sharon Muza, BS, CD/BDT(DONA), LCCE, FACCE, CLE and
Robin Elise Weiss, PhD, MPH, CLC, LCCE, FACCE, AdvCD/BDT(DONA)

Author's note: This chapter is focused on effects of neuraxial (epidural and spinal) analgesia on physiological systems of the laboring person and fetus, and how management of labors may reduce some undesirable effects of neuraxial analgesia. Throughout the book, as applicable, readers will find other information relevant to labor progress with an epidural.

INTRODUCTION: ANALGESIA AND ANESTHESIA—AN INTEGRAL PART OF MATERNITY CARE IN MANY COUNTRIES

After a safe outcome for the birthing person and baby, the management of labor pain is among the most pressing concerns for both parents and the staff who care for them during labor. This concern has driven considerable effort by both low-intervention and high-intervention maternity care providers, as well as the public, to find ways to safely reduce labor pain, pharmacologically and psychophysiologically. The epidural and all the neuraxial approaches have become most popular in industrialized countries, where more than half of all laboring people (or at least those who can afford it) will use it. In this chapter, we explore how a labor and birth with an epidural differs from a physiological labor and birth experience, emotionally and physically for the laboring person, examine the safety and side effects when an epidural is used and explore realistic and practical ways to minimize the adverse effects of the epidural for laboring people who choose to have one, resulting in a more positive experience for all.[1]

NEURAXIAL (EPIDURAL AND SPINAL) ANALGESIA—NEW TERMS FOR OLD APPROACHES TO LABOR PAIN?

The terms neuraxial analgesia and anesthesia are umbrella terms that apply to various pharmacologic pain relief techniques that employ opioids and/or local anesthetics and are injected or continuously infused into the intradural or extradural space. The neuraxis includes the brainstem and the spinal cord. (See the list of different forms of neuraxial analgesia in Box 10.1).

A spirited debate over the scientific validity of studies examining the effects, advantages, disadvantages, benefits, and harms of various forms of epidural and spinal analgesia has raged since the 1960s and 1970s, when they became widely available. The benefits of epidural and spinal anesthesia are excellent pain relief, mental awareness, and therapeutic rest are widely agreed upon. The risks of epidural increased hypotension, motor blockade, fever, urinary retention, longer first and second stages of labor, more oxytocin augmentation, increased rates of instrumental/operative vaginal birth, and increased cesareans for fetal distress although no increase in overall rates of cesarean.[2] A Cochrane review including 40 trials and over 11,000 birthing people found no impact on rates of cesarean section, long-term backache, neonatal Apgar scores or admission to the neonatal intensive care unit.[2] There is disagreement about other potential risks, including breast/chest-feeding difficulties or early cessation; epidurals have been found to both increase and decrease rates.[3,4] Limited information exists about how care providers could use simple protective or corrective measures to reduce these potential adverse effects.

While the risks and benefits of epidurals have been well studied, less is known about indirect risks, benefits, and effects of the management techniques used to ensure an epidural's safety. In other words, not all the problems that occur with epidurals result directly from the anesthesia; some may be created or exacerbated by the management that necessarily accompanies it.

Epidural and other forms of neuraxial analgesia alter the functioning of many bodily systems.[1] It is important to:

1. Focus on the physiology of the maternal-fetal-placental unit in pregnancy and labor.
2. Review alterations in physiology caused by various forms of epidural and spinal analgesia.
3. Consider simple practices or interventions to reduce some of the undesirable effects.
4. Understand the psychological and emotional challenges for laboring people—even when they feel little or no labor pain—to increase their sense of wellbeing during labor, and feelings of accomplishment and satisfaction with their birth experience. While most epidurals are highly effective, one should not assume that a pain-free person needs little attention to their emotional needs.

Box 10.1.   Neuraxial analgesia

This encompasses a variety of techniques, all of which involve the neuraxis, as listed below:2[5]

- Spinal anesthesia
- Intrathecal opioids
- Epidural opioids
- Epidural with both anesthetic and opioids. (May include patient-controlled epidural analgesia, PCEA)
- Combined spinal-epidural anesthesia

In this book we focus on epidural analgesia, since this is the most common neuraxial analgesia used for childbirth; also "epidural" is a more familiar word than "neuraxial" among practitioners and the public. Epidurals are highly desired as an option for pain relief by some pregnant people, while others feel just as strongly about their desire to avoid an epidural. Each pregnant person should be supported by their clinician and support people to make an informed decision that is best for them. The decision to use an epidural may be unnecessarily distressing for some pregnant people. It is important to view epidurals for what they are: a useful tool that some people will want to use, and others will want to avoid.

PHYSIOLOGICAL ADJUSTMENTS THAT SUPPORT MATERNAL-FETAL WELLBEING

The physiological processes of labor, birth, and parent–infant interactions are hormonally regulated, and usually result in a healthy parent and baby who are ready to adjust together to their new life situations.[6] This elegant process is usually reliable and continues functioning, even when the laboring person's activities, such as walking, moving freely, and eating, and drinking, are restricted, and when additional interventions, such as amniotomy, intravenous fluids, synthetic oxytocin, and epidural analgesia, are used. Side effects and trade-offs occur, however, and the challenge with elective interventions is to understand how the normal process is altered, and to recognize what is gained and what is lost.[7] This knowledge may lead to reduction or elimination of some undesired side effects, replacement of the intervention with a more acceptable alternative, or different management to prevent the harmful side effects. Epidural analgesia and all forms of neuraxial analgesia would benefit from this type of analysis.[8,9]

MULTISYSTEM EFFECTS OF EPIDURAL ANALGESIA ON LABOR PROGRESS

Anesthesia is either local—acting only in one area, regional—acting only on some areas, or general, meaning the person is not awake. Epidurals offer regional analgesia; however, many organ systems may be altered. Because the purpose of this book is preventing labor dystocia, how epidural analgesia slows or alters the progress of labor will be discussed and the following systems will be explored: the endocrine system; the central and peripheral nervous systems; the musculoskeletal system; and the genitourinary system.

The endocrine system

The delicate interplay among major hormones, such as oxytocin, beta-endorphins, and catecholamines, play a critical role in labor progress; the birthing person's mental state throughout labor; their level of alertness; pain tolerance; energy; capacity to birth the baby; and mutual regulation between parent and baby; and the birthing person's capacity to feed and connect with the baby after birth. These functions are inhibited or altered by emotional stress, systemic illness, and possibly by some drugs such as synthetic oxytocin, epinephrine, and tocolytics. In addition, it is clear that medications commonly given into the epidural space, such as sufentanil or fentanyl, and the "caine" family of anesthetic agents, can disrupt these hormonal interactions.[6]

Epidural analgesia can often slow normal labor by inhibiting endogenous oxytocin production. First stage labor progress is sometimes also slowed by extreme fear or distress, which is accompanied by high production of catecholamines (the physiologic "fight-or-flight" response). Although normal and beneficial in late labor, high catecholamine levels due to extreme fear, anxiety, or distress earlier in labor can decrease uterine blood flow and prolong labor. In such cases, epidural anesthesia reduces catecholamine production, especially epinephrine, causing, in effect, a "mind-body split," which, according to anecdotal reports, seems to allow progress to improve.[10] A common scenario is one in which the laboring person is having strong contractions for a long time without progress, and the clinician cannot identify a reason. Then the laboring person receives an epidural, gets some rest, and progress improves. In such a case, the epidural is a useful technique to resolve dystocia.

Epidural analgesia may slow normal labor by inhibiting endogenous oxytocin production. The inhibition of the endogenous oxytocin in turn slows contractions further blocking the normal second stage oxytocin surge that then stimulates reflexive pushing.[6] Synthetic oxytocin is often given intravenously to maintain progress. Also, caregivers sometimes resort to prolonged maximal breath-holding and straining by the person (directed bearing down) in the belief that their effort will compensate for less effective contractions. Recent studies have called this into question.[11]

Sometimes instrumental delivery or a cesarean delivery is recommended to expedite the birth. The normal late-labor catecholamine surge, which causes maternal alertness and a burst of energy needed to birth the baby, is blocked by epidural medications. The production of beta-endorphins, the body's own narcotic-like pain relievers, which foster a sense of wellbeing and instinctual behavior, as well as euphoria after birth, may also be blocked by epidural analgesia.[6]

The central nervous system and peripheral nervous system (sensory, motor, and autonomic, including the sympathetic and parasympathetic nervous systems).

Depending on the placement of the anesthetic medications (within the dural sac or extradurally), transmission of sensory and motor impulses is blocked or diminished either from within the central nervous system (as with intrathecal opioids and spinal anesthesia), or within the peripheral nervous system (as with epidural opioids, the segmental or standard epidural block).[12] The combined spinal-epidural analgesia affects transmission in both systems. The opioid agents (e.g., fentanyl or sufentanil), whether given intrathecally or epidurally, also reach the person's brain by means of the circulation and may depress respiration. Nausea, itching, and mild sedation also may result from the opioids reaching the central nervous system. The fetus may also receive these medications and may be impacted after birth, although often neonates are less impacted by an epidural than by systemic narcotic medications. Effects are dose-dependent and studies are conflicting regarding neonatal outcomes.[13]

The pain-relieving success of epidural or intrathecal anesthesia comes from blocking transmission of pain and other impulses over the sensory neurons that connect muscles and organs with the spinal cord and brain. Sensation is blocked throughout the mid-trunk and reduced in the lower body, giving relief from labor pain. The accompanying motor block decreases the birthing person's control over movements in their lower body and decreases pelvic floor muscle tone, though this can vary person to person depending on many factors. Blocking the parasympathetic nervous system results in decreased uterine contractility, alterations in temperature regulation, vasodilation in the affected areas, and reduced ability to dissipate heat because no sweating occurs in the affected areas.[12]

These effects, some of which are dose- and duration-dependent, contribute to maternal and fetal pyrexia and fetal tachycardia.[12,14,15] When maternal temperature reaches clinical fever levels (38 °C or 100.4°F), a caregiver must assess for infection in the laboring person and neonate. Since culturing for infection requires 48 hours for a result, antibiotics are usually begun, with the plan to discontinue if the culture is negative. In the meantime, the infant may be observed in a special care nursery, separated from the family, which can have negative effects on bonding and lactation. (Hospitals using evidence-based practice keep the birthing person and baby together during this waiting period). Then, depending on the culture result, the family will either be reunited or the baby will complete the course of antibiotics. This time is stressful for parents and baby. It may also increase the risks of the failure of initiation of lactation.[16] However, even if the culture is negative, or even if the fever does not reach 38 °C (100.4°F), any increase in maternal temperature during labor, whether from infection or another cause, is potentially harmful to the baby and to labor progress.

Even slight rises in fetal temperature (99.6°F, or higher) markedly increase the likelihood of fetal occiput posterior (OP) position at birth. Osborne, et al., investigated records of 1438 nulliparas, all of whom had an epidural, comparing newborn outcomes of those whose birthing parent developed hyperthermia (99.6°F or 37.5°C, or above; n = 669, or 47%) after receiving the epidural, with those whose parent had no hyperthermia. OP positions were doubled in the fever group. The cesarean rate was 12 times higher in people who had both hyperthermia and a fetus in an OP position than those who had neither.[17] Though disagreement exists as to the cause, other researchers have recently reported that maternal temperature often rises with the length of time the epidural is in place.[18,19,20]

As the birthing person's temperature rises, so does the temperature of the fetus. The fetus is approximately 0.5–0.9 °C warmer than the birthing person. Knowing that infants who are born with a fever are hypotonic at birth, Osborne and others surmise that hypotonia also existed in utero, and compromised the fetus' ability to make the necessary movements to negotiate the irregular pathway through the pelvis.[17] The authors urge further study of this phenomenon.

Another concern about increased fetal/newborn temperature due to epidural analgesia is the need to rule out infection as the cause of the fever. Newborns are often subjected to unnecessary septic workups and antibiotic administration while awaiting results of blood tests. Studies have reported an increase in adverse neonatal outcomes if the birthing person with epidural analgesia has a temperature above 99.5°F.[21]

The repercussions of fever highlight the importance of protecting the fetus from a rise in the birthing person's temperature (caused by epidural, infections, or immersion in water that is too warm).

The musculoskeletal system

The effects of motor nerve blockade depend on the density of the block, and may include loss of all sensation in the laboring person's trunk; reduction or loss of control over their voluntary muscles in the middle and lower trunk; and temporary weakness or complete loss of mobility in the legs. Bearing-down efforts are less effective, even when people are told to hold their breath and strain maximally. Pelvic muscle tone is also reduced, which impairs fetal rotation.

Typically, the laboring person's pelvic floor provides a resilient platform on which the fetal head can rotate, and the muscles lining the pelvis also provide a resilient cushion that encourages rotation. Pressure on these muscles elicits a stretch response that plays an important role in the cardinal movements of descent (flexion, internal rotation, extension, and external rotation). With epidural analgesia, however, the pelvic floor muscles are anesthetized, resulting in a reduction of muscle tone, which may inhibit rotation of the fetal head, and increase the risk of an occiput posterior position at delivery.[22,23] The erroneous solution is to instruct the pushing person to hold their breath and strain as hard and as long as they can through every contraction. Unfortunately, this behavior increases the likelihood of a difficult delivery due to a persistent malposition or a deep transverse arrest.

Delaying bearing-down (sometimes called "laboring down"), efforts for up to two hours or until the fetal head is visible at the introitus allows the fetus more time to "find its way" to an occiput anterior (OA) position and reduces the likelihood of occiput posterior at delivery.[24] While some studies have called this into question, others show benefits, even if it is for maternal satisfaction and/or preference, which is something that should be taken into consideration.[11,25–29]

Recent studies stated that laboring down with an epidural did not indicate any benefits over immediate pushing once fully dilated.[26] Experienced labor and delivery nurses continue to report anecdotally that, for a nullipara with an epidural, delayed pushing until the fetus has descended to a lower station conserves maternal energy reserves and increases maternal satisfaction. One exception may be the fetus in the occiput posterior position. A small RCT showed that having an epidural was associated with an increased risk of fetal malposition.[30]

Use of gravity-enhancing positions and movements may be impossible or possible only with assistance when an epidural is in place. The extent of these effects varies with the type of neuraxial analgesia administered, selection of medication, dosage, and length of time that the epidural has been in place and the use of patient-controlled delivery of small amounts of additional medication.[25]

Injuries to pelvic floor musculature, as well as anal, urinary, and flatal incontinence may be increased by early directed bearing-down efforts (prolonged maximal breath-holding and straining).[31] In addition, fetal malposition increases when epidural analgesia is used; instrumental delivery may be needed. A case control study of 500 birthing people, with 250 in the epidural group and 250 in the control group, demonstrated that having an epidural was associated with an increased risk of fetal malposition.[30] This may also injure the perineum.[23,25,32]

The genitourinary system

The lack of sensation from the laboring person's bladder and inability to void voluntarily increases the possibility of urinary retention or bladder distention during and after labor.[33,34] Labor progress may be slowed by a full, distended bladder, which may crowd the pelvis, impact the efficiency of contractions, and restrict fetal rotation and descent. The laboring person requires careful observation for evidence of bladder distention, monitoring of fluid intake and output, and continuous or periodic catheterization to empty their bladder, which may increase the likelihood of a catheter-associated urinary tract infections (CAUTI).[35] The risk of postpartum hemorrhage is increased with a distended bladder. A randomized control trial of 252 nulliparous birthing people with epidurals were randomized to either indwelling or intermittent bladder catheterization found no difference between groups.[36] Similarly, a meta-analysis of continuous versus intermittent catheterization including 850 birthing people found no difference in rates of postpartum urinary tract infection (UTI), postpartum urinary retention, and postpartum hemorrhage.[37] Despite this, for low-risk laboring people, intermittent bladder catherization with epidural should be considered to facilitate position changes and movement with the epidural.

The chances of perineal trauma are increased, because of the increased need for instrumental delivery, including third- and fourth-degree lacerations. The likelihood of urinary and anal incontinence increases after instrumental delivery.[32]

CAN CHANGES IN LABOR MANAGEMENT REDUCE PROBLEMS OF EPIDURAL ANALGESIA?

Although the debate on true effects of epidural analgesia will and should continue, more attention must be given to other questions. Can some of the disruption in labor physiology be prevented or reversed by a change in labor management? Can different labor management reduce some of the undesired effects of epidural analgesia, improve outcomes, reduce costs, and increase the laboring person's participation and satisfaction in the process? Beneficial effects may result if non-pharmacologic approaches to maintain labor progress and relieve other symptoms were routinely included in management. Following is a four-part management proposal for maternity health practitioners.

1.   Inform the laboring person ahead of time

The pregnant person is informed ahead of time, through information received from comprehensive childbirth education classes, recommended consumer resources, and prenatal discussions with the health care provider, about: (a) the standard information on risks and benefits and alternatives; (b) complete, realistic explanations of how the analgesia is administered; and (c), the routine procedures (often unanticipated to the birthing person in the moment) that are intended to ensure that epidural analgesia is safe (i.e., intravenous fluids and synthetic oxytocin, continuous electronic fetal monitoring, limitation of movement, bladder catheterization, frequent blood pressure monitoring, pulse oximetry, and others). Explanations of common, potentially frightening side effects of epidurals and the clinical actions to correct them should be given to people before labor, e.g., maternal hypotension and fetal bradycardia, inadequate or spotty (windows) pain relief, difficulties or frustrations over pushing with limited to no sensation; newborn care practices if fever has occurred. Distress for the laboring person may be reduced if they are not surprised by the sometimes sudden actions taken to relieve adverse effects.

2.   Shorten the duration of exposure

The rationale for delaying the epidural is that some undesirable side effects develop and may worsen with time, such as: slow labor progress; maternal fever; fetal tachycardia; increasing motor loss in lower limbs (due to cumulative density of the block); persistent fetal malposition, fetal intolerance of labor; and delay in successful breast/chest-feeding. If these potential side effects are of concern to the birthing person or their caregiver, they can try to shorten the duration of exposure by delaying the administration of epidural anesthesia.[24] The best way to do this without causing suffering is for the birthing person to employ non-pharmacologic methods available to relieve labor pain. Childbirth education classes that emphasize comfort measures can be very helpful, because many comfort techniques require mastery before labor. Other techniques can be done during labor by a knowledgeable doula, partner, or caregiver. If labor is intolerable, however, an epidural should not be delayed.[38] As some studies show that timing of epidural placement can be done in early labor.[39] One exception might be if the birthing person has a higher BMI, given that there is increased difficulty in placing the epidural catheter for an increased number of these people, early placement may afford better options and avoid the risks of general anesthesia should cesarean delivery become required. The risks of difficulty rise with increasing BMI.[40,41]

3.   Treat the birthing person as much as possible like a person who does not have an epidural

Adopt practices that maintain or encourage behavior resembling what laboring people do when not anesthetized, for example:

- Employ cooling measures as soon as the birthing person's temperature begins to rise (not until it reaches clinical fever temperature), with cool packs over the parts of their body where sensation is normal, install an electric fan, lower the room temperature and remove blankets. (This suggestion is based on anecdotal evidence only. The practice has not been scientifically evaluated, and controlled investigation of outcomes such as maternal and neonatal fevers, neonatal intensive care unit admission, fetal occiput posterior positions, and antibiotic use should be explored.)[8,17]
- Provide the birthing person with caloric beverages in small amounts for their comfort and sense of normality.[12,42,43]
- Keep the person moving as safety permits; for example, use the "rollover" (Fig. 10.1), in which they spend 30 minutes in each of the following positions:

The use of a small peanut ball between the knees or ankles may reduce labor duration and number of cesarean sections.[44,45] A meta-analysis including 648 birthing people did not show decreased labor length, however there was a trend toward shortened labor duration and fewer cesareans.[46] Further, there is no harm associated with this intervention and possible benefit. Peanut ball use for laboring people with an epidural should be encouraged.

Of course, if the birthing person has too little muscle tone or the fetus does not tolerate one or more positions, avoid it, and use other positions. Pelvic shape and gravity effects are altered with the rollover and more so with the

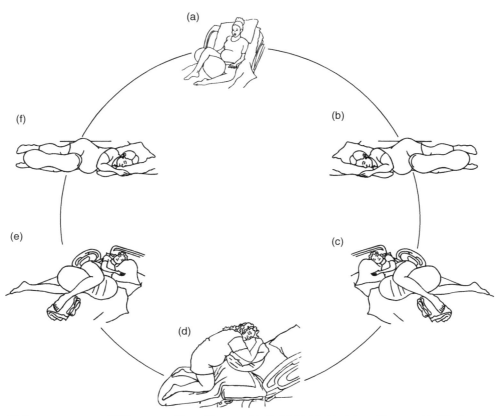

Fig. 10.1. Roll-over sequence. (**a**) Throne position with peanut ball. (**b**) Right side-lying with peanut ball between legs. (**c**) Exaggerated right-side lying with peanut ball between legs. (**d**) Lying over birthing ball, foot of bed dropped. (**e**) Exaggerated left side-lying with peanut ball between legs. (**f**) Left side-lying with peanut ball between legs.

peanut ball. Recruit their support team to help them with position changes. If the laboring person is exhausted and needs sleep, consider less frequent position changes and find a balance between restorative sleep and promoting labor progress through changing positions. Such a protocol has not been studied and deserves scientific evaluation of its effects on fetal position, labor progress, and mode of delivery.

A meta-analysis of 22 studies comparing upright positions during the second stage with supine positions for people with an epidural found that upright postures were associated with fewer instrumental deliveries and episiotomies, but a possibility of greater blood loss.[47] Another more recent review of five randomized controlled trials found no evidence that one position is better than another for people who labor with an epidural.[48] Therefore, people should be encouraged to choose a position of comfort and to change positions periodically (Fig. 10.2).

- Delay maternal bearing down until the fetal head is visible, or the birthing person has an urge to push if that is their preference. (Chart 10.1).[11,25,32,49]
- In the presence of a fetus in a posterior presentation, delayed bearing down may decrease the chance of spontaneous vaginal birth and increase the risk of perineal and vaginal lacerations.[50]
- There is no time limit on the duration of the delay. Maternal and fetal status would be factors in the decision.
- Because the epidural creates such profound alterations of the physiologic labor process, birthing people's participation during second stage will be different from those people with full sensation and normal hormonal and musculoskeletal functioning. If a person begins to feel an urge to push, but can't seem to bear down effectively, they may feel frustrated and anxious ("I can't do it!" "Just get it out!"). They may benefit from assistance in

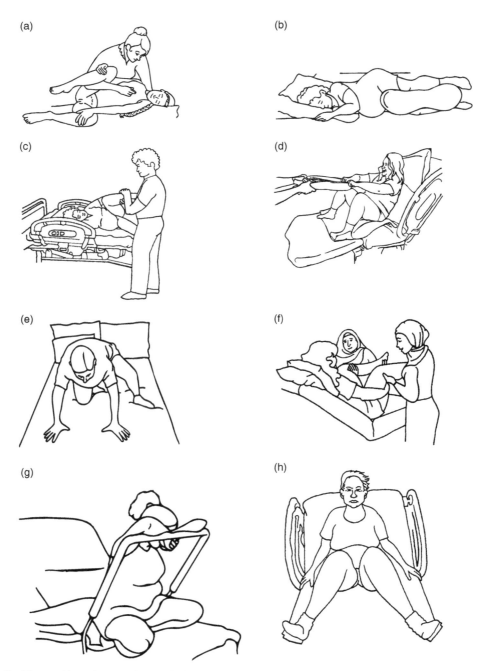

Fig. 10.2. Pushing positions that may be used when people have epidurals side-lying with partner supporting one leg, semi-prone, side-lying with one foot resting on partner's hip, sitting leaning back, kneeling on lowered foot of bed, semi-sitting with support people holding legs, supine with legs in stirrups. (**a**) Left side lying. (**b**) Right side-lying peanut ball. (**c**) Right side lying with foot on partner. (**d**) Tug of war with sheet. (**e**) Runner's lunge in bed. (**f**) Helpers supporting legs while pushing. (**g**) Pushing with squatting bar. (**h**) Closed knee pushing.

bearing down safely and effectively. In such a case, rather than instruct them to hold their breath and strain throughout the contraction, help them to push like a person who does not have an epidural. Based on studies of spontaneous involuntary bearing-down efforts by people who have no epidural, the caregiver's instructions would include: breath-holding that is limited to no more than six seconds, followed by several quick breaths before bearing down again. People repeat this pattern of bearing down followed by short breaths (the repetition of this pattern three to five times per contraction replicates birthing people's spontaneous behavior when they have no anesthesia and no one directs their pushing). Grunting efforts are preferable to the non-evidenced-based, but often used, directed, prolonged breath-holding and straining for slow counts to ten. The caregiver can follow the contractions, either by abdominal palpation or by watching the contraction monitor, and help the birther time their efforts with the peaks of the contractions. If a tocodynamometer is being used, the caregiver can give feedback on how the numbers go up as the birthing person bears down, and how much their efforts add to the intensity of the contractions. This approach is far more motivating and empowering than instruction for directed bearing down, commonly referred to as "count to ten" which the authors of this chapter would not recommend using since evidence of improved outcomes is lacking (see Fig. 11.11).

Descent vaginal birth

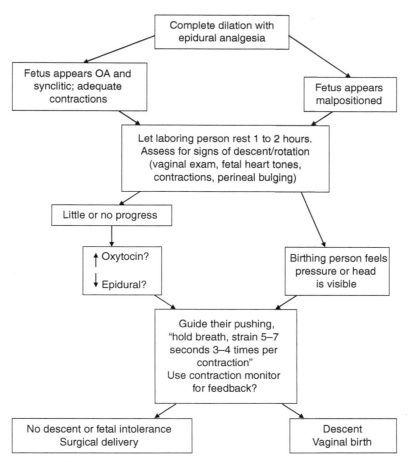

Chart 10.1.   Delayed pushing with an epidural.

Guided physiologic pushing with an epidural

Here are instructions for the person who cannot feel their contractions or is frustrated or wants help. This is how optimal coached physiologic pushing is done:

- Birthing person breathes at onset of the contraction until the intensity has increased by about 20 points (as evidenced on the fetal monitor) or they feel an urge to push; then they bear down for no more than six seconds; "breathes for the baby" several times; and repeats this pattern until the contraction is clearly waning. Some people find it motivating if their support person, doula, or healthcare provider follows the intensity of the contractions on the monitor.

Box (Fig. 10.3) and calls out the numbers, which indicate how much pressure is added by the birthing parent's efforts.[51]

- During labor, avoid twisting the birthing person's torso while helping them change positions. During pushing, if stirrups are used, or if one or both of the birther's legs are being supported and abducted in lithotomy or side-lying positions, their hips, knees, and low back are susceptible to injury due to prolonged pressures or stretching, because they cannot feel the excessive force on these joints and nerves.[52] Caregivers must respect the limits of the hips, knees, and low back, and avoid prolonged excessive flexion, abduction, or external rotation of the hips and knees. Exaggerated lithotomy (thighs severely flexed onto abdomen) should be avoided due to the risk of lumbosacral nerve injury.[12] Thirty to fifty percent of people report backache after childbirth.[53] It is very likely that a portion of backaches are iatrogenic and are thus preventable.[54] Many caregivers who support the limbs of anesthetized patients also experience injuries on the job.[55]
- Place the baby skin-to-skin with the birthing person and conduct assessments and procedures while they are together. Allow plenty of time for unrushed breast/chestfeeding, with minimal instruction or handling of their chest area.[56]

4.   Attend to the emotion needs of a birthing person with an epidural.[57]

The staff and their support team are likely to assume that, because of pain relief from the anesthesia, the birthing person is emotionally content.[58] Birthing people may have conflicting feelings regarding epidural use: they may be very glad for the pain relief, but may still have distress or anxiety over other things or new concerns that occur to them, which may cause them to feel lonely, worried, disappointed, or even mistreated. Here are some examples of emotionally stressful events associated with the use of epidural analgesia:

- Having to wait for an available anesthesiologist once the decision to get an epidural has been made.
- Delay in receiving an epidural while pre-placement procedures are completed.
- Administration of the epidural, especially if the procedure is more difficult than expected.

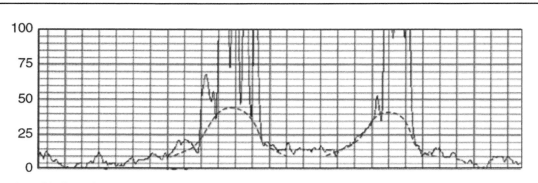

Fig. 10.3.   Monitor strip showing increased pressure when laboring person bears down.

- Surprise or shock over the many safety precautions or interventions (listed earlier in this chapter).
- Feeling alone, if their support team and the staff go out of the room, leaving them with no one to talk to or to ask for small comforts (drinks, extra pillow, hand holding, etc.).
- Thirst and/or hunger.
- Embarrassment from having a urinary catheter.
- Little control over what is done to them, and passive cooperation while the staff and support team facilitate position changes.
- Helplessness and immobility; discomfort with numbness, itching, nausea, breakthrough or windows of pain.
- Concern about labor progress if contractions slow down or space out, or if cervical change seems stalled.
- Distress over the level of feeling they have from the anesthesia. More somatic sensation than anticipated may be concerning. While some may worry about feeling more sensation as labor progresses, others feel more numb than they expected.
- Fear if the staff need to change the laboring person's position to correct fetal bradycardia.
- Worries about the baby's wellbeing.
- Impatience over the length of labor.
- Tension and/or anxiety if their temperature is beginning to rise, or if the baby is becoming tachycardic.
- Worry that they are a burden on their support team.
- Being directed to push when it does not match their desire spontaneous desire to push.
- Feeling incompetent and frustrated over difficulty with pushing; including the length of time that pushing lasts.
- Feelings of disappointment in themselves or from others for requesting an epidural.

Few studies have been done on the emotional responses of the person with epidural analgesia during labor. Wuitchik and colleagues, found that when someone received an epidural, their pain decreased markedly, but their distress levels did not, and were actually similar to those of people without epidurals. In other words, the distress over their pain shifted to concerns over other things after the epidural, such as those listed above.[58]

Another study of nulliparas' experiences of labor with an epidural found that birthing people were pleased with the pain relief and stress reduction it provided, but some felt unsettled or ambivalent afterwards. These experiences were caused by two main factors: the attitudes, actions, and treatment by health caregivers; and insufficient knowledge about side effects and how these are managed. The authors concluded that the epidural "does not guarantee a quality birth experience."[59] The take-home message from these studies is that people still need education and emotional support for satisfaction with childbirth, even if they are free of pain.

Having a doula in this situation can help ameliorate some of the emotional and mental ramifications with an epidural. The staff will have more assessment and monitoring medical aspects to contend to with the presence of an epidural, leaving them with even less time to manage some of these unintended emotional/mental side effects.[60]

CENTERING THE PREGNANT PERSON DURING LABOR

Studies of epidural analgesia have not brought people closer to agreement on its safety, its side effects, and its role—direct or indirect—in increasing the complexity and expense of the care needed to maintain safety, labor progress, and positive family beginnings for healthy birthing people. Supporters of routine use of epidural analgesia in early labor disagree on these effects with those who advocate lower rates, later administration, and alternative ways to manage labor pain. Each side has produced evidence supporting its point of view, but the disagreements are unlikely to be resolved.

The intention here is not to add fuel to the controversy. Rather, it is to suggest that it is time to shift the focus to the whole body and psyche of the birther-infant dyad, and how it is transformed by epidural analgesia. This more holistic perspective provides a context for understanding side effects and encourages constructive efforts to retain the pain-relieving benefit while reducing or preventing at least some undesired effects by preserving normal physiologic function as much as possible. This approach restores the birthing person to a central role. When they become more active in their labor and receive attention to their psychological needs, some outcomes will improve and their satisfaction will be enhanced.

CONCLUSION

This chapter has focused particularly on the impact of epidurals and other types of neuraxial analgesia on the functioning of major organ systems, labor pain, progress, and psychological responses in a healthy, low-risk population. By exploring the typical customary management that accompanies epidural analgesia, we recognize that some policies and practices (rather than the epidural itself), may be responsible for some undesired effects; for example: starting the epidural very early without encouraging the use of non-pharmacologic comfort measures; restriction of movement in the bed; allowing maternal temperature to rise without efforts to reduce it; giving large amounts of intravenous fluids, causing overhydration; and lack of attention to the birthing person's emotional state even when they are free of pain. There are constantly changing ideas and issues being addressed in epidural anesthesia management, so it is important to stay abreast of the topic.[61] Focusing more on minimizing the detrimental effects will increase the efficacy of epidural analgesia.

REFERENCES

1. Simkin P. (2012) Moving beyond the debate: A holistic approach to understanding and treating effects of neuraxial analgesia. *Birth* 39(4), 327–332.
2. Anim-Somuah M, Smyth RM, Cyna AM, Cuthbert A. (2018) Epidural versus non-epidural or no analgesia for pain management in labour. *Cochrane Database of Systematic Reviews*. May 21; 5(5), CD000331. doi: 10.1002/14651858. CD000331.pub4. PMID: 29781504; PMCID: PMC6494646.
3. Newnham EC, Moran PS, Begley CM, Carroll M, Daly D. (2021) Comparison of labour and birth outcomes between nulliparous women who used epidural analgesia in labour and those who did not: A prospective cohort study. *Women Birth*. Sep; 34(5), e435–e441. doi: 10.1016/j.wombi.2020.09.001. Epub 2020 Sep 11. PMID: 32928689.
4. French CA, Cong X, Chung KS. (2016) Labor epidural analgesia and breastfeeding: A systematic review. *Journal of Human Lactation* 32(3), 507–520. doi: 10.1177/0890334415623779
5. Heesen M, Klimek M. (2017) Obstetric analgesia – update 2016. *Journal of Perinatal Medicine* 45(3), 281–289. doi:10.1515/jpm-2016-0118
6. Buckley S. (2015) *Hormonal Physiology of Childbearing: Evidence and Implications for Women, Babies, and Maternity Care.*
7. ACNM, M., NACPM. (2013) A Consensus Statement. Supporting healthy and normal physiologic childbirth. *Journal of Perinatal Education* 22, 14–18 doi: 10.1891/1058-1243.22.1.14.
8. Goer H, Romano, A. (2012) Epidurals and combined spinal-epidurals: The "Cadillacs of analgesia." In: *Optimal Care in Childbirth: The Case for a Physiologic Approach*. Classic Day Publishing, pp. 267–301.
9. Singata M, Tranmer J, Gyte GM. (2013) Restricting oral fluid and food intake during labour. *Cochrane Database of Systematic Reviews* 8. doi: 10.1002/14651858.CD003930.pub3
10. Grant EN, Tao W, Craig M, McIntire D, Leveno K. (2015) Neuraxial analgesia effects on labour progression: Facts, fallacies, uncertainties and the future. *Bjog* 122(3), 288–293. doi: 10.1111/1471-0528.12966
11. Lemos A, Amorim MM, Dornelas de Andrade A, de Souza AI, Cabral Filho JE, Correia JB. (2017) Pushing/bearing down methods for the second stage of labour. *The Cochrane Database of Systematic Reviews* 3(3). doi: 10.1002/14651858. CD009124.pub3
12. Wong C. (2009) Advances in labor analgesia. *International Journal of Women's Health* 1, 139–154. doi: 10.2147/ijwh.s4553
13. Liu ZH, Wang DX. (2020) Potential impact of epidural labor analgesia on the outcomes of neonates and children. *Chinese Medical Journal* 133(19), 2353–2358. 10.1097/CM9.0000000000000900
14. Segal S. (2010) Labor epidural analgesia and maternal fever. *Anesthesia and Analgesia* 111, 1467–1475. doi: 10.1213/ANE.0b013e3181f713d4
15. Sharpe EE, Arendt KW. (2017) Epidural Labor Analgesia and Maternal Fever. *Clin Obstet Gynecol* 60(2), 365–374. doi: 10.1097/grf.0000000000000270
16. Parker LA, Sullivan S, Krueger C, Mueller M. (2015) Association of timing of initiation of breastmilk expression on milk volume and timing of lactogenesis stage II among mothers of very low-birth-weight infants. *Breastfeeding Medicine* 10(2), 84–91. doi: 10.1089/bfm.2014.0089
17. Osborne C, Ecker JL, Gauvreau K, Davidson KM, Lieberman E. (2011) Maternal temperature elevation and occiput posterior position at birth among low-risk women receiving epidural analgesia. *Journal of Midwifery & Women's Health* 56(5), 446–451.

18. Akerman N, Hall W. (2012) Maternal temperature increase. *British Journal of Anaesthesia* 108(4), 699–700.

19. De Orange F, Passini R, Amorim MMR, et al. (2011) Combined spinal and epidural anaesthesia and maternal intrapartum temperature during vaginal delivery: A randomized clinical trial. *British Journal of Anaesthesia* 107(5), 762–767.

20. Khanna P, Jain S, Thariani K, Sharma S, Singh AK. (2020) Epidural Fever: Hiding in the Shadows. *Turk J Anaesthesiol Reanim* 48(5). doi: 10.5152/TJAR.2020.50

21. Greenwell E, Wyshak G, Ringer SA, Johnson LC, Rivkin MJ, Lieberman E. (2012) Intrapartum temperature elevation, epidural use, and adverse outcome in term infants. *Pediatrics* 129(2), e447–e454.

22. Bonica J, Miller F, Parmley T. (1995). Anatomy and physiology of the forces of parturition. In: J Bonica, J McDonald (eds), *Principles and Practice of Obstetric Analgesia and Anesthesia*, (Second edn). Williams & Wilkins.

23. Lieberman E, Davidson K, Lee-Parritz A, Shearer E. (2005) Changes in fetal position during labor and their association with epidural analgesia. *Obstetrics & Gynecology* 105(5, Part 1), 974–982.

24. Goer H. (2014) Epidural analgesia: To delay or not to delay, that is the question. *Connecting the Dots.* https://www.lamaze.org/Connecting-the-Dots/Post/TitleLink/Epidural-Analgesia-To-Delay-or-Not-to-Delay-That-Is-the-Question

25. Brancato R, Church S, Stone P. (2008) A meta-analysis of passive descent versus immediate pushing in nulliparous women with epidural analgesia in the second stage of labor. *Journal of Obstetrics, Gynecology and Neonatal Nursing* 37(1), 4–12.

26. Cahill A, Srinivas SK, Tita ATN, et al. (2018) Effect of immediate vs delayed pushing on rates of spontaneous vaginal delivery among nulliparous women receiving neuraxial analgesia: A randomized clinical trial. *JAMA* 320(14), 1444–1454. doi: 10.1001/jama.2018.13986

27. Goer H. (2018 November 20). Should we abandon "Laboring Down" with epidurals? A closer look at new evidence. [Blog post]. Should We Abandon "Laboring Down" with Epidurals? A Closer Look at New Evidence. *Connecting the Dots.* Retrieved from: https://www.lamaze.org/Connecting-the-Dots/Post/should-we-abandon-laboring-down-with-epidurals-a-closer-look-at-new-evidence (accessed April 21, 2021).

28. Hofmeyr GJ, Singata-Madliki M. (2020) The second stage of labor. *Best Practice and Research in Clinical Obstetrics and Gynaecology* 67, 53–64. doi: 10.1016/j.bpobgyn.2020.03.012

29. Roberts J and Hanson L. (2007) Best practices in second stage labor care: Maternal bearing down and positioning. *Journal of Midwifery & Women's Health* 52, 238–245. doi: 10.1016/j.jmwh.2006.12.011

30. Menichini D, Mazzaro N, Minniti S, Ricchi A, Molinazzi MT, Facchinetti F, Neri I. (2021) Fetal head malposition and epidural analgesia in labor: A case-control study. *Journal of Maternal-Fetal and Neonatal Medicine* 21, 1–10. doi: 10.1080/14767058.2021.1890018

31. Cahill AG. (2017) Identifying the best way to manage labor. *Missouri Medicine* 114(3), 160–162.

32. Albers L, Borders N. (2007) Minimizing genital tract trauma and related pain following spontaneous vaginal birth. *Journal of Midwifery and Women's Health* 52(3), 246–253.

33. ObsGyae & Midwifery News (2011, December 29). Post-partum bladder care: Background, practice and complications. http://www.ogpnews.com/2011/12/post-partum-bladder-care-background-practice-and-complications/444.

34. Kearney R, Cutner A. (2008) Postpartum voiding dysfunction. *The Obstetrician & Gynaecologist* 10(2), 71–74.

35. Richens Y. (2016) Urinary catheterisation: Indications and complications. *British Journal of Midwifery* 24, 164–168. doi: 10.12968/bjom.2016.24.3.164

36. Dempsey A, Krening C, Vorgic L. (2020) Multisite randomized controlled trial of bladder management in labor with epidural analgesia/anesthesia. *Journal of Obstetric, Gynecologic & Neonatal Nursing* 49(6), 564–570. doi: 10.1016/j.jogn.2020.07.005

37. Li M, Xing X, Yao L, Wang X, He W, Wang M, Li H, Xun Y, Yan P, Hui X, Yang X, Yang K. (2019) The effect of bladder catheterization on the incidence of urinary tract infection in laboring women with epidural analgesia: A meta-analysis of randomized controlled trials. *International Urogynecology Journal* 30(9), 1419–1427. doi: 10.1007/s00192-019-03904-1

38. Simkin P, Hull K. (2011) Pain, suffering and trauma in labor and prevention of subsequent posttraumatic stress disorder. *Journal of Perinatal Education* 20(3), 166–176.

39. Lipschuetz M, Nir EA, Cohen SM, Guedalia J, Hochler H, Amsalem H, Karavani G, Hochner-Celnikier D, Unger R, Yagel S. (2020) Cervical dilation at the time of epidural catheter insertion is not associated with the degree of prolongation of the first or second stages of labor, or the rate of instrumental vaginal delivery. *Acta Obstetricia et Gynecologica Scandinavica* 99(8), 1039–1049. doi: 10.1111/aogs.13822

40. Dalbye R, Gunnes N, Blix E, Zhang J, Eggebø T, Nistov Tokheim L, Øian P, Bernitz S. (2021) Maternal body mass index and risk of obstetric, maternal and neonatal outcomes: A cohort study of nulliparous women with spontaneous onset of labor. *Acta Obstetricia et Gynecologica Scandinavica* 100(3), 521–530. doi: 10.1111/aogs.14017

41. González-Tascón C, Díaz EG, García IL. (2021) Epidural analgesia in the obese obstetric patient: A retrospective and comparative study with non-obese patients at a tertiary hospital. *Brazilian Journal of Anesthesiology* 21. doi: 10.1016/j.bjane.2021.02.054

42. Carlson N, Barukh R. (2016) New recommendations on oral intake in labor. *Journal of Obstetric, Gynecologic & Neonatal Nursing* 45, 253–261.

43. Harty C, Sproul E, Bautista MJ, et al. (2015, October 24–28). A review of fasting and the risk of aspiration in labor. *Anesthesiology* 2015, San Diego, CA.

44. Tussey CM, Botsios E, Gerkin RD, Kelly LA, Gamez J, Mensik J. (2015) Reducing length of labor and cesarean surgery rate using a peanut ball for women laboring with an epidural. *The Journal of Perinatal Education* 24(1), 16–24. doi: 10.1891/1058-1243.24.1.16

45. Hickey L, Savage J. (2019) Effect of peanut ball and position changes in women laboring with an epidural. *Nursing for Women's Health* 23(3), 245–252. doi: 10.1016/j.nwh.2019.04.004

46. Grenvik JM, Rosenthal E, Saccone G, Della Corte L, Quist-Nelson J, Gerkin RD, Gimovsky AC, Kwan M, Mercier R, Berghella V. (2019) Peanut ball for decreasing length of labor: A systematic review and meta-analysis of randomized controlled trials. *European Journal of Obstetrics, Gynecology, and Reproductive Biology* 242, 159–165. doi: 10.1016/j.ejogrb.2019.09.018

47. Gupta J, Sood A, Hofmeyr GJ, Vogel JP. (2017) Position in the second stage of labour for women without epidural anaesthesia. *Cochrane Database of Systematic Reviews* 5. doi: 10.1002/14651858.CD002006.pub4

48. Kibuka M, Thornton JG. (2017) Position in the second stage of labour for women with epidural anaesthesia. *Cochrane Database of Systematic Reviews*. doi: 10.1002/14651858.CD008070.pub3

49. Osborne K, Hanson L. (2014) Labor down or bear down. *Journal of Perinatal & Neonatal Nursing* 28(2), 117–126.

50. Saad H, Maged AM, Meshaal H, Hassan SM, Kamel A, Salah E. (2021) Delayed versus early pushing during the second stage of labour in primigravidas under epidural anaesthesia with occipitoposterior malposition: A randomised controlled study. *Journal of Obstetrics and Gynaecology* 23, 1–5. doi: 10.1080/01443615.2020.1867973

51. Simkin P. (2018) *In the Birth Partner: A Complete Guide to Childbirth for Dads, Doulas, and All Other Labor Companions*, 5th edn. Harvard Common Press, p. 322.

52. Reynolds F. (2011) Peripheral neuropathy. In: D Gambling, J Douglas, R McKay (eds), *Obstetric Anesthesia and Uncommon Disorders*. Cambridge University Press, pp. 215–228.

53. Wong C, Scavone B, Dugan S, et al. (2003) Incidence of postpartum lumbosacral spine and lower extremity nerve injuries. *Obstetrics & Gynecology* 101(2), 279–288.

54. Simkin P, Bolding A. (2008) Supporting the laboring woman without injuring your self. *International Journal of Childbirth Education* 22(4), 17–21.

55. Stichler J, Feiler J, Chase K. (2012) Understanding risks of workplace injury in labor and delivery. *Journal of Obstetric, Gynecologic & Neonatal Nursing* 41, 71–81. doi: 10.1111/j.1552-6909.2011.01308.x

56. USA B. (2010) *The Ten Steps to Successful Breastfeeding*. Retrieved December 29 from: www.babyfriendlyusa.org

57. Jepsen I, Keller KD. (2014) The experience of giving birth with epidural analgesia. *Women and Birth* 27(2), 98–103.

58. Wuitchik M, Baka D, Lipshitz J. (1990) Relationships between pain, cognitive activity and epidural analgesia during labor. *Pain* 41(2), 125–132.

59. Hidaka R, Clark-Callister L. (2012) Giving birth with epidural analgesia: The experience of first-time mothers. *Journal of Perinatal Education* 21(1), 24–35.

60. Bohren M, Hofmeyr G, Sakala C, Fukuzawa RK, Cuthbert A. (2017) Continuous support for women during childbirth. *Cochrane Database of Systematic Reviews* (7). doi: 10.1002/14651858.CD003766.pub6

61. Toledano RD, Leffert L. (2021) What's new in neuraxial labor analgesia. *Current Anesthesiology Reports*, 1–8. doi: 10.1007/s40140-021-00453-6

Chapter 11

Guide to Positions and Movements

Lisa Hanson, PhD, CNM, FACNM, FAAN and Emily Malloy, PhD, CNM

Many techniques are designed to reduce pain and enhance relaxation without the use of pain medications. With reduced reliance on pain medications also comes reduced exposure to potential side effects of the medications (including immobility, changes in hormone balance, and other factors that interfere with labor progress, as well as adverse effects on pregnant person or baby).

This chapter focuses on maternal positions and movements. Evidence suggests that maternal positions, especially when chosen by the laboring person, increase comfort and, by altering pelvic shape and gravity effects, improve labor progress.[1,2]

MATERNAL POSITIONS AND HOW THEY AFFECT LABOR

This section contains descriptions of positions and specific features of each. We have arranged the positions in categories. The positions in each category cause similar physical changes. For example:

- Semisitting and side-lying positions are restful and gravity neutral. They may help an exhausted laboring person save their energy, especially if they have been up and walking for a long period. Also, if progress is rapid, neutralizing gravity may slow the labor to a more manageable pace.
- Upright positions take advantage of gravity to apply the presenting part to the cervix, improve the quality of the contractions, and enhance the descent of the fetus.[1,3]
- Positions in which the laboring person leans forward are thought to enhance fetal rotation or help maintain the favorable occiput anterior (OA) position, and reduce back pain.[3-6]
- Asymmetrical positions, in which the laboring person flexes one hip and knee, change the shape of the pelvis, enhance rotation, and reduce back pain.
- The exaggerated lithotomy position, used for several contractions in the second stage, may facilitate the passage of a "stuck baby" beneath the pubic symphysis.
- Dorsal positions tend to cause supine hypotension and increase back pain. Contractions are more frequent and painful, yet less likely to improve labor progress![1,3]
- Recently the use of knees together pushing has been suggested.

Side-lying positions

Side-lying and semiprone

When: During first and second stages.

How to use side-lying: The laboring person lies on their side with both hips and knees flexed and a pillow between their legs, or with their upper leg raised and supported (Figs. 11.1 through 11.4).

How to use semiprone: The laboring person lies on their side with lower arm behind (or in front of) their trunk, their lower leg extended, and their upper hip and knee flexed 90 degrees or more, supported by one or two pillows or a peanut-shaped ball. They roll partly toward their front (Fig. 11.5 through 11.7).

See below regarding which side the laboring person should lie on.

What these positions do

- Allow tired people to rest.
- Are safe if pain medications have been used.
- Are gravity neutral (can be used with a very rapid first or second stage).
- May relieve hemorrhoids.
- May resolve fetal heart rate problems, if due to cord compression or supine hypotension.

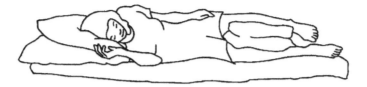

Fig. 11.1.   Side-lying.

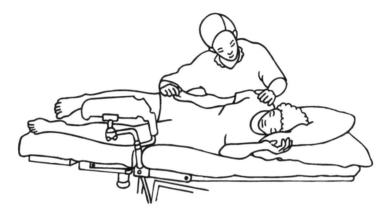

Fig. 11.2.   Side-lying with leg in leg rest.

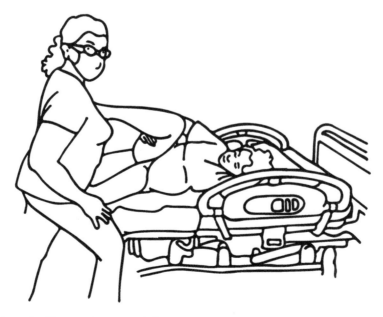

Fig. 11.3.   Side-lying to push with upper leg supported.

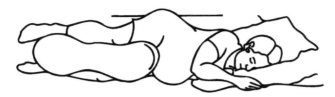

Fig. 11.4.   Side-lying with peanut shaped ball.

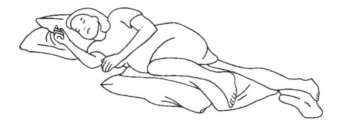

Fig. 11.5.   Semiprone, lower arm forward.

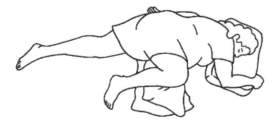

Fig. 11.6.   Semiprone, lower arm behind.

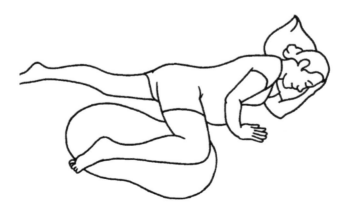

Fig. 11.7.   Semiprone, with use of peanut ball.

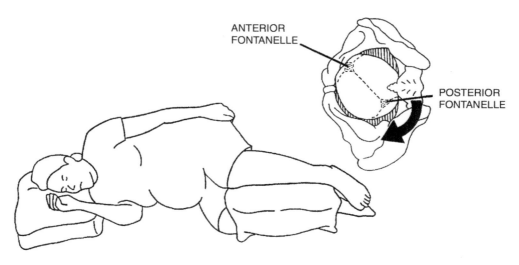

ANTERIOR FONTANELLE

POSTERIOR FONTANELLE

Fig. 11.8. Side-lying on the "correct" side, with fetal back toward the bed.

- Help to lower high blood pressure (especially left lateral positions).
- May promote progress when alternated with walking.
- Avoid pressure on sacrum (unlike sitting and supine positions).
- In second stage, because there is no pressure on the sacrum (as there is with sitting), these positions allow posterior movement of the sacrum as the fetus descends.
- May enhance rotation of an occiput posterior (OP) baby.

Note: Gravity effects are different when a laboring person is side-lying versus semiprone.

If side-lying, the laboring person with a known or suspected OP fetus should lie on the same side as the fetal occiput and back ("baby's back toward bed"; Fig. 11.8). This helps shift the fetus from OP to occiput transverse (OT). Ask the laboring person with an OP fetus to lie on the same side as the occiput for 15 to 30 minutes to encourage rotation from OP to OT; then ask them to change to kneeling and leaning forward for 15 to 30 minutes (to encourage rotation from OT to OA). As can be seen in Fig. 11.9, side-lying on the side opposite the fetal occiput actually tends to take the fetus into direct OP.

If the laboring person is semiprone they should lie on the side opposite the fetal occiput ("baby's back toward ceiling;" Fig. 11.10) for at least 15 to 30 minutes. In this position, their pelvis is rotated so that the pubis is pointing more toward the bed than with straight side-lying. This alters the effects of gravity so that the fetal trunk is encouraged to rotate to transverse and then to anterior. If the position of the occiput is uncertain use trial and error, rotating through the eight positions of the "roll-over," using progress or comfort in each position as an indicator of progress (Fig. 11.11).

When to use side-lying positions

- As long as labor continues to progress well and the laboring person wants to use them.
- When supine hypotension occurs.
- When the laboring person has been given narcotics or an epidural.
- When the laboring person has gestational hypertension.
- May resolves some fetal heart rate problems.
- When the laboring person finds it comfortable in first or second stage.

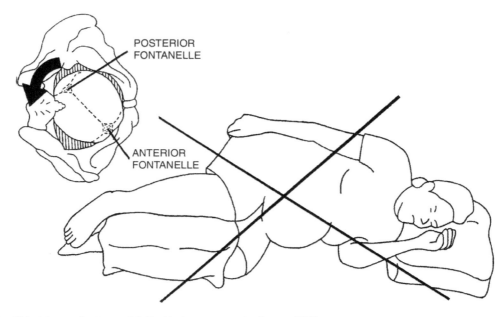

Fig. 11.9.   Side-lying on the "wrong" (left) side for suspected or known ROP.

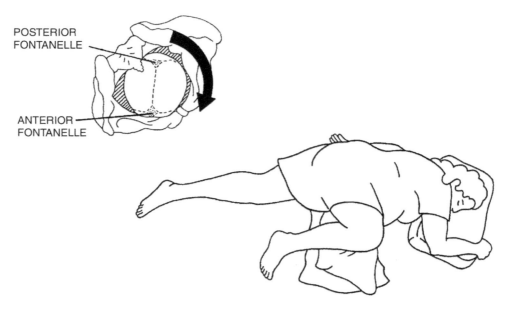

Fig. 11.10.   Laboring person with an OP fetus, in semiprone on the "correct" side with fetal back "toward the ceiling."

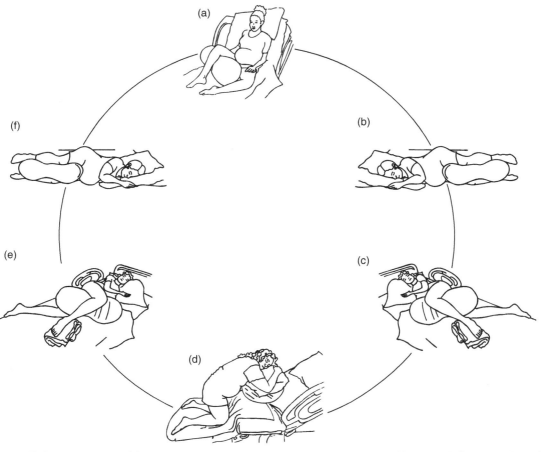

Fig. 11.11. Roll-over sequence. (a) Throne position with peanut ball. (b) Right side-lying with peanut ball between legs. (c) Exaggerated right-side lying with peanut ball between legs. (d) Lying over birthing ball, foot of bed dropped (e) Exaggerated left side-lying with peanut ball between legs. (f) Left side-lying with peanut ball between legs.

- When the laboring person is tired.
- In second stage, if hemorrhoids are painful in dorsal positions.
- In a rapid second stage, to neutralize gravity effect.

When not to use side-lying positions

- When the laboring person is unwilling, due to increased pain or preference for another position. However, if it is explained that this position may improve labor progress, the person may be willing to try it.
- When a gravity advantage (a vertical position) is needed to aid descent, especially if second stage progress has slowed.
- When they have been in side-lying for more than an hour without progress.

The "semiprone lunge"

When: During first and second stages.

How: With the laboring person in a semiprone position, the partner or doula stands facing the bed and places the laboring person's upper foot against the partner's hip.

During contractions, the partner leans slightly against the laboring person's foot to flex their hip and knee more and hold the leg in a flexed position (Fig. 11.12). It is important that the partner does not lean excessively, as this might overstretch the ligaments in the laboring person's sacroiliac or hip joint and cause later pain or poor function. This is especially problematic if the laboring person has an epidural and is unable to feel discomfort from stretching. A peanut ball can be used to support the laboring person in a semi-prone lunge (Fig. 11.13).

What this position does

- Changes the shape of the pelvis, slightly opening the upper sacroiliac joint, and giving more room on the upper side of the pelvis.
- Increases chances of rotation of an OP or asynclitic fetus.
- Is comfortable and effortless for the laboring person.

When to use the semiprone lunge

- When dilation or descent has slowed.
- If a fetal malposition is suspected.
- When the laboring person has an epidural, which does not allow them to maintain their upper leg in the flexed position without help and limits the positions she can use.
- If the laboring person is too tired to do the kneeling or standing lunge, and it is desirable to alter pelvic shape.

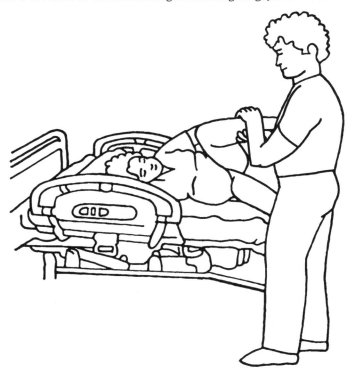

Fig. 11.12. Semiprone lunge.

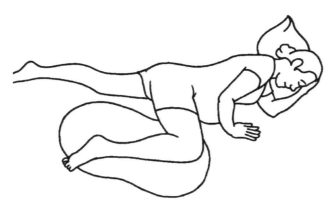

Fig. 11.13.   Semiprone lunge with peanut ball.

When not to use the semiprone lunge

- When a gravity advantage (a vertical position) is needed to aid descent, especially if second stage progress has slowed.
- When the laboring person has been in the position for more than an hour without progress.

Side-lying release

When: May be used twice a week prior to labor (for about 2½ minutes on each side) or during labor, to correct any of these: a stall in labor contractions, contractions with no progress, malpositioned baby, or pain in one or both hips or in the pelvis.

This technique was developed by Carol Phillips, DC, who has encouraged its utilization by birth workers during pregnancy and birth to correct soft-tissue tension and torque in the pelvis and surrounding structures, which can increase labor pain and slow labor progress. It is now featured as an important part of the whole Spinning Babies Approach (C. Phillips, personal communication, September 25, 2016, Tully 2018; Tulley 2019).

How to do it (see Fig. 11.14):

- Use a fairly firm surface above the floor. It should be long enough for the laboring person to stretch out. A hospital bed, massage table, or a couch works well. The laboring person does this with the aid of a helper (doula, nurse, partner, midwife).
- The laboring person chooses which side they will lie on first.
- They lay on their side, with a pillow beneath their head, and their head level and in line with the straight spine.
- The helper stands in front of them, leaning with one side of the helper's body or hip against the edge of the bed to keep the laboring person from falling. A chair can be placed beside the bed for the laboring person to hold onto, or they can grasp the bedrail on a hospital bed.
- The laboring person scoots themselves right to the edge of the bed, with their hips about 2 inches (5 cm) from the edge. For a person in the third-trimester of pregnancy or a laboring person, the pregnant belly extends beyond the edge of the bed.
- It is very important that the laboring person's hips and shoulders are in balance, and aligned vertically so that neither the top hip nor the shoulder is tipping further back or forward than the lower hip or shoulder.
- Body alignment may be improved if the laboring person extends her top arm above their head, resting it on a cheek and the side of their head.
- The helper curves both hands (one on top of the other) over the top and front of the laboring person's hip—over the anterior superior iliac spine (ASIS bone)—using enough pressure to keep the laboring person's hip

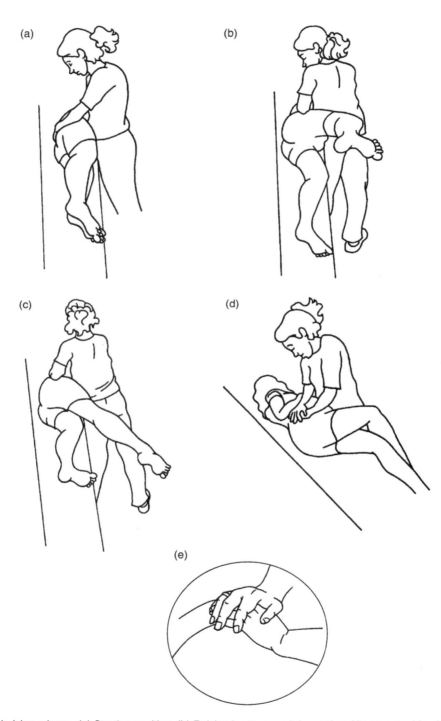

Fig. 11.14. Side-lying release. (**a**) Starting position. (**b**) Raising leg to move it forward and hang over side of the bed. (**c**) Top leg hanging over side of bed. (**d**) Helper's hand cupped over top front of hip—over the hip bone (anterior superior iliac spine)—seen from above (**e**). Same as (d), seen from behind the mother.

from leaning forward out of alignment. She or he may rock their hip gently to encourage relaxation of the muscles in the area.
- The laboring person straightens their lower leg (without help from the helper), with their feet and toes dorsiflexed (flexed toward their knee).
- While the helper assists the laboring person to maintain a perfect side-lying position, the laboring person (without help) raises their leg, about 30 degrees, and moves it forward beyond the edge of the bed, then slowly lowers it so that it is hanging down loosely in front of them. They maintain that position, relaxing their leg, for 2 to 20 minutes or until the leg relaxes and lengthens a bit. Nothing should touch or support their leg; the leg should be free to hang.
- The helper makes sure the pregnant person's back remains straight, with their top shoulder and hip aligned directly above the lower shoulder and hip, and presses down on the hip and back enough to keep the hips aligned vertically.
- This technique is then repeated on the other side. It is important to use the side-lying release on both sides, to establish and maintain balance in the pelvic joints and muscles.

What this technique does

- It relaxes and lengthens muscles that support the pelvis, including the pelvic floor. This helps relieve back pain.
- The weight of the leg causes a gentle stretch and release of tension in the muscles around the hip and pelvis, potentially creating more space within the pelvic basin and increased flexibility of pelvic joints, allowing the baby's head to move into a more favorable position.

When to use the side-lying release

- During pregnancy twice per week, to gently stretch hip and pelvic muscles, or to relieve pelvic or hip pain.
- During labor if contractions stall or slow down once the labor is established.
- If there are contractions with no progress.
- If there is a suspected malpositioned baby.
- If there is pain in one or both hips or in the pelvis.

When not to use the side-lying release

- If the laboring person is unwilling (however, once it is explained that this technique might reduce pain and improve labor progress, they may be willing to try it).
- If labor is progressing well.

Note: If the laboring person has joint disease, unexplained bleeding, previous injury involving the hips and/or pelvis, or limited movement in the selected joints, consult with an appropriate specialist before using, or avoid this technique. (This description of side-lying release is adapted from the writings of Gail Tully.[8,9])

Sitting positions

Semisitting

When: During first and second stages.
  How: The laboring person sits with their trunk at a greater than 45-degree angle with the bed (Fig. 11.15)

What this position does

- Provides some gravity advantage, compared with supine.
- May be better than supine for:
  ○ increasing pelvic inlet dimensions;
  ○ improving fetal oxygenation.
- Is an easy and restful position to assume.
- Pressure on sacrum and coccyx may impair enlargement of the pelvic outlet, especially when the laboring person sits on a firm surface.

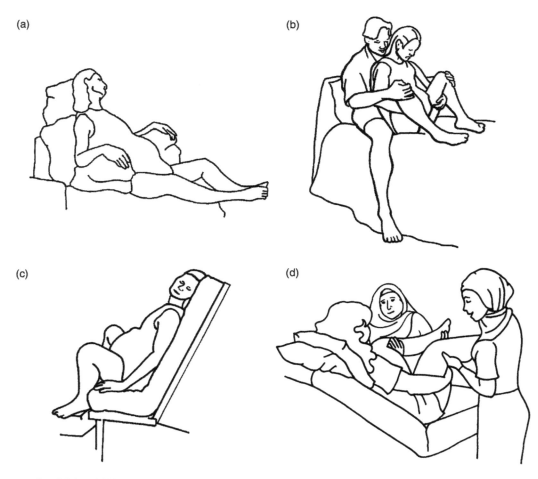

Fig. 11.15.   Semisitting. (**a**) To rest. (**b**) To push. (**c**) With bed back raised. (**d**) With leg support.

When to use semi-sitting positions

- If progress is good, and the laboring person prefers it.
- When the laboring person needs rest.
- When an epidural is in place, as an alternative to supine or side-lying.
- When the birthgiver wants to see the birth.
- For caregiver's convenience during second stage, in viewing perineum.

When not to use semisitting positions

- With known or suspected OP fetus.
- If fetal heart rate reacts adversely.
- If laboring person has hypertension and this position exacerbates it.
- When the laboring person refuses, due to increased pain or preference for another position. However, once it is explained that this position might improve labor progress, the laboring person may be willing to try it.

Sitting upright

When: During first and second stages.
   How: The laboring person sits straight up on a bed, chair, or stool (Fig. 11.16).

What this position does

- Provides gravity advantage.
- Allows a tired laboring person to rest if they are well supported.
- Allows for placement of hot pack on shoulders, low back, or lower abdomen or cold pack on low back.
- Enables the laboring person to rock or sway in rocking chair or on birth ball.

When to use upright sitting positions

- When the laboring person needs to rest.
- When the laboring person has back pain.
- When the laboring person finds it comfortable in first or second stage.
- When active labor progress has slowed; sitting up is thought to be especially beneficial if their knees are lower than their hips.[5]

When not to use upright sitting positions

- When the laboring person is unwilling, due to increased pain or a preference for another position. However, if it is explained that there is a chance that this position will improve progress, the laboring person may be willing to try it.

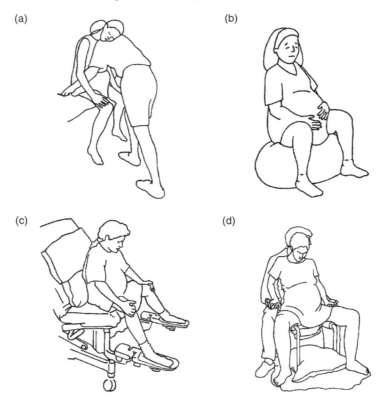

Fig. 11.16. Sitting upright. (**a**) With partner support in first stage. (**b**) On a birth ball. (**c**) To push. (**d**) On a birthing stool.

- When fetal heart rate is compromised in that position.
- When the person has an epidural and insufficient trunk strength to maintain position.

Sitting, leaning forward with support

When: During first and second stages.

How: The laboring person sits with feet firmly placed, knees apart, and leans forward, arms resting on thighs or on a prop in front of them (Figs. 11.17a, 11.17b), or they straddles a chair or toilet and rests their upper body on the back (Figs. 11.17c, 11.17d).

What this position does

- Provides gravity advantage.
- Is restful if the laboring person is well supported.
- Relieves back pain.

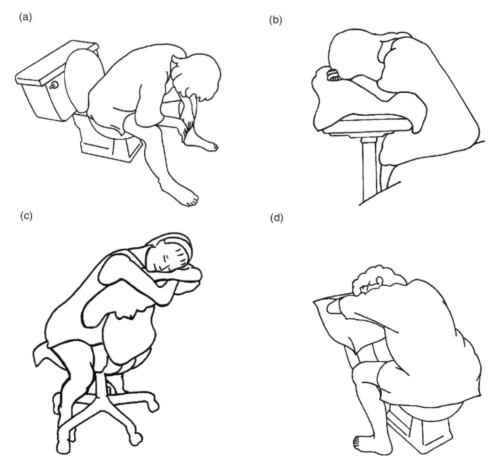

(a)   (b)   (c)   (d)

Fig. 11.17.   Sitting, leaning forward. (**a**) On a toilet. (**b**) On a tray table. (**c**) Straddling a chair.

- May enhance rotation from OP (better than supine and semisitting positions).
- Aligns fetus with pelvis (see Fig. 2.2).[7]
- Enlarges pelvic inlet (compared with supine).
- Allows easy access for backrub.

When to use sitting and leaning forward

- If the laboring person is semisitting and labor is not progressing, to shift the weight of the fetal torso off the spine.
- When the laboring person has back pain.
- When the laboring person finds it comfortable in first or second stage.
- When active labor progress has slowed.

When not to use sitting and leaning forward

- When the laboring person is unwilling, due to increased pain or a preference for another position. However, if it is explained that this position may improve labor progress, the laboring person may be willing to try it.
- If pain and discomfort does not improve after six to eight contractions in this position.
- If epidural or narcotics interfere with their ability to maintain this position.

Standing, leaning forward

When: During first and second stages.

How: The laboring person stands and leans on the partner, on a raised bed, over a birth ball placed on the bed, or on a wall rail or countertop (Fig. 11.18). They may sway from side to side.

What this position does

- Provides gravity advantage.
- Enlarges pelvic inlet (compared with supine or sitting).
- Aligns fetus with pelvic inlet.[5,7]
- May promote flexion of fetal head.
- May enhance rotation from OP or OT, especially if combined with swaying movements.[5]
- Causes contractions to be less painful but more productive than in supine or sitting.[3]
- Relieves back pain by reducing pressure of the fetal presenting part on the laboring person's sacrum.
- May be easier to maintain than hands-and-knees position.
- If the laboring person is embraced and supported in the upright position by their partner, the embrace increases their sense of wellbeing and may reduce catecholamine production.
- May increase their urge to push in second stage.

When to use standing and leaning forward

- When labor progress is slow or arrested.
- When contractions space out or lose intensity.
- When the laboring person has back pain.
- When the laboring person finds it comfortable in first or second stage.

When not to use standing and leaning forward

- When the laboring person is unwilling, due to increased pain or a preference for another position. However, if it is explained that this position may improve labor progress, the laboring person may be willing to try it.
- When labor progress is adequate in less strenuous positions.
- When birth is imminent and the attendant is unable or unwilling to deliver the baby in this position.
- When epidural or narcotics interfere with the laboring person's motor control.

(a)   (b)

(c)   (d)

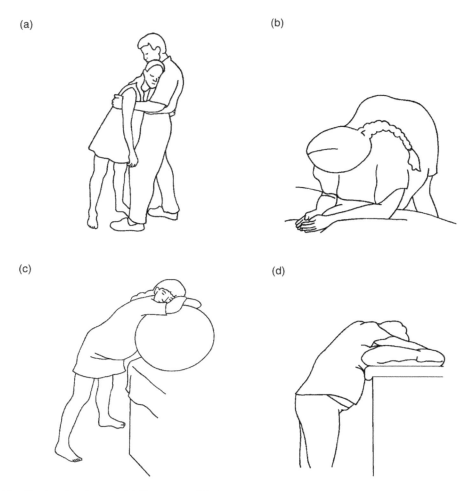

Fig. 11.18.   Standing leaning forward. (**a**) On partner. (**b**) On a bed. (**c**) On a birth ball. (**d**) On a counter.

Kneeling positions

Kneeling, leaning forward with support

When: During first and second stages.
   How: The laboring person kneels on bed or floor (possibly with knee pads or pillow beneath knees), leaning forward onto back of bed, on a chair seat, birth ball, or other support (Fig. 11.19).

What this position does

- Takes advantage of the benefits of gravity.
- Aligns fetus with pelvic inlet.
- Enlarges pelvic inlet more than side-lying, supine, or sitting.
- Allows easy access for back pressure.
- Relieves strain on hands and wrists compared with hands and knees.

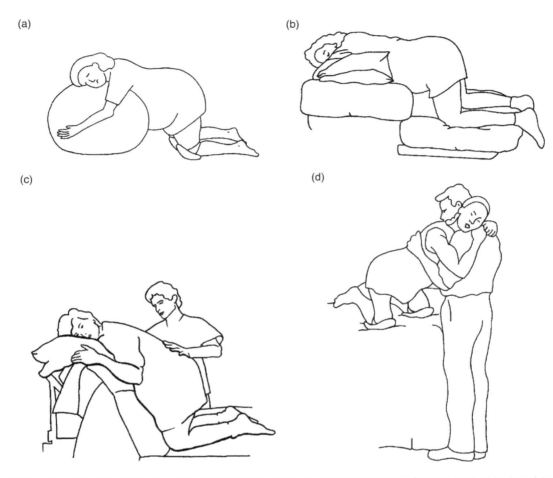

Fig. 11.19. Kneeling. (**a**) Leaning on a ball with knee pads. (**b**) On the foot of the bed. (**c**) Over the back of the bed. (**d**) With partner support to push and knee pads.

- Allows easy movement (swaying, rocking).
- May resolve some fetal heart rate problems.
- May cause soreness in knees (to prevent this, the laboring person can kneel on a soft pillow or wear kneepads, such as those made for sports or gardening).

When to use kneeling and leaning forward with support

- When fetus is thought or known to be OP or otherwise malpositioned.
- When the laboring person has back pain.
- When labor progress has slowed in first or second stage.
- When the laboring person is in a bath or pool, if space allows.
- When non-reassuring or indeterminate fetal heart tones are noted with supine or side-lying position.
- When fetus is at a high station.
- If the laboring person finds it comfortable.
- To alternate with other positions for back pain.

When not to use kneeling and leaning forward

- When the laboring person has pain in their knees or legs.
- If the laboring person is very tired.
- When first or second stage is not progressing in the position.
- If epidural or narcotics impair their motor control.
- When the laboring person is unwilling, due to increased pain or a preference for another position. However, if it is explained that this position may improve labor progress, the laboring person may be willing to try it

Hands and knees

When: During first and second stages.

How: The laboring person kneels (preferably on a padded surface), leans forward, and supports themselves on either the palms of their hands or their fists (the latter being more tolerable if she has swollen hands or carpal tunnel syndrome)

What this position does

- Aids fetal rotation from OP or OT.[7]
- May aid in reducing an anterior lip in late first stage.
- Reduces back pain.[7]
- Allows swaying, crawling, or rocking motion to promote rotation and increase comfort.
- Relieves hemorrhoids.
- May resolve fetal heart rate some fetal heart rate problems.
- Allows easy access for counterpressure or double hip squeeze.
- As a part of the measures used to relieve shoulder dystocia.
- Allows access for vaginal exams.
- May cause the laboring person's arms to tire; to relieve this, she rests upper body and head on a pile of pillows, chair seat, or birth ball.

When to use hands and knees (Fig. 11.20)

- When labor progress has slowed in first or second stage.
- When fetal heart tones are non-reassuring or indeterminate.
- When the laboring person has back pain.
- When the fetus is thought or known to be OP.
- When the laboring person finds it comfortable in first or second stage.
- When an anterior lip slows progress.

When not to use hands and knees

- When the laboring person is unwilling, due to increased pain or a preference for another position. However, if it is explained that this position may improve labor progress, the person may be willing to try it.
- When epidural or narcotics impair their motor control.

Open knee–chest position

When: During prelabor, first and second stages.

How: The laboring person goes to hands and knees, then lowers their chest to the floor, so that their buttocks are higher than their chest. In the open knee–chest position (Fig. 11.21a–c) their knees are together and their hips are less flexed (>90-degree angle) than in the usual closed knee–chest position (Fig. 11.22). This more open position puts the buttocks higher and the pelvis at a very different angle compared to when the knees are spread or drawn up under the trunk.

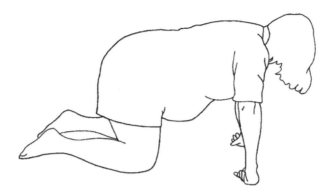

Fig. 11.20. Hands and knees.

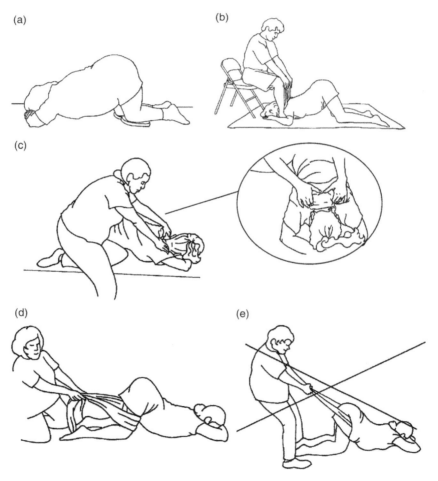

Fig. 11.21. Open knee–chest position. (**a**) With knee pads. (**b**) With shoulders leaning against partner's padded shins. (**c**) With shoulder support by partner. (**d**) With shawl around thighs and partner pulling back. (**e**) An *Unsafe* way to use the shawl. See caution box below.

> **Caution:** DO NOT wind the shawl into a narrow band and pull back with it beneath the laboring person's abdomen. This can restrict circulation through the groin area. Instead, fold the rebozo to a width of 8–10 inches (20–25 cm). Spread it over their thighs, and when pulling, pull back (parallel to the floor or bed) rather than up, to keep the shawl from narrowing and putting pressure in the groin.

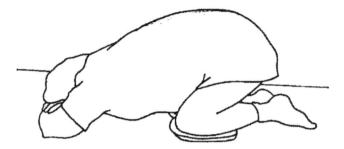

Fig. 11.22. Closed knee–chest position.

What this position does

- May protect against fetal hypoxia/anoxia when employed during management of a prolapsed cord.
- If used during the latent phase or any time before engagement, it allows repositioning of the fetal head. The laboring person may need to hold this position for 8 to 10 contractions in a row or 30 to 45 minutes for this purpose. Gravity encourages the fetal head to "back out" of the pelvis and rotate or flex before re-entering.
- May resolve some fetal heart rate problems.
- May reduce an anterior lip.
- May Reduces back pain.
- May relieve pressure on hemorrhoids.

This position may be tiring if maintained for 30 minutes or more. It can be made easier if: (1) pillows are used beneath their chest; (2) they kneel and place their head between their partner's ankles (see Fig. 11.21b), allowing their shoulders to lean against the partner's shins (place padding on shins, for comfort); (3) partner pulls back against the laboring person's thighs using a shawl spread wide over their thighs (see Fig. 11.21d); or (4) partner pulls back on the laboring person's shoulders while leaning back (see Fig. 11.21c). All these techniques reduce the effort required by the laboring person to remain in the position (Fig. 11.21d, 11.21e).

When to use the open knee–chest position

- As a part of emergency management of prolapsed cord.
- When one suspects OP during prelabor or early labor; contractions "couple" (come in pairs close together), followed by a longer interval; or when they are short, frequent, irregular, and painful, especially in the low back and are not accompanied by dilation.[8] This position may be alternated with semiprone (exaggerated runner's lunge) position.
- When the laboring person has back pain.
- To deminish the laboring person's premature urge to push.
- When the laboring person has a swollen cervix or anterior lip.
- If the caregiver is about to perform a digital or manual rotation of an OP head during first or second stage.

When not to use the open knee–chest position

- If the laboring person becomes short of breath or has gastric upset or other discomfort.
- If epidural or narcotics interfere with motor control.
- When the laboring person is unwilling, due to increased pain or a preference for another position. However, if it is explained that this position may improve labor progress, the laboring person may be willing to try it.

Closed knee–chest position

When: During first and second stages.

How: The laboring person kneels and leans forward, supporting themselves on their hands, then lowers their chest to the bed, with their knees and hips flexed and abducted beneath their abdomen (see Fig. 11.22).

What this position does

- Reduces back pain.
- Is less strenuous than hands-and-knees or "open" knee–chest position.
- Spreads ischia, enlarging pelvic outlet (bispinous and intertuberous diameters).
- Relieves hemorrhoids.
- May resolve some fetal heart rate problems.
- Is an antigravity position, which may help reduce an anterior lip.

When to use the closed knee–chest position

- When the laboring person has back pain.
- When the laboring person has a swollen cervix or anterior lip.

When not to use the closed knee–chest position

- In prelabor or early labor when fetal rotation is desired (instead, try open knee–chest with hips at >90-degree angle).
- When the laboring person objects, due to increased pain or a preference for another position. However, if it is explained that this position may improve labor progress, the laboring person may be willing to try it.
- If the laboring person becomes short of breath or has gastric upset or other discomfort.
- During a normally progressing second stage (works against gravity).

Asymmetrical upright (standing, kneeling, sitting) positions

When: During first and second stages.

How: The laboring person sits, stands, or kneels, with one knee and hip flexed, and foot elevated above the other (Fig. 11.23). Comfort guides the laboring person in which leg to raise. She should try both sides; one side may be much more comfortable than the other; the more comfortable side is probably the one to use.

What these positions do

- Exert a mild stretch on adductor muscles of the raised thigh, causing some lateral movement of one ischium, thus increasing pelvic outlet diameter. This is more pronounced when the laboring person raises their leg to the side rather than forward.
- May aid rotation from OP.
- Reduce back pain.
- Provide gravity advantage.
- Allow the laboring person to "lunge" in this position, thereby causing the pelvic outlet to widen even more on that side.

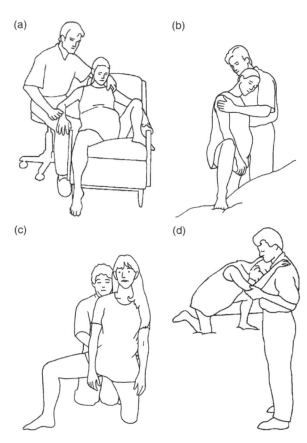

Fig. 11.23. Asymmetrical upright positions. (**a**) Sitting. (**b**) Standing. (**c**) Kneeling. (**d**) Kneeling with partner support.

When to use asymmetrical upright positions

• When the laboring person has back pain.
• When active labor progress has slowed.
• When rotation is desired in first or second stage.
• When the fetus is suspected to be asynclitic or otherwise malpositioned.

When not to use asymmetrical upright positions

• When the laboring person finds that these positions increase pain in their knees, hips, or pubic joint.
• When she has an epidural or narcotics that may weaken their legs or impair their balance.

Squatting positions

Squatting

When: Primarily during second stage, but any time the laboring person finds it comfortable.
   How: The laboring person lowers themselves from standing into a squatting position with their feet flat on the floor or bed, using their partner, a squatting bar, or their support for balance, if necessary (Fig. 11.24).

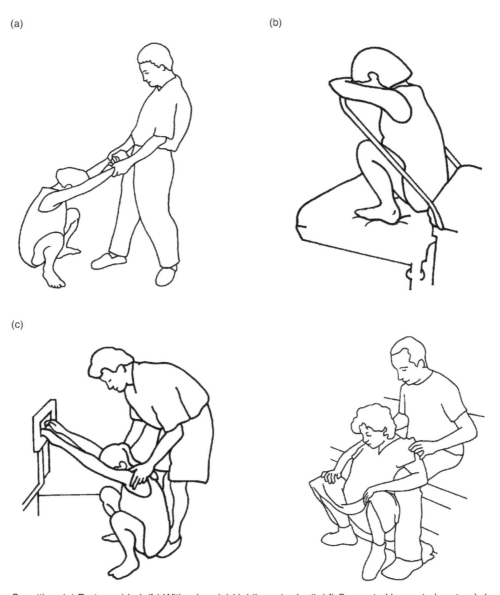

Fig. 11.24. Squatting. (**a**) Partner-aided. (**b**) With a bar. (**c**) Holding a bed rail. (**d**) Supported by seated partner's legs.

What this position does

- Provides gravity advantage.
- Enlarges pelvic outlet by increasing the intertuberous diameter.
- Allows the sacrum to move freely.
- May require less bearing-down effort than horizontal positions.
- May enhance urge to push.
- May enhance fetal descent.

- May relieve back pain.
- Allows freedom to shift weight for comfort.
- Provides mechanical advantage: upper trunk presses on fundus more than in many other positions.
- If continued for a prolonged period, squatting compresses the blood vessels and nerves located behind the knee joint, impairing circulation and possibly causing entrapment neuropathy. As long as the laboring person sits back or rises to standing after every contraction or two, such problems are avoided. Similarly prolonged squatting can lead to perineal edema which can be relieved by a change to another position. Note: People for whom squatting is a customary resting position do not have these potential nerve and circulation problems.

When to use squatting

- When more space within the pelvis is desired during second stage, especially when fetus is in a plus station and OA.
- When descent in late second stage is inadequate.

When not to use squatting

- When there is lower extremity joint injury, arthritis, or weakness.
- When an epidural has caused motor or sensory block in the legs.
- We recommend support of spontaneous pusing. The combination of prolonged breath-holding and squatting could increase the risk of perineal damage.

Supported squatting ("dangling") positions

When: During second stage.

How to do the supported squat: During contractions, the laboring person leans with their back against their partner, who places forearms under her arms and holds their hands, taking all their weight (Fig. 11.25a). They stand, bearing their weight, between contractions. (Caution: This requires a good deal of strength in the partner, who should be sure not to lean forward, as it could cause injury to the back. The partner should remain upright or lean against a wall for support.)

How to do the "dangle": This may be easier on the partner than the supported squat. The partner sits on a high bed or counter, feet supported on chairs or footrests, with thighs spread. The laboring person stands between the partner's legs with their back to their partner, and places their flexed arms over the partner's thighs. During the contraction the laboring persons lowers themselves slowly, and their partner presses on the sides of their chest with their thighs; their full weight is supported by their arms on his thighs and the grip of their thighs on their upper trunk (Fig. 11.25b). If the partner places their feet directly beneath his knees, the laboring person's weight is borne by their bones, rather than having them rely totally on their muscle strength. The laboring person bears down with their urge to push, and then stands between contractions.

A "birth sling," suspended from the ceiling, may also be used to support the laboring person (Fig. 11.25c). The dangle or use of a birth sling is much easier for the partner than the supported squat.

How to make a birth sling: A birth sling may be constructed from a length of sturdy cloth, folded to about 2 feet (60 cm) wide. It is looped so that each end is attached to an eye bolt in 10 the ceiling or another strong support. It should be long enough that the laboring person can place it around their shoulders like a shawl and lower themselves so that their knees are flexed and the sling bears all their weight. The laboring person grasps each side of the sling as she lowers themselves. They can avoid direct pressure on their armpits by wearing the sling like a shawl and flexing their elbows (Fig. 11.25c).

Ensure safety by checking that the sling will not give way when there is weight in it, and be sure there is someone standing by the laboring person whenever they are using the sling.

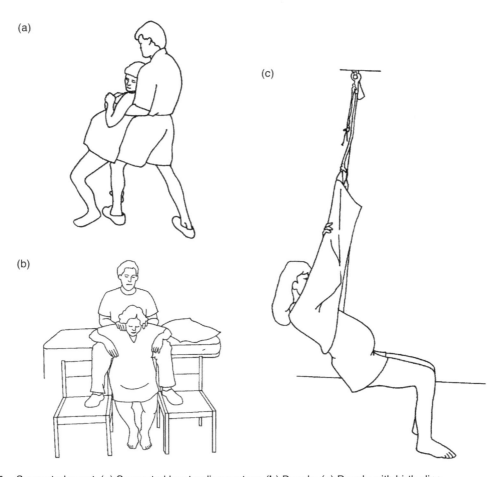

Fig. 11.25. Supported squat. (**a**) Supported by standing partner. (**b**) Dangle. (**c**) Dangle with birth sling.

What this position does

- Provides gravity advantage.
- Elongates the laboring person's trunk: may help resolve asynclitism by giving the fetus more room to reposition the angle of the head in the laboring person's pelvis.
- Allows more mobility in pelvic joints than in other positions, as there are no direct pressures pulling or pushing on the pelvis (except for the baby's presenting part!).
- Allows fetal head to "mold" the laboring person's pelvis as needed.
- Enables the laboring person to feel secure and supported by the partner or sling, which may reduce catecholamine production.
- Using the supported squat or dangle for a prolonged period may cause paresthesia (numbness, tingling) in the laboring person's hands, from pressure of the partner's arms or thighs in their armpits (causing nerve compression in the brachial plexus). To prevent this, the laboring person should stand up and lean on their partner between contractions or try the dangle instead. The dangle allows the partner's legs or the birth sling to support all of the laboring person's weight; if done properly (with the partner pressing his or their thighs against the laboring person's rib cage), the numbness and tingling should not occur. The dangle is also less tiring for the partner than the supported squat.
- The dangle leaves the partner's hands free to stroke or hold the laboring person.

When to use supported squatting positions

- When more mobility of pelvic joints is needed.
- When lengthening of the laboring person's trunk seems desirable, as with an asynclitic fetus.
- In second stage, when fetal head is thought to be large, asynclitic, OP, or OT.
- When descent is slow or not taking place.

When not to use supported squatting positions

- When the laboring person is unwilling, due to increased pain or a preference for another position. However, if it is explained that this position may improve labor progress, the laboring person may be willing to try it.
- If the laboring person has weakness or pain in their shoulder joints.
- When birth is imminent, unless the caregiver has agreed that delivery can take place in this position.
- When the laboring person has an epidural or narcotics that interfere with their balance or the use of their legs.
- When no one is available who is strong enough to support the laboring person or there is no birth sling available.

Half-squatting, lunging, and swaying

When: During first or second stage.

How: The laboring person stands and, holding onto a supporting device suspended from above (Fig. 11.26a), lowers their body and leans back so that she is in a half-squat (Fig. 11.26b). She may raise one leg, as in the standing lunge (Fig. 11.35a) or sway from side to side with a feeling of security (Fig. 11.26c).

What this position and swaying movements do

- Provide gravity advantage.
- Alter pelvic dimensions when the laboring person goes from standing to half-squatting, and when she sways from side to side in a half-squatting position, or with one leg raised.
- May facilitate fetal rotation and descent.
- May be difficult for the laboring person to use if she is exhausted or has upper body weakness.

When to use the half-squat with lunging or swaying

- When more mobility of pelvic joints is needed.
- When the laboring person is unable to do a full squat.
- When the fetal head is thought to be large, asynclitic, OP, or OT.
- In second stage, when descent is not taking place.

When not to use the half-squat with lunging or swaying

- If the laboring person is unwilling.
- When birth is imminent, unless the caregiver agrees that delivery can take place in this position.
- When the laboring person has an epidural or narcotics that interfere with their balance or the use of their legs.

Lap squatting

When: During second stage for four to six contractions followed by another position.

How: The partner sits on an armless straight chair; the laboring person sits on their partner's lap, facing and embracing their partner and straddling their partner's thighs. Their partner embraces them and, during contractions, spreads his or her thighs, allowing the laboring person's buttocks to sag between them. The laboring person keeps from sagging too far by bending her knees over her partner's thighs. The partner sits up straight and does not lean forward (Fig. 11.27). This position requires two support people, strength and caution to prevent injury.

(a)

(b)

(c)

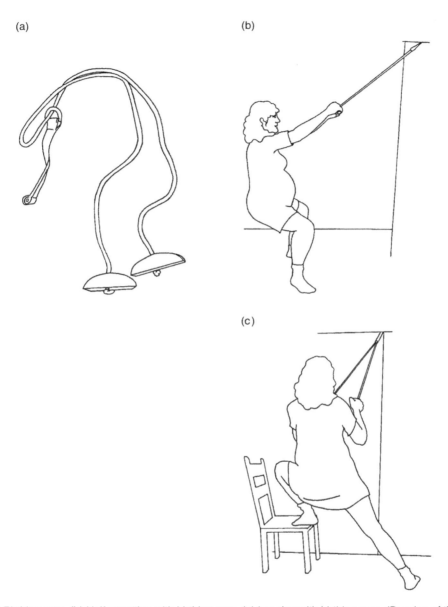

Fig. 11.26. (**a**) Birthing rope. (**b**) Half-squatting with birthing rope. (**c**) Lunging with birthing rope. (Drawing of the rope based on PrePak Products, Inc.)

Note: The birthing rope shown here, originally designed to aid upper body stretching, attaches over a sturdy door, which remains closed during use. The apparatus hangs on the side of the door opposite the direction in which the door opens. The supportive rope enables the laboring person to maintain positions that would not be possible without it. Caution: A support person should remain close by to aid the laboring person with balance.

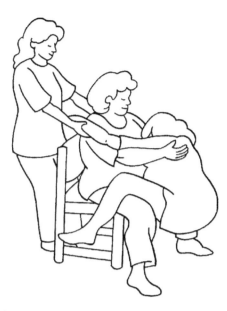

Fig. 11.27.   Lap squat, with three people.

What this position does

- Provides all the advantages of squatting (gravity, enlarging pelvic diameters) without the laboring person having to bear all their weight in the squatting position.
- Allows the laboring person to rest between contractions, while they are held by both their partner and the laboring person holding their wrists or hands.
- Passively enlarges the pelvic outlet.
- Requires less bearing-down effort than many other positions.
- Relaxes the pelvic floor.
- May enhance descent if fetus is OA, or help reposition a non-OA fetus.
- Mechanical advantage when baby is low in the pelvis: upper trunk presses on fundus more than in other positions.
- May enhance the laboring person's sense of security, as she is held closely.
- Is awkward for the caregiver (who must get on floor to view progress).
- May be tiring for the support laboring person who bears the laboring person's weight. The second support laboring person's help in supporting the laboring person is an important safety precaution.
- May be less effective if fetus is asynclitic.

When to use lap squatting

- When second stage progress has arrested.
- When the laboring person has joint problems that make other squatting positions impossible.
- When the laboring person is too tired to squat or dangle.
- When all other positions have been tried.
- Can be used with a light epidural. To do this, the laboring person sits on the side of the bed with their legs dangling and spread apart. The partner sits on a rolling stool and rolls to the edge of the bed, which should be lowered to just above the level of the partner's lap. The partner faces the laboring person, with his or their arms encircling their hips, and the partner slides the laboring person off the bed onto his or their lap. The laboring person holds their partner around the neck and their partner holds them around their waist and rolls away from the bed. The doula (or another support person) assists with the transfer of the laboring person from bed to the

partner's lap, and then, standing behind the partner, takes the laboring person's hands, and the laboring person and doula hold each other's wrists securely.

When not to use lap squatting

- When the laboring person finds it impossible or much more painful.
- When there is no strong support laboring person available, or the laboring person is too heavy to be supported.
- When there is no third laboring person available to help.
- When the laboring person has a dense epidural and has no use of her legs.

Supine positions

Supine

When: We do not recommend routine use of supine positions during first and second stage of labor. There are times when supine positions may be useful for assessments or interventions. The supine position is overused has never been shown to be the preferred labor pushing or birthing position of human beings. It became popular and overused because of the preference of birth attendants. It allows easy viewing of the perineum. If needed for an intervention we would recommend limiting the time the laboring person is supine. Raising the head of the bed to greater than 30 degrees preventions the hemodynamic changes associated with the use of the supine position (supine hypotention). If supine is needed for a specific reason, a rolled towel can be placed under the back on the left or right side, to prevent supine hypotension.

How: The laboring person lies flat on their back or with their trunk slightly raised (<45 degrees). The legs may be out straight, bent with their feet flat on the bed, in leg rests, or drawn up and back toward their shoulders (Fig. 11.28).[10]

What this position does

- Allows easy access for vaginal exams.
- Allows access if instruments are needed for delivery.

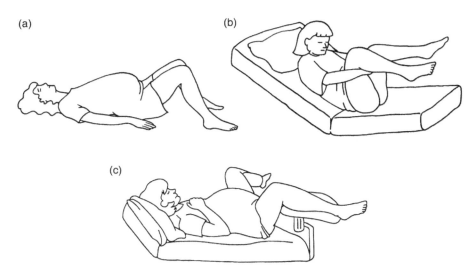

(a)   (b)

(c)

Fig. 11.28. (**a**) Supine with hips and knees flexed. (**b**) Supine, head of bed somewhat elevated. (**c**) Supine with leg supports.

Unintended consequences: Supine positions may:

- Increase the laboring person's perception of pain.
- Make the laboring person feel less active (and more passive) in the labor and birth process.
- Cause "supine hypotension" in the laboring person, with resulting reduction in oxygen to the fetus with subsequent fetal heart rate abnormalities. This can be quickly corrected with a position change to right or left side.
- Places the fetus in an unfavorable drive angle in relation to pelvis. This may lead to illusion of cephalopelvic disproportion due to the reduced pelvic diameters characteristic of this position (often corrected by changing positions).
- Impede rotation from OP or OT to OA.
- Requires the laboring person to push against gravity.
- Causes contractions to become more painful, but less effective than when the laboring person is vertical.

When to use the supine position

- When necessary for medical interventions that cannot be done with the laboring person in another position.

When not to use the supine position

- When medical interventions are not needed.
- Research has shown that Women prefer nonsupine positions.
- We do not recommend the routine use of suppine positions for second stage labor.

Sheet "pull-to-push"

When: During second stage, during contractions (Fig. 11.29).

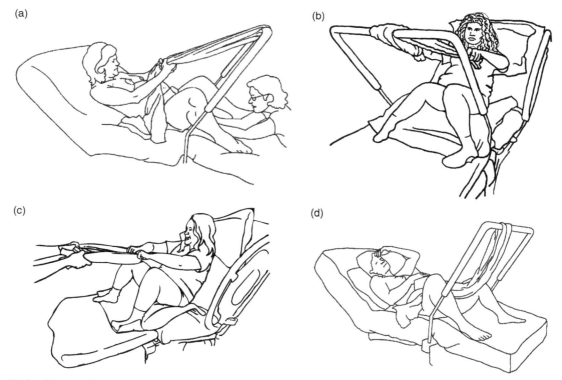

Fig. 11.29.   Sheet pull-to-push. (**a**) Pulling during contractions knees apart. (**b**) Pulling during contraction knees-together. (**c**) Tug of war. (**d**) Resting between contractions.

How: The laboring person lies on their back with their trunk raised to at least 30 degrees. Their knees are flexed and their feet are either flat on the bed or braced on the uprights of the squatting bar. A sheet or long shawl is looped either around the squatting bar, or around a bar at the foot of the bed, or it may be grasped at one end by a nurse, partner, or doula. The other end is held by the laboring person.

When the contraction begins, the laboring person holds the sheet tightly and pulls on it while lifting their head and bearing down. It is important that she does not pull themself to sitting but remains quite flat. This maximizes use of their abdominal muscles and gives them leverage to bear down effectively. If the laboring person pulls their self to sitting upright, it reduces significantly their use of their abdominal muscles and defeats the purpose of the activity. If another laboring person is holding the other end of the sheet, he or she should brace himself or themself so as not to get pulled over! At the end of the contraction, the laboring person lies back and rests.

What sheet pull-to-push does

- Aids a laboring person to push effectively.

When to use sheet pull-to-push

- When the laboring person is unable to push effectively, especially with an epidural.
- When, because of custom or hospital policy, the laboring person is restricted to a horizontal position for pushing.
- When little progress has been made with other positions.

When not to use sheet pull-to-push
- When the fetal heart tones are non-reassuring.
- When the laboring person does not have upper body strength.

Exaggerated lithotomy (McRoberts' position)

When: During second stage labor.

How: The laboring person lies flat on their back, legs abducted, and knees pulled toward their shoulders (by their self or by two other people, each one drawing one leg up toward one of their shoulders; Fig. 11.30).

What this position does

- May cause supine hypotension, with resulting reduction in oxygen supply to the fetus.
- Removes any positive effects of gravity.
- Is awkward and tiring for the laboring person.
- Puts fetus in an unfavorable drive angle, with exceptions (see later).
- May be beneficial if the fetal head is "stuck" and cannot pass beneath the pubic arch when the laboring person is in other positions. Pulling the laboring person's knees toward their shoulders rotates their pelvis posteriorly, flattening their low back and moving their pubic arch toward their head.[11,12] This position may allow the fetus to slip under the arch and continue its descent (see Fig. 11.30).

> **Precaution:** If the laboring person has an epidural, there is danger of injuring their pubic symphysis or sacroiliac joints by forcing their legs back beyond safe limits. Without sensation, the laboring person cannot feel the joint pain that would otherwise signal impending damage. Those supporting their legs should resist the temptation to force their legs back, as they could cause serious long-term damage.[13]

When to use exaggerated lithotomy

- As an intervention, when gravity positions and positions to enlarge pelvic diameters have been tried, but the fetus remains "stuck" at the pubis.
- As an intervention only for people laboring without epidurals and only brief periods.
- For the management of shoulder dystocia.

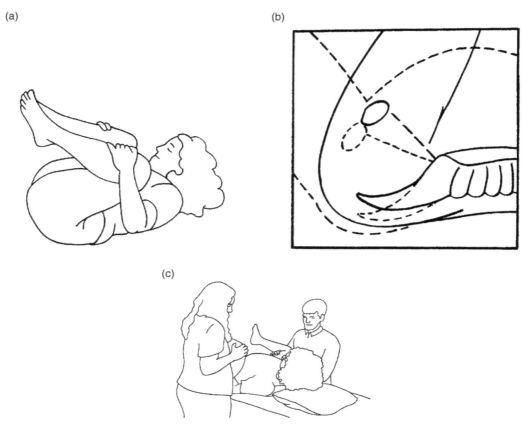

Fig. 11.30. **(a)** Exaggerated lithotomy (McRoberts' position). **(b)** Exaggerated lithotomy (detail). **(c)** Exaggerated lithotomy (McRoberts') with people supporting the laboring person's legs.

When not to use exaggerated lithotomy

● Not recommended as a routine second stage labor position.
● Not recommended when the laboring person has an epidural as its use has been associated with lumbo-sacral nerve damage.

MOVEMENTS IN FIRST AND SECOND STAGES

Sometimes specific movements by the laboring person improve their comfort and help the baby find its way through the birth canal. This section contains descriptions of movements by the laboring person that may:

● May help resolve a fetal malposition such as OP, persistent OT, or asynclitism.
● Enhance fetal descent by continually altering the shape and size of the laboring person's pelvic basin.
● Reduce labor pain by allowing the laboring person to find more comfortable positions and movements, to enable them to cope with the hours of contractions needed to dilate the cervix and press the fetus through the pelvis.
● Increase the laboring person's active participation, and decrease their emotional distress, thus contributing to fetal wellbeing.

Some of these movements will not be usable by some laboring people; for example, those with joint problems that do not allow these movements, or who have anesthesia that prevents them from moving in these ways, or if the fetal heart rate response is non-reassuring when the laboring person tries a particular movement.

Pelvic rocking (also called pelvic tilt) and other movements of the pelvis

When: Primarily early first stage, but any time, if desired.

How: On hands and knees, the laboring person "tucks their seat under" by contracting their abdominal muscles and arching their back, and then relaxes, returning their back to a neutral position (Fig. 11.31). It is done slowly and rhythmically throughout contractions when they has back pain and presumed OP or other malposition.

It will be easier on their arms and wrists if they do not bear weight on their hands but rests their upper body on a support, such as a bean bag, chair seat, birth ball, or adjustable bed (Fig. 11.32).

Other pelvic movements, such as swaying hips from side to side, are also helpful. The birth ball allows the laboring person to roll their upper body on the ball—forward and back, side to side, and in circles—almost effortlessly.

Why pelvic rocking helps:

If the laboring person kneels and leans forward on ball or chair, gravity may encourage rotation of the fetus from OP to OA. The pelvic rocking movement around the fetal head may help to dislodge the head, fostering rotation to OA[4,7] or correcting asynclitism. The position and movement reduce back pain, possibly by easing pressure of the fetal occiput on the laboring person's sacroiliac joint. For many, this position is the only one they can tolerate when back pain is severe.

Advantages

- Gravity plus movement helps alter the position of the fetus's head within the pelvis, and encourages rotation from OP.
- Relieves back pain.
- If the presumption of OP is in error, this exercise will not lead to malpositioning.

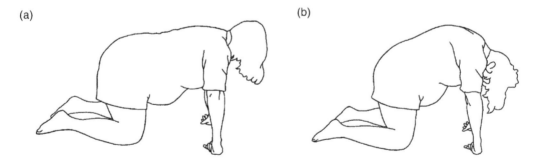

(a)   (b)

Fig. 11.31.   **(a)** Pelvic rocking, first position: flat back. **(b)** Pelvic rocking, second position: flexed back with "seat tucked under".

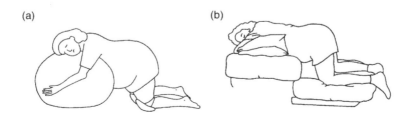

(a)   (b)

Fig. 11.32.   Pelvic rocking with support. **(a)** Resting upper body on ball. **(b)** Resting upper body on bed, with foot of bed lowered.

Disadvantages

- The laboring person's knees may become tired or sore. Knee pads may help.
- If continuous fetal monitoring is being use, the belts may slip. A support person or caregiver may have to hold the transducer in place or monitor intermittently. With some monitors, it is possible to insert a washcloth between the belt and the transducer in order to press the transducer more snuggly against the abdomen to keep it from slipping.

Hip sifting

When: When OP is suspected or the laboring person finds it comfortable.

How: With the laboring person on hands and knees, the caregiver or support person drapes a sheet over the laboring person's hips, twists the fabric next to their hips (Fig. 11.33a), and pulls forward with one hand and back

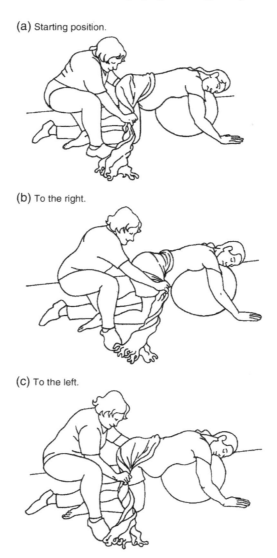

(a) Starting position.

(b) To the right.

(c) To the left.

Fig. 11.33. (**a**) Hip sifting, starting position. (**b**) Hip sifting to the right. (**c**) Hip sifting to the left.

with the other, about 4–5 inches (10–12 cm) in each direction. These alternating movements help the laboring person to sway their hips from side to side (Figs. 11.33b, 11.33c). This may also be done by alternating pulling up and down. The movements are quick so that the laboring person feels their hips are "jiggling." They relax their trunk and hips to allow the "sifting" or jiggling to occur. This can be done during or between contractions, according to the laboring person's preference. The rhythmic movement is comforting, and may help a malpositioned fetus move into a better position. Other advantages and disadvantages of hip sifting are similar to those of the pelvic rocking movement.

Flexion of hips and knees in hands and knees position (Fig. 11.34)

When: Mostly during second stage, when descent is very slow.

How: The laboring person begins on hands and knees with their knees spread apart, and slowly moves their trunk back so that their buttocks are above their heels and their knees and hips are flexed as much as possible. They may hold that position during the contraction while pushing; then they slowly return to the starting position until the next contraction. They repeat this slow rocking motion for several contractions.

Why hip and knee flexion helps

The hip and knee flexion while on hands and knees causes posterior tilting of the pelvis, and nutation of the sacroiliac joints—posterior rotation of both the lower sacrum and the anterior superior iliac spine (ASIS), which increases the anterior-posterior diameter of the pelvic outlet.[14]

(a) Starting position for Flexion and rocking on hands and knees.

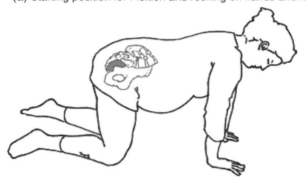

(b) Hips and knees fully flexed.

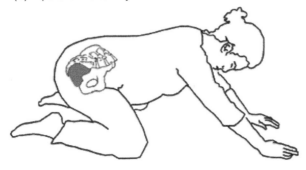

Fig. 11.34. Flexion and rocking on hands and knees. (**a**) Starting position. (**b**) Hips and knees fully flexed.

When to use this position

- When second stage descent is delayed.
- When a fetal malposition is suspected.
- If the laboring person wants to do it.

When not to use flexion and rocking on hands and knees

- If joint problems do not allow these movements.
- If fetal heart rate response is non-reassuring.
- If anesthesia prevents the laboring person from moving in this manner.
- When the laboring person is unwilling, due to increased pain or a preference for another position. However, if it is explained that this position may improve labor progress, the person may be willing to try it.

The lunge

When: Primarily first stage, but also second stage if desired.

How: Stabilize a chair so that it will not slide. The laboring person stands, facing forward with the chair at their side. They raise one foot, places it on the chair seat, and rotates their raised knee and foot to a right angle from the direction toward which they are facing (Fig. 11.35a). Keeping their body upright, they shift their weight sideways (lunges), abducting their hip and flexing their raised knee, and then returns to upright, continuing these rhythmic sideways lunges through each contraction. They repeat throughout several contractions in a row. They should feel a stretch in one or both inner thighs; if not, they should widen the distance between the foot on the floor and the foot on the chair. Their partner helps them with balance.

The lunge can also be done on a bed in the kneeling position (Fig. 11.35b).

Caution: It is important to keep moving while lunging: the laboring person should not pause when their knee is maximally flexed, which could cause strain on ligaments supporting the knee joint. Continuous movement protects against such injury.

Deciding direction in which to lunge

If the fetus is known to be OP, the laboring person should lunge in the direction of the occiput (e.g., if the fetus is ROP, it lunges to the right).

Even if the baby is not believed to be OP and if the laboring person has no back pain, the lunge may be useful at any time when active labor progress has slowed. The changes in pelvic shape caused by the lunge may correct subtle fetal positional problems. The laboring person will probably find that lunging to one side feels better than the other. The side that feels better is probably the one that gives more room for the occiput to adjust.

Why the lunge helps

The elevated femur acts as a lever at the hip joint, "prying" one ischium outward. This creates more space in that side of the pelvis for the posterior occiput to rotate or the asynclitic occiput to resolve its position. Lunging also uses gravity to advantage.

When to do the lunge

- Whenever labor progress is slow or has stopped, despite continuing contractions.
- If a fetal malposition is suspected or confirmed.

When NOT to do the lunge

- If the laboring person has balance problems, injury or pain in the hip, knee, or pubic symphysis.
- When narcotic or epidural analgesia renders it unsafe.
- If the laboring person is exhausted and in need of a rest.
- When the laboring person is unwilling, due to increased pain or a preference for another position. However, if it is explained that this position may improve labor progress, the person may be willing to try it.

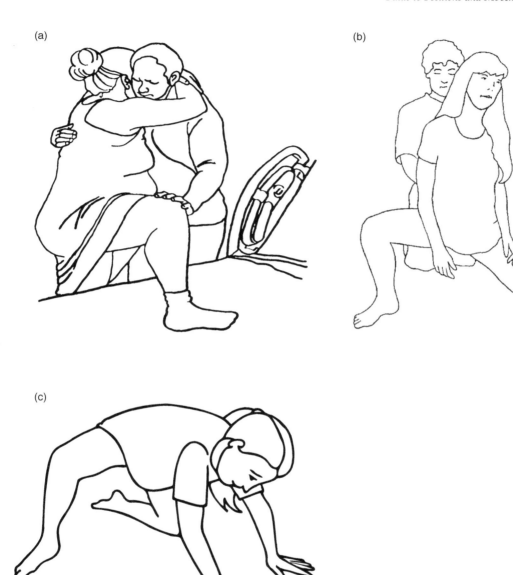

(a)

(b)

(c)

Fig. 11.35. (**a**) Standing lunge. (**b**) Kneeling lunge. (**c**) Runner's lunge.

Walking or stair climbing

When: Primarily first stage, but also second stage if desired.

How: The laboring person walks or climbs stairs (Fig. 11.36), continuing during contractions if possible. If not, they lean on their partner or the railing. If they spread their feet wide apart on each stair, in effect they are "lunging" and climbing stairs at the same time.

Alternatively, they may face the railing and climb the stairs sideways, one or two steps at a time.

(a)   (b)

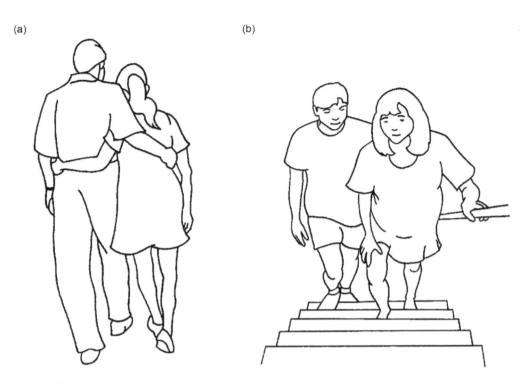

Fig. 11.36. (**a**) Walking. (**b**) Stair climbing.

Why walking and stair climbing help

Slight but repeated changes in the alignment of pelvic joints occur with each step (more so with stair climbing), encouraging fetal rotation and descent. Walking and stair climbing also use gravity to advantage, and may improve morale, especially if it provides a change of scene.

When to use walking and stair climbing

- Whenever labor progress is slow or has stopped, despite continuing contractions.[1]
- If a fetal malposition is suspected or confirmed.
- When the laboring person's spirits might benefit from a change of scene and some distraction.
- Any time the laboring person wishes to walk.

When NOT to use walking or stair climbing

- Same circumstances as when the lunge should be avoided (see above).
- When stairs are inconveniently located.
- When continuous electronic fetal monitoring is indicated and telemetry is not feasible.

Slow dancing

When: Primarily first stage, but also second stage if desired.

   How: The laboring person stands facing their partner and leans on them, and they sway slowly from side to side. The partner embraces them and presses on their low back. The laboring person puts their arms around the partner's neck, or lets them hang relaxed at their sides possibly hooking their thumbs into their partner's back pockets or waistband. They rest their head on their partner's shoulder or chest. The partner remains upright; leaning

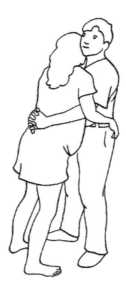

Fig. 11.37. Slow dancing.

forward for long periods may cause back pain. They shift their weight from foot to foot with their favorite music, and they can breathe in the rhythm of the "dance." This is the most relaxing and least tiring way to maintain an upright position, since the laboring person is partially supported (Fig. 11.37).

Between contractions, they may continue slow dancing, or walk together, or the laboring person might sit until the next contraction.

It is important that the laboring person's partner does not bear a lot of their weight; they should lean on them, not hang from them. They might not be able to bear their weight for very long!

Why slow dancing helps

Slight but repeated changes in the pelvic joints occur as the laboring person sways, encouraging fetal rotation and descent. This vertical position uses gravity to advantage.

Advantages

- The partner's embrace and support may reduce emotional stress and catecholamine production, enabling the uterus to work more efficiently.
- The partner, who knows and loves them more than anyone else, provides a kind of support that no one else can give, as well. For partners who want to help but feel at a loss to know how, this is most gratifying.
- Rhythmic swaying movements are comforting and may enable trunk and pelvic muscle relaxation.
- The partner can press on laboring person's lower back, providing some counterpressure to relieve back pain.
- Can be done beside the bed, with monitors and intravenous lines attached to the laboring person's body.
- Good substitute for walking.

Disadvantages

- The laboring person needs a partner with whom they feel comfortable "slow dancing." Laboring people without an intimate partner may not feel comfortable slow dancing with support people.
- A large height discrepancy between the laboring person and their partner may make slow dancing challenging or impossible.
- Similar physical benefits can be gained if the laboring person leans and sways over a birth ball placed on a table or birth bed. They can also lean and sway on the bed, counter, or wall.

Abdominal lifting

When: Primarily first stage, but also second stage if desired.

How: The laboring person stands upright. During the contraction, they interlock the fingers of both hands beneath their abdomen and lifts their abdomen upward and inward, while bending their knees to tilt their pelvis[15] (King, 1993) (Fig. 11.38). They maintain the lift throughout the contraction. The partner may assist with abdominal lifting by placing a woven shawl (Fig 11.38b)—5 to 6 feet (150–180 cm) long, 18 or more inches (~45 cm) wide, and folded in half or in thirds—around the laboring person, beneath their abdomen, crossing it in the back and lifting their abdomen for their, while the laboring person bends their knees. They can give feedback on whether it feels that his lift is similar to theirs. If not, the shawl and the angle of the lift can be adjusted.

> ***Caution:*** In the rare instance that the umbilical cord is located low and anterior in the uterus, the abdominal lift might compress the cord. If so, the fetus may "protest" by increasing activity, and the abdominal lift should be discontinued. The laboring person should be told that if they try the abdominal lift in early labor before there is a nurse or caregiver present, they should discontinue it if their fetus becomes notably more active ("The baby doesn't like it."). It is also wise to periodically check the fetal heart tones during a contraction while the abdominal lift is being done. If the heart rate declines, discontinue the abdominal lift.

> ***Caution:*** After abdominal lifting, rapid progress sometimes occurs suddenly. It should not be done when the laboring person is having strong active labor contractions, until they are where they intend to give birth.

(a)   (b)

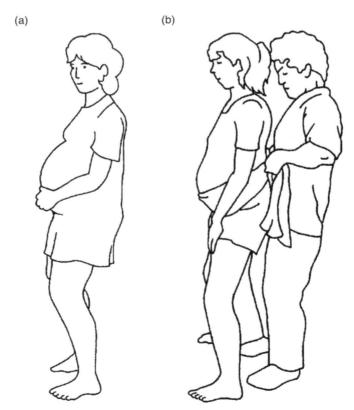

Fig. 11.38. **(a)** Abdominal lifting. **(b)** Abdominal lifting with a shawl.

Why abdominal lifting helps

Though this technique has not been studied for its effectiveness, anecdotes of better labor progress along with decreased back pain have made this technique quite popular. Abdominal lifting can relieve back pain and help align the long axis of the fetus with the axis of the pelvic inlet. This improves fetal positioning and the efficiency of contractions.

Abdominal lifting seems to be particularly helpful for those laboring people with:

- Back pain in labor associated with a fetal OP position or such maternal conditions as:
- A pronounced curve in the low back ("swayback");
- Pendulous abdomen (weak abdominal muscles);
- A short waist (from iliac crests to lowest ribs);
- Some previous low back injuries.

Advantages

- Reduces back pain.
- Provides gravity advantage.
- May be done at any stage of labor, from prelabor into the second stage.
- Sometimes leads to rapid labor (especially in multiparas or those with pendulous abdomens).

Disadvantages

- Is tiring for the laboring person if used over a long period.

Abdominal jiggling with a shawl

The "jiggle" (also known as baby sifting or shawl sifting) maneuver involves the use of a woven shawl 5 to 6 feet (150–180 cm) long and about 18 or more inches (45 cm) wide. The use of the shawl for many purposes during pregnancy and birth began with traditional midwives in Latin America.[16–18].

When to use abdominal jiggling

First or second stage, if progress has slowed, laboring person has backache, or if fetal malposition is suspected.

How to use abdominal jiggling

- The laboring person kneels and leans forward from the hips (on hands and knees, over a birth ball or chair seat).
- The shawl is folded to 12 to 18 inches (30–45 cm) wide and is placed under the laboring person's mid-abdomen (with the center of the shawl over the center of their abdomen and the ends held behind their).
- The midwife or other caregiver stands straddling the kneeling laboring person (Fig. 11.39) or just behind the standing laboring person, holding the ends of the rebozo, so that they are perpendicular to the laboring person's trunk.
- The caregiver then pulls on both ends of the rebozo to lift the laboring person's abdomen slightly toward their back. This will probably feel very good to the laboring person.
- Between or during contractions (whichever the laboring person prefers), the caregiver gently jiggles the laboring person's abdomen by alternately and rhythmically pulling up on one end of the rebozo and then the other, while the laboring person relaxes their trunk. The caregiver can try doing this slowly or rapidly, so that they are "jiggling" the laboring person's belly.
- Over a period of a time (perhaps 30 to 45 minutes, or as tolerated by the laboring person), the fetus may resettle in a more favorable position.

Why It Helps

If the laboring person is very tense, the jiggling enhances relaxation of the trunk and may ease the baby into a more favorable position. There are no known research studies of this technique, only anecdotal reports of success, and no known harmful effects.

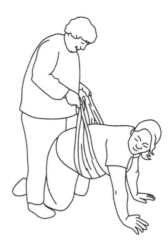

Fig. 11.39. Abdominal jiggling (also known as "shaking the apple tree")

Advantages

Partner or other companion can be shown how to do this on the spot. Can be done at any time in labor, except close to delivery.

Caution: We recommend that doula or partner use abdominal jiggling only with the approval of the doctor or midwife. Periodic fetal heart tone checks by the maternity professional will indicate whether the fetus is tolerating the procedure. If the laboring person tires of it, or it seems ineffective, it is time to try something else.

Disadvantages

May be tiring for the laboring person; knees may become sore (knee pads help). Over time, this technique becomes tiring for both the laboring person and the caregiver, who may wish to have another laboring person take over.

The pelvic press

When: Second stage.

How: With the laboring person standing, the partner, doula, caregiver, or preferably two people stand behind or beside their, and during a contraction, the laboring person or laboring persons press their iliac crests very firmly toward each other (Fig. 11.40). This should cause some movement in the pelvis, slightly narrowing the upper pelvis. The ilia pivot at the sacroiliac joints, causing the mid-pelvis and the pelvic outlet to widen. Combining the pelvic press with the squatting position may give the greatest chance of increasing space within the pelvis. Within three or four contractions, there may be some evidence of rotation or descent.[5]

How the pelvic press helps: The pelvic press is a technique for enlarging the mid-pelvic and intertuberous diameters in second stage. The added room may allow fetal rotation and descent in cases of a malposition or "tight fit" at the pelvic outlet.

When to use the pelvic press

- In second stage, when there is a delay in descent or a caput forming (due to malposition or cephalopelvic disproportion).
- In second stage, when a laboring person reports severe back pain.
- In second stage, if the laboring person is unable to squat.

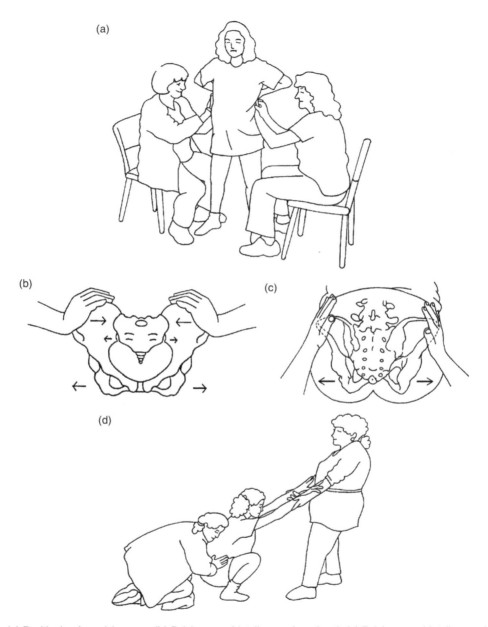

Fig. 11.40.   (**a**) Positioning for pelvic press. (**b**) Pelvic press (detail, seen from front). (**c**) Pelvic press (detail, seen from rear). (**d**) Pelvic press, Laboring person squatting.

When NOT to use the pelvic press

- When the pelvic press causes severe bone or joint pain, as it might if the laboring person has arthritis or a previous injury to their pelvis.
- When the laboring person has an epidural, because without sensation, joints could be damaged.

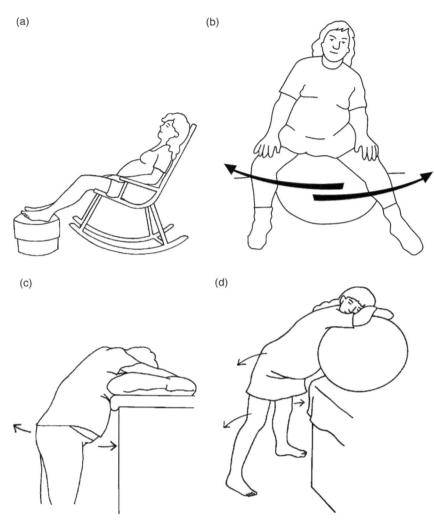

Fig. 11.41.   (**a**) Sitting in a rocking chair. (**b**) Swaying on a birth ball. (**c**) Rocking, leaning on a counter. (**d**) Standing, swaying with a ball.

Other rhythmic movements

When: First or second stage.

How: Moving their bodies rhythmically often seems to occur instinctively in people who are coping well in labor. Rocking in a chair (Fig. 11.41a) or swaying while sitting on a birth ball (Fig. 11.41b) or while standing and leaning over a tray table (Fig. 11.41c) or birth ball that is placed on a bed (Fig. 11.41d) are examples of such rhythmic bodily movements. Furthermore, some people find rhythmic stroking or rocking by someone else or by themselves—stroking their own leg or hair, or their partner's arm, or an object—to be soothing. Moaning or self-talk in rhythm is similarly helpful. These behaviors are not planned. They occur spontaneously and instinctively when the laboring person feels safe. If a person with slow labor progress is not spontaneously moving as described here, the caregiver might suggest that they try it, and guide their in rhythmic movements, so that they might adopt or adapt them as they becomes used to doing it.

Why rhythmic movements help Rhythmic movements tend to be calming.

• Rhythmic movements may alter the relationships among fetus, pelvis, and gravity to promote progress.
• When spontaneous, rocking is often an indication that the laboring person is coping well.

REFERENCES

1. Lawrence A, Lewis L, Hofmeyr G, Styles C. (2013) Maternal positions and mobility during first stage labour. *Cochrane Database of Systematic Reviews* (8), Art. No.: CD003934. doi: 10.1002/14651858.CD003934.pub3
2. Gizzo S, Di Gangi S, Noventa M, Bacile V, Zambon A, Nardelli GB. (2014) Women's choice of position during labour: Return to the past or a modern way to give birth? A cohort study in Italy. *BioMed Research International* Article ID 638093, 7. doi: 10.1155/2014/638093
3. Simkin P, O'Hara M. (2002) Nonpharmacologic relief of pain during labor: Systematic reviews of five methods. *American Journal of Obstetrics and Gynecology* 186, S131–S159.
4 Hunter S, Hofmeyr G, Kulier R. (2009) Hands and knees posture in late pregnancy or labour for fetal malposition (lateral or posterior). *Cochrane Database of Systematic Reviews* (4), Art. No.:CD001063. doi: 10.1002/14651858.CD001063.pub3
5. Sutton J. (2001) *Let Birth Be Born Again: Rediscovering and Reclaiming Our Midwifery Heritage.* Bedfont, Middlesex, UK: Birth Concepts.
6. Fenwick L, Simkin P. (1987) Maternal positioning to prevent or alleviate dystocia in labor. *Clinical Obstetrics and Gynecology* 30(1), 83–89.
7. Stremler R, Hodnett E, Petryshen P, Stevens B, Weston J, Willan A. (2005) Randomized controlled trial of hands and knees positioning for occipitoposterior position in labor. *Birth* 32, 243–251.
8. Tully G, Spinning Babies Approved Trainers. (2015) How to do the side-lying release. In: *Spinning Babies Quick Reference Guide: Solutions in Your Birth Bag.* Bloomington, MN: Maternity House Publishing, Inc.
9. Tully G. How to do the side-lying release. Available at: http://spinningbabies.com/?s=side-lying+release (accessed August 25, 2016).
10. Gupta JK, Hofmeyr GJ, Shehmar M. (2012) Position in the second stage of labour for women without epidural anaesthesia. *Cochrane Database of Systematic Reviews* (5), Art. No.: CD002006. doi: 10.1002/14651858.CD002006.pub3
11. Gherman R, Tramont J, Muffley P, Goodwin T. (2000) Analysis of McRoberts' maneuver by Xray pelvimetry. *Obstetrics & Gynecology* 95, 43–47.
12. Henderson C, MacDonald S. (2013) *Mayes' Midwifery: A Textbook for Midwives*, 14th edn. Baillière-Tindall.
13. Health T, Gherman R. (1999) Symphyseal separation, sacroiliac joint dislocation transient lateral femoral cutaneous neuropathy associated with McRoberts' maneuver. A case report. *Journal of Reproductive Medicine* 44(10), 902–903.
14. Steffes S. (2015) Laboring personal communication with Penny Simkin.
15. King JM. (1993) *Back Labor No More!!!* Dallas, TX: Plenary System.
16. Tully G. Rebozo sifting. Spinning Babies. Available from: http://spinningbabies.com/learn-more/techniques/the-fantastic-four/rebozo-sifting (accessed August 25, 2016).
17. Trueba G. (2001) Comfort measures for childbirth: The Rebozo Way [DVD]. Available from: Guadelupe Trueba (email:).
18. Cohen S, Thomas C. (2015) Rebozo technique for fetal malposition in labor. *Journal of Midwifery and Women's Health* 60, 445–451.

Chapter 12

Guide to Comfort Measures

Emily Malloy, PhD, CNM and Lisa Hanson, PhD, CNM, FACNM, FAAN

Simkin's Labor Progress Handbook: Early Interventions to Prevent and Treat Dystocia, Fifth Edition. Edited by Lisa Hanson, Emily Malloy, and Penny Simkin.

INTRODUCTION: THE STATE OF THE SCIENCE REGARDING NON-PHARMACOLOGIC, COMPLEMENTARY, AND ALTERNATIVE METHODS TO RELIEVE LABOR PAIN

Nonpharmacologic, complementary and alternative pain management option have been used for centuries. Scientific evidence continues to grow. The purpose of this chapter is to present evidence and techniques that are often desired by birthing people.

GENERAL GUIDELINES FOR COMFORT DURING A SLOW LABOR

We recommend the following comfort guidelines when labor progression is slow.

- Frequent position changes (about every 20 to 30 minutes) may shorten labor and reduce the laboring person's pain and enhance coping. When progress is adequate and the laboring person and fetus tolerates the contractions well, there is no need to change anything.
- Rhythmic movement reduces pain and anxiety and enhance coping.
- There are various effective techniques reduce back pain.
- Heat and cold, as shown later in this chapter, reduce various types of pain.
- Hydrotherapy, reduces muscle tension, pain, and anxiety. Immersion in water also provides buoyancy (reducing the effect of gravity on the laboring person.
- Techniques such as relaxation, rhythmic breathing and moaning patterns, and spontaneous bearing-down efforts give many people a sense of mastery over their pain and help them get through a long, potentially worrisome labor.

NON-PHARMACOLOGIC PHYSICAL COMFORT MEASURES

Heat

How

- Apply a warm moist towel, heating pad, heated silica gel pack, heated rice pack, or hot-water bottle to the lower abdomen, groin, thighs, lower back, shoulders, or perineum, or
- Direct a warm shower onto the laboring person's shoulders, abdomen, or lower back, or suggest they immerse in warm water (see "Hydrotherapy" below) or
- Apply a warmed blanket that covers the entire body.

How heat helps: Heat (Fig. 12.1) increases local skin temperature, circulation, and tissue metabolism. It reduces muscle spasm and raises the pain threshold.[1,2] Heat also reduces the "fight-or-flight" response (as evidenced by trembling and "goose bumps").[3,4] Local heat or a warm blanket calms the laboring person and also may increase their receptivity to a stroking type of massage that they cannot tolerate when skin is sensitive or sore due to the fight-or-flight response.

Please note: Rice-filled microwaveable packs can be purchased in many department stores, or they can easily be made by the laboring person by filling a large tube sock with 1.5 pounds (0.68 kg) of dry uncooked rice and stitching or tying close the top of the sock. Placing the rice pack for 3 to 5 minutes in a micro- wave oven set on "high" or for 10 minutes in a covered ceramic dish in a 180°F (82 °C) oven provides moist heat for up to 30 minutes. Adding lavender seeds or flowers to the rice may appeal to some people. Rice packs can be reheated and reused for the same laboring person but should not be reused by others.

Caution: If the rice pack is being reheated in a microwave oven that is also used to heat food, caution should be exercised to avoid contaminating the oven with the laboring person's body fluids. Place the rice pack in a glass

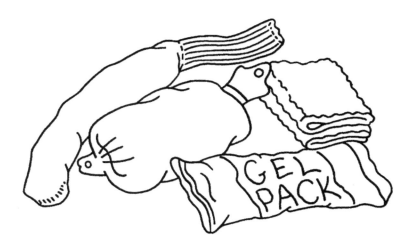

Fig. 12.1. Heat.

or plastic container or consult your infection control department if this is a concern. Rice packs can also be frozen for use as cold packs.

A further caution: Compresses should not be uncomfortably hot to the person applying them. People in labor may have an altered perception of temperature and may not react to excessive heat even if it is causing a burn. Wrap one or two (or more) layers of toweling or a plastic disposable bed pad around the source of heat as needed to ensure it is not too hot. The caregiver should test the temperature on their own inner arm to make sure it is tolerable.

Special cautions on the use of heat with a laboring person who has an epidural

- One side effect of epidural analgesia is an alteration in thermoregulation (an imbalance between the generation of body heat by the contracting uterus and the body's ability to dissipate it), which may lead to temperature elevation and associated effects on the fetus.[5,6] If the laboring person's temperature is elevated, covering them with a warm blanket may provide comfort.
- Because a laboring person with an epidural lacks sensation, never place a hot or warm compress on the area of the body affected by the epidural (even if they report pain in that area). It may cause a burn. See Chapter 9 for further discussion of labor management when an epidural is used.

When to use heat

- When the laboring person reports or shows pain in a specific area.
- When the laboring person reports or shows signs of anxiety or muscle tension.
- When the laboring person reports feeling chilled.
- In the second stage, warm compresses on the perineum enhance relaxation of the pelvic floor and reduce pain.

When not to use heat

- When the laboring person reports feeling uncomfortably warm or has a fever.
- If staff are worried about potential harm from the heat.

Heat should be avoided on parts of the laboring person's body where sensory perception is altered.

(a)   (b)

(c)   (d)

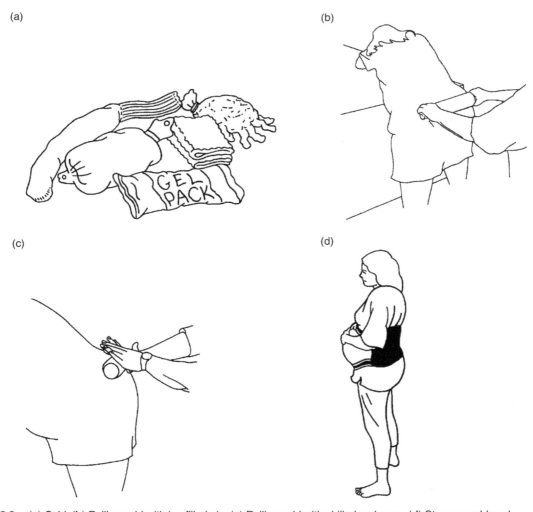

Fig. 12.2.   (**a**) Cold. (**b**) Rolling cold with ice-filled pin. (**c**) Rolling cold with chilled soda can. (**d**) Strap-on cold pack.

Cold

How

- Apply cold compresses to lower back, or perineum, using an ice bag, frozen gel pack or rice pack, latex glove filled with ice chips, frozen wet washcloth, cold can of soft drink, plastic bottle of frozen water, or another cold object (Fig. 12.2a–c).
- Provide a large strap-on gel pack (available from sports medicine suppliers) for the low back (Fig. 12.2d). This allows the laboring person to move or walk around.
- Use a cold moist washcloth to cool a sweating laboring person's face, hands, or arms.
- Place a cold gel pack or plastic bottle of cold water against the anus to relieve painful hemorrhoids in second stage (unless they have no sensation in the area).

Caution: Always put one or two layers of fabric or a disposable bed pad between the cold item and the laboring person's skin. This avoids the sudden discomfort that would occur with the direct application of cold to the skin and allows for a gradual and well-tolerated shift from feeling cool to feeling cold.

How cold helps: Cold is especially useful for musculoskeletal and joint pain.

Cold decreases muscle spasm (works longer than heat). It reduces sensation in the area by lowering tissue temperature, which slows the transmission of pain and other impulses over sensory neurons (explaining the often-noted numbing effects of cold). Cold also reduces swelling and is cooling to the skin.[3,7]

When to use cold

- When the laboring person reports back pain in labor.
- When the laboring person feels overheated, is sweating, or has a fever during labor.
- When hemorrhoids cause excessive pain.
- After the birth, as a cold compress on the laboring person's perineum to relieve swelling or stitch pain.

When not to use cold

- When the laboring person is already feeling chill. Use heat first in this case.
- When the laboring person is from a culture in which the use of cold is perceived as a threat to the laboring person's wellbeing during labor or postpartum. Ask if they prefer a hot pack, a cold pack, or neither.
- When the laboring person reports that the use of cold is not helping or is irritating.
- When the laboring person has an epidural, do not place a cold pack on the area of body affected by the epidural.

One study found that alternating heat and cold on the low back and lower abdomen during the first stage and on the perineum during the second stage reduced people's labor pain.[8]

Hydrotherapy

How   *Shower:* The laboring person stands or sits in the shower (Fig. 12.3), with water at a comfortable temperature, and directs the shower spray where they wants it (on their back or front). A hand-held shower head is more versatile in directing the spray than a fixed shower head.

   Bath: They sit, kneel, or recline in a tub of deep warm water, preferably with enough space for them to change position and perhaps for their partner to get in (Fig. 12.4a–d).

   Caution: Water temperature in the bath should not exceed 98–100°F (37–37.5 °C), because warmer water may raise the laboring person's temperature and cause fetal tachycardia.[9,10] The laboring person should leave the bath after 1.5 hours or so for 30 minutes. This ensures the greatest benefits of the bath. The laboring person can return to the bath after 30 minutes or so.[1,9,11,12]

How hydrotherapy helps   Hydrotherapy (shower or bath) reduces muscle tension, pain, and anxiety dramatically for many people.

   The effects of immersion in water may be summarized as follows: Bathing provides buoyancy and warmth, both of which often bring immediate pain relief, relaxation, lowering of catecholamines, increase in oxytocin, lowering of elevated blood pressure,[13] and more rapid active labor progress. The extent of these effects depends on many variables, such as the water depth and temperature, the duration of the bath, cervical dilation on entry, the laboring person's cultural perceptions, and psychological factors. Benefits seem to be greatest if the water is at shoulder depth and at body temperature, if the laboring person waits until active labor before entering the bath, and if they remain in the water for a period up to about 1 to 1.5 hours.

Why the laboring person should leave the water periodically   Fluid balance is altered by immersion in deep water. The hydrostatic pressure on the immersed parts of the laboring person's body (which increases with the depth of the water) presses tissue fluid into the intravascular space.[9] This increases their blood volume, especially in their chest, which triggers the gradual release of a fluid-regulating hormone, ANF (atrial natriuretic hormone).

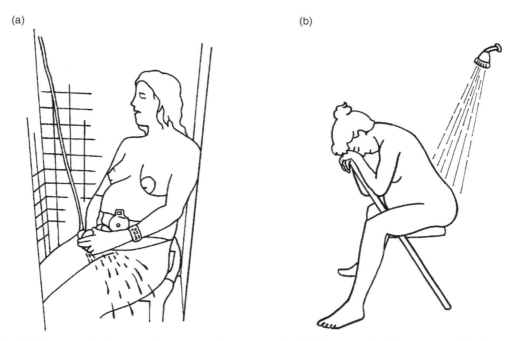

Fig. 12.3. **(a)** Shower on laboring person's abdomen (with telemetry). **(b)** Shower on the laboring person's back.

Over time, ANF inhibits functioning of the posterior pituitary gland, including production of vasopressin (another fluid-regulating hormone) and oxytocin.[9] Of course, the decrease in oxytocin production leads to slowing of labor. Leaving the water for 30 minutes after 1 to 1.5 hours reverses this effect.

How to monitor the fetus in or around water

With a hand-held Doppler device, use models designed for underwater use. If these are not available, the laboring person must lift their abdomen out of the water or step out of the shower as needed for intermittent monitoring (Fig. 11.4d). The older wired electronic fetal monitoring tocodynamometers and ultrasound transducers ("belt monitors") are used underwater with telemetry units held out of the water in some hospitals with people who are monitored continuously (Fig. 11.4b). These belt monitors are highly water resistant, and because the battery-powered telemetry units operate on a very low voltage, many hospitals consider them safe for the laboring person and fetus.[12]

The sensors are usually covered with waterproof gloves or long plastic bags (these covers are used more to protect the equipment than the laboring person).

Please note: Before trying this, please contact your hospital's biomedical services or engineering department regarding both safety and any potential equipment damage connected with underwater use of the specific equipment used in your hospital.

The wireless remote waterproof tocodynamometers and ultrasound sensors can be used for continuous monitoring in the shower or bath. They are attached by belts to the laboring person's abdomen but are self-contained and have no wires attached, as shown in Figs. 12.3a and 12.4a. These cause minimal interference with rest, bathing, or movement by the laboring person.

Guide to Comfort Measures

12

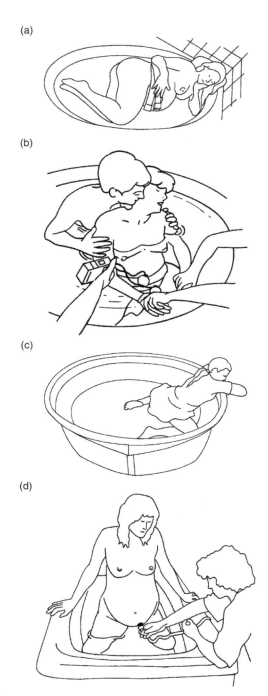

(a)

(b)

(c)

(d)

Fig. 12.4.   Water immersion. (**a**) Side-lying with wireless monitor. (**b**) NEW sitting with hand-held telemetry unit. (**c**) Kneeling in birth pool. (**d**) Monitor out of water.

When to use hydrotherapy

• As a possible alternative to bedrest in labor for people with gestational hypertension.

Showers: Use in any phase of first stage labor or early second stage.

Immersion in bath: Use after active labor is established (with one exception—see later). Because immersion in water often slows contractions when used before active labor,[9] a bath is sometimes recommended to stop preterm contractions or to slow exhausting prelabor contractions and give the laboring person some temporary rest. Entrance into the water before 5 cm dilation, however, has been associated with longer labor and greater need for oxytocin augmentation.[10] Barbara Harper, an American expert on water birth, suggests a less strict approach to timing of entry into the bath than awaiting 5 cm dilation—leaving the decision up to the laboring person. If the labor slows when they are in the water, then recommend that they get out until labor becomes reestablished, which might occur before or after 5 cm dilation.[14]

• Immersion in deep water when one is in preterm labor, prelabor, or latent labor often stops contractions temporarily through the mechanism described earlier. This may be desirable if the laboring person is having preterm labor contractions or an exhaustingly long prelabor; otherwise, it is not desirable because it could suppress early labor progress. If the laboring person awaits active labor before entering the bath, dilation often speeds up and pain is reduced.[9]

When not to use hydrotherapy
Showers

• When the laboring person's balance or ability to stand is unreliable, due to medication or other reasons.
• When there is a medical contraindication requiring restriction to bed.

Immersion in a bath

• Before active labor is established (unless slowing of labor or temporary cessation of contractions is desired).
• When there is a medical contraindication such as bleeding or fetal distress.
• When birth is imminent (unless the laboring person and practitioner are planning a water birth).
• When the laboring person has received narcotic medications or an epidural for pain.[15,16,17,18]

Touch and massage

How
Various forms of touch, including patting or holding the laboring person's shoulder or hand, stroking their cheek or hair, even if brief, can convey to the laboring person a sense of caring, reassurance, understanding, or nonverbal support. Cultural views of this kind of touch vary, especially if it is not given by a family member, close friend, or a female. Personal comfort with touch also varies, so the caregiver must be tactful, ask permission, or observe for signs that the laboring person wants comforting touch (i.e., reaching for the caregiver's hand, responding positively to a fleeting pat after a clinical procedure). Caregivers may not always feel comfortable giving this kind of touch and, if not, they should not do it.

Massage during labor is formalized touch with the intention of enhancing relaxation and relieving pain.[1] It may involve a specific part of the body, such as the hands, feet, scalp, shoulders, or back. It may involve light or firm stroking, kneading, or still pressure. It may include the use of the hands or any of a variety of massage devices. It may be done with or without oils, lotions, or powders.

When to use touch or massage

• When the laboring person seems tense, frightened, or anxious.
• When the laboring person describes pain in a specific area (i.e., the back, thigh, and abdomen).
• When the laboring person's arms, legs, or feet ache or are tired from great effort.
• When the caregiver wants to express empathy, or reassurance.

When not to use touch or massage

- When the caregiver is uncomfortable or unskilled in its use.
- When the laboring person does not want it, or it is not helping.
- When there are cultural proscriptions against its use.

Effectiveness of touch and massage: Two trials of massage by the person's partner, who were taught to give 20- to 30-minute massages to the people several times during labor, found that the massage groups had less pain and anxiety and reported greater satisfaction with their childbirths than the control groups.[19] A fourth trial used a pain questionnaire to compare labor pain in one group of laboring people who received usual nursing care plus massages at three times in the first stage of labor, with a similar group who received usual care only. The massage group reported less pain up to 7 cm of dilation, at which time pain was assessed as the same in the two groups.[20]

How to give simple brief massages for shoulders and back, hands, and feet

A laboring person may appreciate one or more brief (1–3-minute) massages of their shoulders, back, hands, or feet. It will soothe them and offer a little comfort break.

Follow these general guidelines:

- Always ask for permission and describe the massage you would like to do.
- Be sure your hands are clean and warm and that they are comfortable.
- Use unscented massage oil. Squirt a little on your hands and rub them together briskly to warm your hands.
- Once you begin, do not remove both hands until you are done. It is unsettling for the person to relax into a massage, only to have the massager's hands disappear, and not know when or where they will touch them next.

Three-part shoulder mini-massage
When to use it

- Anytime during labor if they are tense—during or between contractions.

When not to use it

- When they do not want to be touched or do not like the massage.

How: The laboring person sits up, or leans forward and rests their head on their arms or a pillow. You stand behind them.

Part 1: Place your hands comfortably on their shoulders near the neck. Stroke firmly from the neck to the shoulders, then over the shoulders to her upper arms. Knead the upper arms a few times (let them tell you how firmly to stroke and knead), and stroke firmly back toward the neck. Do that three or four times.

Part 2: With your hands molded over the tops of their shoulders, "knead" or squeeze and release their shoulder muscles as firmly as they like (ask them for feedback) for 1 to 2 minutes.

Part 3: Using the middle three fingertips of one hand, make some brief deep circle massages on spots on the tops of their shoulders and small areas along the spine. Circle in one area for 15 to 30 seconds, then move to another. They'll tell you their preferred places.

"Criss-cross" massage over the small of her back
When to use

- Anytime during or between contractions.

How (Fig. 12.5)   The laboring person kneels on the bed or the floor leaning over the birth ball or other support. (If they are on the bed, you will be able to adjust the height of the bed so you can reach her back without strain.) Because support person's knees may get sore fairly quickly, it is a good idea for them to wear knee pads or to kneel on a soft pad or pillow. (The foam pads made for gardeners work very well.)

Begin by facing the laboring person's side. Look at their back and notice the place where their waist is narrowest. That is where you will place your hands—on each side at the narrowest part, below the ribs. Be sure not to press

(a)

(b)

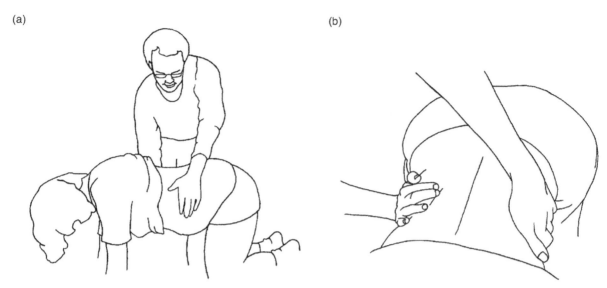

Fig. 12.5. **(a)** "Criss-cross" back massage. **(b)** Close-up view of "criss-cross" back 11 massage. (Source: Simkin P. [2008]. The Birth Partner: A Complete Guide to Childbirth for Dads, Doulas, and All Other Labor Companions, 3rd edition. Boston, MA: Harvard Common Press. Reprinted with permission.)

on their ribs. It is uncomfortable. Place your right hand on their side farthest from you, fingers pointing down. Place your left hand on their near side, fingers pointing up. Press their sides in quite firmly. The laboring person should like that feeling. Then, using a slow steady rhythm, stroke firmly with your hands moving up and across their back toward each other. Cross one hand over the other and move to the original starting spots on her sides. Maintaining the same pressure, press their sides in again, and repeat the crossover movement over and over as long as they want. The inward pressure on their sides brings much relief. You may do this during or between contractions for as long as the laboring person likes.

Hand massage "pressure and friction" (Fig. 12.6) This massage relaxes the hand all the way up the arm, while still giving them pain-relieving benefits of pressure on the palms of the hands.

When to do it

• During or between contractions.
• If they have been clenching their fists during contractions, or gripping the sheet or bedrail.

How: Stand or sit facing the laboring person, a little above them. Ask them to relax their arms, and take one of their hands in both of yours. Grasp it so that your thumbs, including the bases of your thumbs, are placed side by side on the back of their wrist. The pads of your fingers (not your fingernails) press into their palm.

Then, without moving your hands, increase your grip gradually and ask them to tell you when you are squeezing "hard enough." You may be surprised at how much pressure the laboring person likes. When they says it is enough, maintain that pressure, and firmly and slowly slide your hands (including the tips of your thumbs all the way to the fleshy bases below your thumbs) apart and off their hand (Fig. 12.6). You are combining pressure on their palm with friction over the back of their hand. Replace your thumbs in the starting position and repeat 10 times or so.

Caution: If their hands are very swollen or if they have carpal tunnel syndrome (tingling or numbness that worsens with pressure), they will want very little pressure or will not want you to do this massage at all.

(a)   (b)

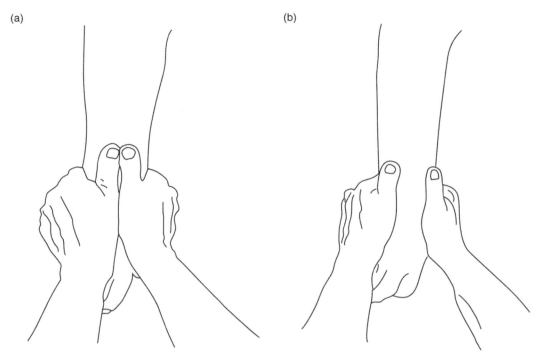

Fig. 12.6.   (**a**) Hand massage, thumbs together. (**b**) Hand massage, thumbs apart. (Source: Simkin P. [2008]. The Birth Partner: A Complete Guide to Childbirth for Dads, Doulas, and All Other Labor Companions, 3rd edition. Boston, MA: Harvard Common Press. Reprinted with permission.)

Three-part foot massage   *The purpose:* to restore circulation and relieve foot aches and fatigue caused by prolonged standing and walking.

When to do it

•   Between contractions and if they complain that her feet are hurting or getting tired.

How: Part 1: "Pressure and friction" (Fig. 12.7): This is similar to the hand massage above. The laboring person sits on the bed with her feet extended, and you grasp one of their feet with both hands. Grasp it so that your thumbs, including the bases of your thumbs, are touching each other. The pads of your fingers (not your fingernails) press into the sole of their foot. Squeeze until they say that is firm enough. You may be surprised at how much pressure they want. Maintain that pressure, and slowly slide your thumbs apart and off their foot (see Fig. 12.7). You are combining pressure on the sole of their foot with friction over the back of the foot. Replace your thumbs in the starting position and repeat 10 times or so.

    Part 2: "Squeezing the apple" (Fig. 12.8): If massaging their right foot, use your right hand, and press the heel of your hand firmly into the arch of her foot and grasp the heel. Don't press your fingertips into their heel. Squeeze and release it several times, as if you were squeezing an apple or tennis ball.

    Part 3: Deep circle massage with fingertips (Fig. 12.9): (This description applies to massage of their left foot. You can adapt it to apply to the right.) Hold the sole of the left foot in your left hand. With the pads of the three middle fingers of your right hand, give a deep circle massage in the "magic spot," on the top of their foot just below her ankle. The spot is slightly off center toward the outside of their foot. Ask if you are rubbing a spot that feels good. Move around as necessary. Your fingers do not move on their skin; rather, you are moving their skin over their underlying muscles and bones. Do this for 30 to 60 seconds.

    Once you have completed all three steps on one foot, repeat with the other foot. Then they will be ready to walk some more.

(a)   (b)

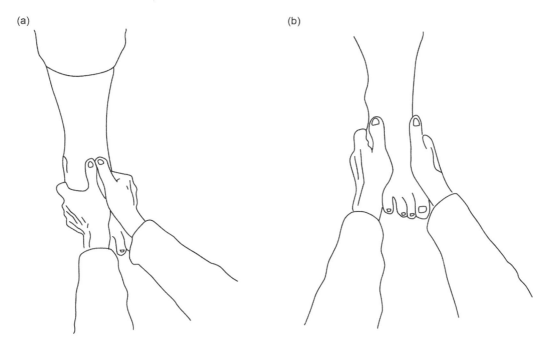

Fig. 12.7. **(a, b)** "Pressure and friction" foot massage. (Source: Simkin P. [2008]. The Birth Partner: A Complete Guide to Childbirth for Dads, Doulas, and All Other Labor Companions, 3rd edition. Boston, MA: Harvard Common Press. Reprinted with permission.)

With a bit of practice, these massages are easily mastered and equip you to give comfort and attention in a short time.

Acupuncture

The ancient Eastern healing art of acupuncture is used to relieve pain from a variety of conditions, including labor. In traditional Chinese medicine, acupuncture involves the balance of *qi* energy along the body's 14 meridians (pathways for energy flow). Acupuncture involves the insertion of fine disposable needles into the skin that stimulate specific points along the meridians (Fig. 8.9). Pain relief can occur immediately or within a 15–20-minute period. It is theorized that pain relief is achieved through several mechanisms including enhanced blood flow, decreasing pain perception, and the release of beta-endorphins (endogenous analgesics).[21] No risks from acupuncture have been identified when it is practiced by trained practitioners using disposable needles.

There is limited evidence from individual studies concerning the efficacy of acupressure for pain relief in labor.[21] Smith and colleague conducted a systematic review of acupuncture and acupressure including 28 trials that included 3960 laboring people.[22] Thirteen trials included acupuncture as an intervention. This systematic review was limited by the variation in outcomes studied reduced the certainty of the findings; acupuncture probably decreased the use of pharmacologic analgesia, and may have increased satisfaction with pain relief, but did not significantly reduce pain intensity when compared to sham acupuncture. More research is needed to demonstrate the effectiveness of acupuncture for labor pain relief including ideal point selection and techniques.[21]

When to use acupuncture: When a trained acupuncturist is available, and the laboring person wishes to use it for pain relief.

When not to use acupuncture: When a trained acupuncturist is not available.

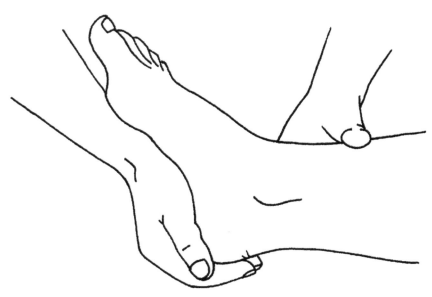

Fig. 12.8. "Squeezing the apple" foot massage.

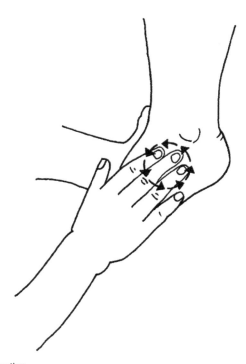

Fig. 12.9. Deep massage with fingertips.

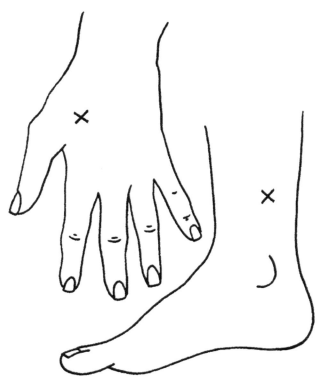

Fig. 12.10.   Acupressure points: hoku point (Liver 4) on hand (on the back of the hand, where the metacarpal bones of the thumb and the index finger come together); Spleen 6 point on ankle (on the tibia), four finger widths above the medial malleolus (inner ankle bone): apply pressure on the tibia and diagonally forward; this point will be very tender.

Acupressure

Acupressure can be used to stimulate specific points used in acupuncture but does not require specific training. Pressure on the points illustrated in Fig. 12.10 during labor is thought to enhance contractions, and possibly to reduce labor pain.

- Press firmly with a finger on the point for 10 to 60 seconds. Then rest for an equal length of time.
- Repeat this cycle for up to six cycles. Contractions may speed up during that time.

How acupressure helps

Acupressure is based on acupuncture theory, which states that specific health problems, including poor progress or excessive pain in labor, arise when there is a blockage of energy flow along particular meridians in the body. By releasing the blockage, harmony and smooth functioning return.

When to use acupressure

- When labor induction is considered necessary within a few days. The laboring person might try self-help measures to start labor, in hopes of avoiding induction, but only after discussing this with her doctor or midwife.
- In labor, when more frequent contractions are desired or needed.
- When contractions are very painful but not accompanied by labor progress.

When not to use acupressure

- During pregnancy before term (unless induction is being planned), because it may result in preterm labor contractions. We also suggest that the laboring person does not even experiment with it on themselves before labor.
- If they have not consulted their doctor or midwife.[23,24,25]

Continuous labor support from a doula, nurse, or midwife

Until the late 20th century, nurses and midwives, along with people's partners, were designated as the main people to provide support to laboring people. Professional staff were expected to add labor support to their long list of other tasks, and it was assumed that any knowledgeable professional could easily do this without instruction. People's partners were assumed to be calm and capable enough to "coach" a laboring person through labor. More recently, doula research has shown that effective non-clinical labor support cannot be an "add-on" to other duties, nor can a loved one provide all the support a laboring person needs.[26,27] A doula is a person (usually a laboring person), trained and experienced in childbirth, who accompanies laboring people and their partners throughout labor and birth (Fig. 12.11). They provide continuous emotional support, physical comfort, and non-clinical advice and assists the laboring person in getting the information needed to make informed choices regarding options. They are usually a lay person, although some nurses and childbirth educators have become doulas.

How the doula helps

The doula focuses on the laboring person through each contraction, offering calm reassurance, praise, encouragement, and comfort, as needed and appropriate. They also guide, assist, and reassure the laboring person's partner. They rarely take a break and remains with the laboring person until after the birth. Doulas usually do not work in shifts. The doula performs no clinical tasks. Rather their sole responsibility is the laboring person's and partner's emotional wellbeing and the laboring person's physical comfort. Some hospitals and health agencies have doulas on staff to help people, beginning when they are admitted, but most doulas contract privately with clients. Some work as volunteers; most charge a fee.

In North America, doulas are certified by DONA International (formerly Doulas of North America), the International Childbirth Education Association (ICEA), To Labor, and the Childbirth and Postpartum Professional

(a)   (b)

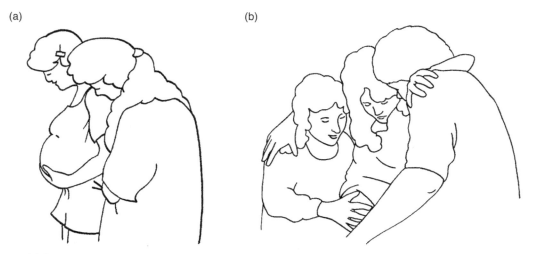

Fig. 12.11. (**a**) Doula supporting a laboring person. (**b**) Doula supporting a couple.

Association (CAPPA). The concept of the doula is growing rapidly in Europe, Australia, New Zealand, and parts of Asia. Doulas UK represents and supports doulas in the United Kingdom.

When to use a doula

• A doula should be used whenever one is available and the laboring person wants their services. There are no known harmful effects when doulas, as described earlier, are in attendance.

When not to use a doula

• A doula should not be used when the laboring person prefers not to have one.

Effectiveness of doulas   A recent systematic review of 22 randomized controlled trials of continuous labor support from 16 countries, included more than 15,000 women.[28] The researchers found that women who received continuous labor support benefited, but the greatest benefit was found in the trials in which the support provider was not a hospital staff member with clinical care responsibilities, nor someone from the laboring person's social network. Care by doulas and other non-clinical personnel resulted in 28% fewer cesareans; 31% less use of synthetic oxytocin to speed labor; 9% of mothers less likely to use any pain medication; and 34% less likely to rate their birth negatively. Another systematic review of randomized controlled trials of continuous support by doulas or nurses only in North America reported similar results.[29] Support begun in early labor provided greater benefit than support begun in active labor. The laboring people who benefited most were those whose care was provided by doulas rather than by nurses, whose support was begun during early rather than inactive labor, and those who were not accompanied by a loved one rather than those who were accompanied by a loved one.

What about staff nurses and midwives as labor support providers?

"There are two common barriers to be overcome before nurses can provide skilled labor support to their patients: lack of time and lack of knowledge."[30]

Although nursing students learn about labor support basics, few have an opportunity to provide support to a laboring person. While many maternity nurses enjoy and are skilled in the labor support role, others have little knowledge of these skills. Nurses, many of whom are dedicated to supportive care, are often frustrated at the demands that take them from the laboring person's side. They tend to be very busy with multiple tasks and are often assigned more than one laboring person in labor. Also, they must give priority to their clinical responsibilities. These factors combine to leave many laboring people with little skilled emotional support or guidance for a low-intervention birth.

The largest randomized controlled trial evaluating the effectiveness of nurses as labor support providers included 6915 women who gave birth in 13 hospitals in the United States and Canada. All the participating hospitals had high rates of medical interventions. The supported group received continuous support from a specially trained nurse who had volunteered to provide the extra support. The control group received "usual care." There were very few differences in outcomes between the groups, except for slightly less use of continuous fetal monitoring, and more indicators of satisfaction with their births at 7 weeks postpartum in the supported group. The authors propose that the lack of differences in outcomes between the supported and the usual care groups may be due to the fact that the settings for the trial were highly interventive, relying heavily on continuous electronic monitoring, epidural analgesia, and induction and augmentation of labor.[31] The fact that the nurses were hospital employees who were accustomed to functioning within a high-intervention setting may also have influenced the lack of differences between the groups' outcomes.[29,32]

What about midwives? Labor support is a core value of midwifery education (ACNM Core Comptencies; ICM website definition of midwives). Continuous one-to-one care by midwives who focus on psychosocial aspects of childbirth has been shown to produce more favorable outcomes when compared with the usual care by obstetricians.[33] Sometimes midwives, particularly those who practice in hospital environments, have clinical responsibilities that take them away from the bedside of laboring people. In North America, although the numbers of midwives and doulas are increasing, there are still relatively few of either group. Thus the favorable outcomes achieved by midwives are available to very few North American laboring people, while in many other countries midwives are the primary care providers for the vast majority of childbearing people.

Assessing the laboring person's emotional state[34]

It is not always possible to assess a laboring person's sense of wellbeing by observing their external façade. For example, a laboring person who is still and quiet during contractions may be as peaceful and confident as they appear, or they may feel as if they are "screaming inside" or "barely keeping the lid on"—moving a muscle or letting out a sound will open the dam of emotions and cause them to lose all sense of control. Another laboring person who is vocal and active may feel calm and safe as long as they can express and release their feelings or, as one laboring person said, "shout down the pain." Sometimes the best way to assess the laboring person's wellbeing is to ask them. Occasionally ask between contractions, "What was going through your mind during that contraction?" The answer may tell much about their emotional needs and whether they are coping well or is distressed. This knowledge will help others provide appropriate emotional support. One unique and important study found that when people answered this question with indications of distressing thoughts (as opposed to answers that indicated that they were coping) during the latent phase (possibly indicating excessive catecholamine production), they were at increased risk for prolonged labor, non-reassuring fetal heart tones, intolerance of labor, and all the interventions that accompany such problems. This was not true when the people indicated distressing thoughts during active labor or transition. "We conclude that latent labor is a critical phase in the psychobiology of labor and that pain and cognitive activity [thoughts] during this phase are important contributions to labor efficiency and obstetric outcome."[35] Therefore, checking the laboring person's thoughts and eliminating or reducing stressors are worthwhile goals, especially in early labor when a laboring person has little need for clinical care. The following are specific ways to reduce stress and enhance the laboring person's emotional well-being.

Provide reassuring or comforting sensory stimuli

- music that the laboring person likes;
- massage, backrub, touch, holding their hand;
- lighting that suits the laboring person;
- juice or frozen juice bars in a flavor they like;
- pleasant-smelling hand cream or massage oil;
- if continuous electronic fetal monitoring is needed, making the heart tones audible if the laboring person finds it reassuring; otherwise, turning them down.

Provide reassurance and praise

- Ask what sensations the laboring person is having. Explain what causes them and reassure them that these sensations are normal. "Your body knows just what it's doing"; "I know this is difficult. It's because you're making good progress."
- Suggest comfort measures to the laboring person and their partner.
- Compliment them: "You're doing so well!"; "Don't change a thing"; "You're perfect"; "That's the way!"
- If they are interested, explain monitor tracings to the laboring person. Respect their wishes regarding information.
- Explain that the vocal laboring person next door says it helps them cope or push when they yell. And, if culturally appropriate, you might add, "You might also find that helpful at some point."
- Help them reframe distressing thoughts, especially in early labor: "Can you imagine your strong contractions doing exactly what they are supposed to do—open your cervix and bring your baby to you?"

Encourage Effective Coping Behaviors

- Encourage and reinforce the laboring person's spontaneous coping behaviors, such as rhythmic movements, sounds, and position changes. ("You are good at finding the positions and sounds that work for you.")
- If you are not sure whether a specific behavior is helping the laboring person or is simply a sign of distress, ask non-judgmentally—e.g., "Does it help to shake your hands during the contraction?"
- Encourage the use of hydrotherapy. Many people "let go" in the shower or bath.
- If the laboring person is silent, in their own world, try not to disturb hem with questions or procedures.

- If the laboring person loses rhythm in their movements, breathing, or vocalizing, help them get it back with eye contact, speaking in soothing rhythmic tones, nodding your head, or moving your hand rhythmically, so that they can follow the rhythm that you give them (which should mimic closely the rhythm they had).

Create and Protect the Labor and Birth Environment

These suggestions are applicable for hospital and birth centers, since those who give birth at home are in their own environment.

- Keep curtain and/or door closed.
- Knock before entering and encourage other staff to do the same.
- Close the door of any other laboring persons who are vocal.
- Minimize interventions if the laboring person does not want them (especially painful or invasive ones).
- Avoid bringing unnecessary staff members into the laboring person's room.
- Ask other staff to make sure they cannot possibly be overheard by any laboring people when discussing their patients. Information and vocabulary that are emotionally neutral to staff members may be frightening to the laboring person.
- If the laboring person is accompanied by someone who seems to make them anxious, ask privately if they would like that person to leave the room. Send him or her on an errand, or suggest they get a snack. If necessary, ask that person to wait elsewhere.
- If children are present, assure that each child has their own adult helper. If a child wants or needs to leave the room, their adult helper can accompany them without removing support from the laboring person.
- Provide a more private, less-inhibiting environment:
- Sometimes people need privacy, a small space, and freedom from disturbances to adjust psychologically to the demands of labor. Encourage the laboring person to spend some time in the bathroom with the door closed. Labor progress sometimes improves after some private time. Many people who are "holding back" during second stage can relax their pelvic floors on the toilet.
- If you are concerned that the baby may be born suddenly, instruct the laboring person to push the call light in the bathroom if they feel a lot of pressure.
- Remember that nudity or being scantily clad is threatening or embarrassing for some people. Offer an extra gown or robe to cover the laboring person's back.
- Some people feel more like themselves if they wear their own clothing in labor, while some want to remove all clothing.

TECHNIQUES AND DEVICES TO REDUCE BACK PAIN

Counterpressure

How

- The laboring person's partner applies steady pressure throughout the contraction on the laboring person's sacral area with an open hand or a fist (Fig. 12.12).
- The laboring person tells the partner where to push (wherever the pain is most intense) and how hard to push.
- If needed, the partner places their other hand on the front of the laboring person's hip (over the anterior superior iliac spine) to help them keep maintain balance.

How counterpressure helps

- It is not clear exactly how or why counterpressure eases back pain in labor.

It may change the shape of the pelvis enough to ease pain caused by the pressure of the occiput posterior or asynclitic baby's occiput on the sacroiliac joints. Judging from its popularity with people, every caregiver should know and be able to teach partners how to do counterpressure.

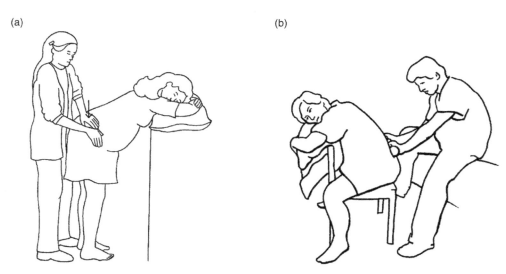

(a)   (b)

Fig. 12.12. (**a**) Counterpressure. (**b**) Counterpressure with tennis balls.

When to use counterpressure

• When the laboring person reports back pain.

When not to use counterpressure

• When the laboring person reports that counterpressure is not helping, or when they find it annoying.

The double hip squeeze

How: One or two people may perform the double hip squeeze. If there is one partner, they place their hands on the outsides of the laboring person's hips, over the gluteal muscles (well below the iliac crests, over the "meatiest" part of the buttocks), and presses inward toward the center of the pelvis with the whole palm of their hands (not just the heels of the hands) steadily throughout the contraction (Fig. 12.13). As with counterpressure, the laboring person decides how much pressure they need and exactly where the partner should place their hands. This is hard work for the partner. If this is too difficult to continue for as long as the laboring person needs it, it helps to have another person there to do the two-person double hip squeeze (see later). If there is no other person to help, then one-handed counterpressure may be used for a few contractions to allow the partner a break. Then they should resume the double hip squeeze if the laboring person finds it more helpful.

The two-person double hip squeeze. The laboring person kneels over a birth ball, the seat of a chair, or on the lowered foot portion of a birthing bed over a pile of pillows placed on the mid-portion of the bed. Two people stand, one on either side of the laboring person. Each support person places one open hand on the side of the hip above and medial to the hip joint. Their other hand covers the first hand. Then, at the same time, they lean in to put bilateral pressure on both hips (Fig. 12.13c). The pressure remains steady and equal through the contraction. Between contractions, they remove their hands and rest. The two-person double hip squeeze is much easier for those who must do it.

Note: This is different from the "pelvic press," which is used in cases of deep transverse arrest, persistent occiput posterior, or borderline cephalopelvic disproportion.

How the double hip squeeze helps   It is not clear how or why the double hip squeeze eases back pain in labor. The pressure may change the shape of the pelvis as does counterpressure (see previous section). It may slightly reduce the stretch in the sacroiliac joints, easing the strain on those ligaments caused by internal pressure of the malpositioned fetal head.

(a)

(b)

(c)

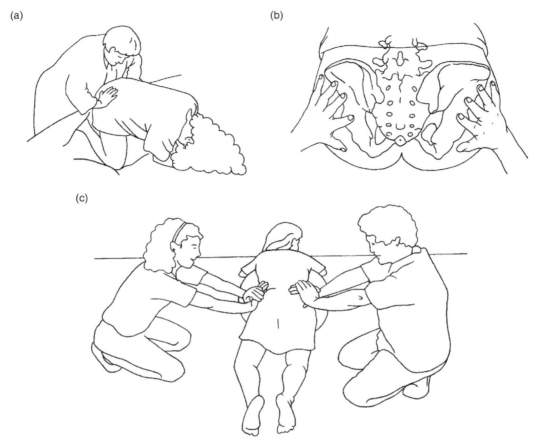

Fig. 12.13. (a) Double hip squeeze. (b) Double hip squeeze (detail, seen from rear). (c) Double hip squeeze with two support people.

Note: The authors consider it a poor prognosis if the back pain does not decrease considerably between contractions, and/or the laboring person needs maxi- mum pressure in the double hip squeeze (i.e., requiring all the strength of her partner) to obtain relief. We believe that such extreme pressure may indicate that the fetal head is deeply engaged in its malposition or complicated by an accompanying problem, such as a nuchal hand, making it less likely to self- correct spontaneously than when moderate or minor pressure is sufficient to relieve pain. In fact, one may wonder if the extreme hip pressure might decrease the volume in the pelvic basin and actually impair self-correction of the malposition. This possibility should be researched because the double hip squeeze seems very effective in relieving back pain, but it should not come at the cost of preventing rotation!

Other measures—e.g., the open knee–chest position abdominal lifting, the knee press, or the use of cold or heat, or the pelvic press in second stage or an epidural—may be preferable to maximal pressure in the double hip squeeze.

When to use the double hip squeeze

• When the laboring person reports back pain.

When not to use the double hip squeeze

• When the laboring person reports that it is not helping.

The knee press

How If the laboring person is seated: The laboring person sits upright on a straight chair with their low back against the back of the chair. They place their feet flat on the floor and with knees a few inches apart. (If their feet do not reach the floor, books or other supports can be placed beneath each foot—Fig. 12.14.)

The partner or doula kneels on the floor in front of the laboring person and cups their hands over the laboring person's her knees. Locking their elbows in close to the trunk, and rising off their haunches, the partner leans toward the laboring person throughout each contraction, allowing their upper body weight to apply pressure on her knees, directed from their hands straight back toward her the laboring person's hip joints. The laboring person feels a slight release in her low back and relief of back pain.

If the laboring person is side-lying, with one or two pillows supporting them upper knee: Two partners are needed. Only the upper knee is pressed. The laboring person flexes their upper knee and hip joints to 90-degree angles. One partner presses on the laboring person's sacrum during contractions to stabilize them. The other partner cups the laboring person's top knee in their hand and presses on that knee directly toward the hip joint.

How the knee press helps: Pressure directed via the femur straight into the joint of the flexed hip alters the configuration of the pelvic basin, releasing the sacroiliac joints and relieving low back pain.

When to use the knee press

• When the laboring person has back pain.

(a)

(b)

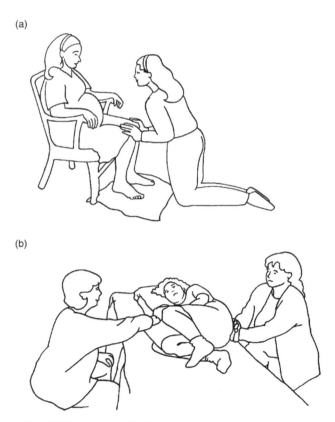

Fig. 12.14. **(a)** Knee press, seated. **(b)** Knee press, lateral.

When not to use the knee press

- When the laboring person reports the knee press is not reducing her their pain.
- When the laboring person has joint pain, inflammation, or damage in her their knee joints.

Cook's counterpressure technique No. 1: ischial tuberosities (IT)

Authors' note: We are grateful to Lisa-Marie Sasaki Cook, RN, for teaching us the following two counterpressure techniques. The following descriptions are adapted from her unpublished manuscript.[36]

How

- The laboring person lies on one side or on hands and knees with hips flexed to 90 degrees, which allows partner or caregiver to palpate the IT ("sit-bones") and then apply pressure on both spots with thumbs, heels of the hands, fists, or tennis balls during or between contractions. The laboring person gives feedback on where and how hard to press. If the laboring person is on their hands and knees position they can also "lean" into the pressure as feels comfortable (Fig. 12.15).

How: Cook's IT counterpressure helps   The ITs are points of attachment for many muscles, including hamstring muscles, hip rotators, and adductors. Also, three major pelvic ligaments are connected to the ITs. As the fetal head descends through the pelvis, these muscles and ligaments undergo significant pressure, resulting in

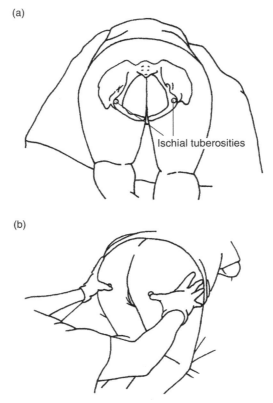

(a)

Ischial tuberosities

(b)

Fig. 12.15.   (**a**) Bony landmarks for Cook's ischial tuberosity (IT) counterpressure. (**b**) Hand placement for Cook's IT counterpressure.

pelvic pain, especially during contractions. Direct manual counter-pressure to the ITs provides an opposing force, decreasing the pain in the pelvis.

When done between contractions, people may be better able to relax within the pelvis. In Chinese medicine, the IT points are known as acupuncture points UB36 (Urinary Bladder 36) or by the Chinese name Chengfu, which translates into English as "receiving support." UB36 is described as being located at the midpoint of the inferior gluteal fold. This point, when activated, is said to alleviate pain in the lower back and gluteal region, sciatica, and other conditions.

When to use Cook's IT counterpressure No. 1

- During any phase of labor—early, active, transition, and second stage prior to crowning, especially when a laboring person complains of back pain or pelvic pressure, with or without an epidural.
- When a laboring person has a premature urge to push before complete dilation with a cervical lip or swelling.

When not to use Cook's IT counterpressure No. 1

- When the laboring person states that this counterpressure is not helping or is unpleasantly distracting.
- When the laboring person complains that it causes discomfort.
- When they have the following contraindications:
  - pre-existing symphysis pubis problems;
  - past pelvic trauma (accident, violence, obstetric trauma, etc.) that may have damaged the pelvic girdle area.

Cook's counterpressure technique No. 2: perilabial pressure

Late in the second stage, the caregiver presses externally with thumbs or fingers just outside the laboring person's labia against both inferior pubic rami to counteract the forces of the fetal head against the pubic arch and pelvic musculature.

Note: It is not appropriate for the doula to use this technique unless they are asked to do so by the laboring person and caregiver.

How: With the laboring person in a semi-sitting position with knees drawn up and spread apart, or side-lying, or squatting, the caregiver uses thumbs or index fingers from both hands or, in a single-handed technique, one thumb and index or middle finger to provide counterpressure just outside the external labia toward the inferior rami of the pubic arch (Fig. 12.16). The points can be located by palpating the prominent adductor longus tendons and pressing just posterior to their insertion sites against the bony inferior pubic rami.

The laboring person tells the caregiver how hard to press and whether it is more effective when used during or between contractions. With the two-handed technique, the care provider is still able to support the perineum while providing pain relief using counterpressure with the upper hand to the descending rami.

How Cook's perilabial counterpressure No. 2 helps: As the fetal head descends toward the pelvic outlet and approaches crowning, the perineal muscles and ligaments of the pelvic floor and the skin and mucosa of the vagina are stretched, causing burning and stinging in her vagina (the "rim of fire"). The counterpressure at the inferior rami counteracts the force of the fetal head against the pubic arch and soft tissue to decrease the pain.

When to use Cook's perilabial counterpressure No. 2

- During or between contractions or continuously.
- When the laboring person has an uncontrollable premature urge to push before complete dilation with a cervical lip or swelling.
- During late second stage when the laboring person is pushing and the head is approaching crowning.
- At crowning when the laboring person is trying not to push in order to protect them perineum from lacerations.

When not to use Cook's perilabial counterpressure No. 2

- When the laboring person states that this counterpressure is not helping or is unpleasantly distracting.

(a)

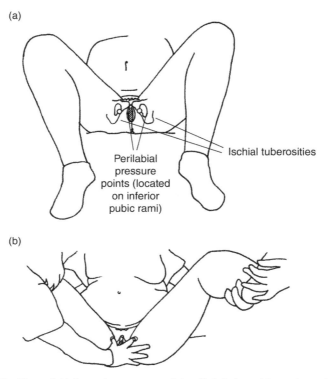

Ischial tuberosities

Perilabial
pressure
points (located
on inferior
pubic rami)

(b)

Fig. 12.16. (**a**) Location of Cook's perilabial counterpressure points with inferior pubic rami as reference points. (**b**) Placement of caregiver's fingers for the one-handed Cook's perilabial counterpressure technique.

- When the laboring person complains that it causes discomfort.
- When they have the following contraindications:
  - pre-existing symphysis pubis problems;
  - past pelvic trauma (accident, violence, obstetric trauma, etc.) that may have damaged the pelvic girdle area.

TECHNIQUES AND DEVICES TO REDUCE BACK PAIN

Cold and heat

Cold and heat may be used to relieve back pain. Following are brief instructions for their use. See "Non-Pharmacologic Physical Comfort Measures" earlier in this chapter for rationales and complete explanations on heat and cold.

Any cold or warm compress should be wrapped in a towel or pad, and before placing it on the laboring person's skin, the caregiver should test the temperature of the compress on their inner forearm to be sure the cold or heat is tolerable (Fig 12.17).

- If the laboring person has received an epidural, do not place a cold or warm compress on any part of their body where sensation is altered.

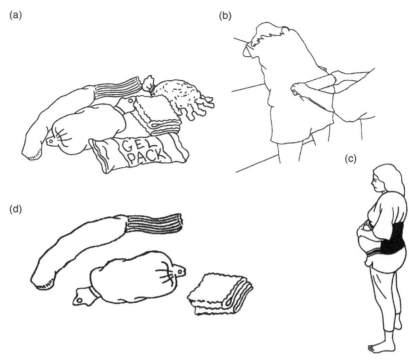

(a)

(b)

(c)

(d)

Fig. 12.17.   (**a**) Sources for cold: Cold gel pack, cold wash cloths, ice-filled glove. (**b**) Rolling cold. (**c**) Strap-on cold pack. (**d**) Sources for heat: Warm rice-filled sock, hot water bottle, warm wash clothes.

Cold and rolling cold

Note: Always place one or two layers of cloth between the laboring person's skin and the cold object to protect their skin from possible damage and to avoid the sudden shock of a freezing object directly placed on their skin.

Pressing and rolling a cold can of juice or soft drink over the laboring person's low back is sometimes appreciated more than steady pressure in one area.

When to use cold for back pain

- When the laboring person has musculoskeletal pain (especially low back pain).

When not to use cold for back pain

- If the laboring person is already chilled.
- If they do not want cold used (for personal or cultural reasons).
- If they prefer heat.
- If the laboring person has an epidural, do not place a cold object on any area with altered sensation (cool cloths would be safe).

Warm compresses

See "Non-pharmacologic physical comfort measures" earlier in this chapter for more information.

When to use warm compresses

• If the laboring person has low back pain and prefers a warm pack to a cold pack.

When not to use warm compresses

• If the laboring person has a fever.

Caution: The laboring person's temperature sense may be distorted when they are in labor.

Hydrotherapy

Note: Hydrotherapy (Fig. 12.18) often results in dramatic pain reduction and may enhance labor progress. See earlier in this chapter for instructions on hydrotherapy.

Maternal movement and positions

A variety of positions, and movements can be used to improve comfort and coping (Fig 12.19) and are discussed in detail in Chapter 11.

Birth ball

The birth ball (Fig. 12.20) is an excellent aid to movement and relaxation during labor. It is a physical therapy ball. Unlike large balls made for children's use, physical therapy balls are made to support adult weights. Such balls usually have a 300-lb (136-kg) weight limit, but you should check with the seller or manufacturer if this information is not included with the ball. The most widely used sizes are 65 cm and 75 cm in diameter. For people less than 5 feet 3 inches (160 cm) tall, a 55-cm ball is a good size; for those between 5 feet 3 inches and 5 feet 9 inches (175 cm), the 65-cm ball is a good size; for those taller than 5 feet 10 inches (178 cm), a 75-cm-diameter ball is a better choice.

Birth balls can be inflated to varying degrees of firmness and differing diameters, according to the laboring person's comfort. (Unfortunately, there is wide variation in the actual inflated size of the balls from one manufacturer to another. One manufacturer's "65-cm ball" may be much smaller than another manufacturer's. To some extent, this can be corrected by the amount of inflation. Furthermore, the balls stretch over time and with use.)

(a)   (b)

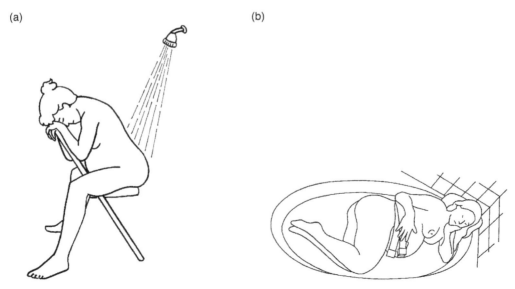

Fig. 12.18.   (**a**) Shower on laboring person's back. (**b**) Bath.

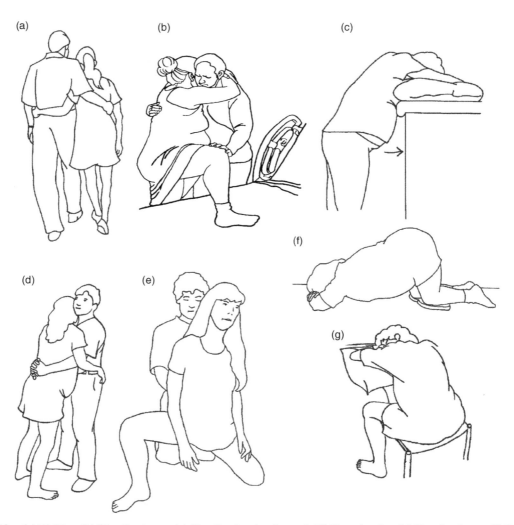

Fig. 12.19.   (**a**) Walking. (**b**) Standing lunge. (**c**) Standing leaning forward. (**d**) Slow dancing. (**e**) Kneeling lunge. (**f**) Open knee chest. (**g**) Straddling a chair.

The round shape of the ball makes swaying (while sitting on it or leaning over it) almost effortless. It is a comfortable alternative to the hands-and-knees position. Cover the ball with a waterproof bed pad, towel, or blanket. The ball can be cleaned with the same disinfectant used on the birthing bed mattress.

Other inflated devices—peanut- or egg-shaped—are available, but they are limited in versatility compared with the ball. A peanut ball is especially useful to prop the laboring person's upper leg while side-lying or semiprone.

Caution: The first few times a laboring person sits on the ball, they may feel a bit unsteady. They should hold on to the bed or their partner until they are totally secure. Also, as they lower to sit on the ball, they should keep a hand on it to be sure it does not roll away! Once they are seated, their feet should be in front of them and, about 2 to 2.5 feet (60–75 cm) apart. If they are insecure while sitting on the ball, they can still use it while kneeling or standing, as shown in Figs. 12.20b and 12.20c. Some childbirth classes provide balls to try before labor. Some hospitals also have them to use during labor.

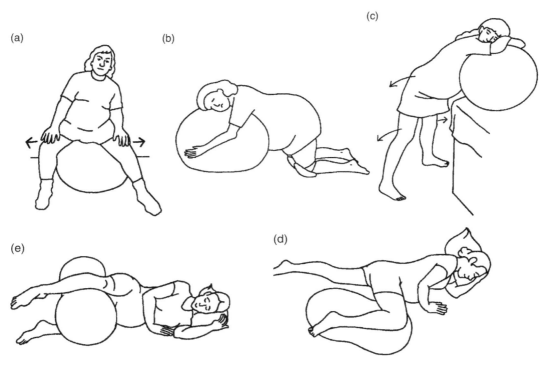

Fig. 12.20. (**a**) Sitting, swaying on a birth ball. (**b**) Kneeling on a birth ball, with knee pads. (**c**) Standing, swaying with ball. (**d**) Semiprone with peanut ball. (**e**) Side-lying with peanut ball.

Many parents buy a ball for their own use in labor and afterward. The ball is very useful for soothing a fussy baby, when the parent sits on the ball with the baby nestled into their shoulder and bounces gently. This is much easier on the parent's back than walking with the baby. It is also a useful aid for postpartum exercise.

Transcutaneous electrical nerve stimulation (TENS)

A TENS unit is a hand-held battery-operated device that causes transmission of mild electrical impulses through the skin where they stimulate nerve fibers. TENS units (Fig. 12.21) are available for sale or rent from physical therapy clinics and from medical equipment rental companies and, in many countries, from chemists or drugstores.
How: The four reusable stimulating pads, or electrodes, are placed on the low back on the paraspinal muscles on either side of the spine, two with their top edges at the level of the lowest ribs and two with their bottom edges slightly above the level of the gluteal cleft (Fig. 12.21a), and held in place by adhesive on the pads.
TENS units have adjustable parameters that vary with the model used: the most common British units, designed for childbirth, are simple and can be adjusted for intensity and for mode (continuous or burst, off and on). Alternating the mode after a contraction helps keep the laboring person from habituating to one kind of stimulation, which diminishes its effectiveness over time. The unit comes with instructions. Other more versatile and complex units, with more adjustable parameters, are also available. The laboring person or their partner increases the intensity of the nerve stimulation during contractions, and then decreases it and changes the sensation between contractions. In the UK model, this is all done with a thumb switch. (American models do not come with the thumb switch, which is awkward because the partner must turn two dials to change the stimulation between and during contractions.) The laboring person feels a "buzzing," prickly or tingling sensation, that is always kept below painful levels.

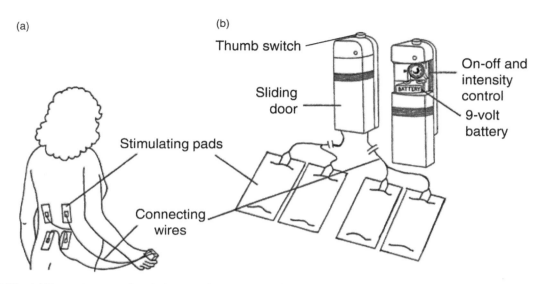

Fig. 12.21. (**a**) Transcutaneous electrical nerve stimulation (TENS) in use. (**b**) British TENS unit designed for childbirth.

Fetal monitoring: Rarely, the TENS unit interferes with transmission of ultrasound fetal monitor signals. If this is a problem, it can be dealt with by discontinuing the stimulation temporarily so that clear signals are obtained or discontinuing the monitoring if there is no medical reason to have continuous fetal monitoring.

How TENS helps   TENS stimulates tactile nerve endings and inhibits awareness of pain, as described in the gate control theory of pain.[37] TENS may also increase local endorphin production. It appears to have greater benefit if started early in labor, especially if the laboring person has back pain.

TENS allows the laboring person complete mobility, and a sense of control, in that they or their partner controls the use of TENS.

When to use TENS

- TENS is more effective when started in early labor, so it makes sense for the laboring person to obtain a TENS unit and be instructed in its use before labor begins. Then they can begin using it early in labor before going to the hospital or birth center.
- Throughout labor if the laboring person finds it helpful.
- TENS appears to be most beneficial those who have back pain.

When not to use TEN

- When using hydrotherapy (although the laboring person may remove the electrodes while in the water and replace them when they get out).
- When the laboring person reports that the TENS is not helping. (They may want to turn it off for a while without removing it. They may discover that the contractions are more painful without it.)
- If there is any irritation of the laboring person's skin at the sites of the electrodes.

Effectiveness of TENS   A systematic review of trials of TENS for management of labor pain (19 randomized trials, 1671 women) included 15 trials where TENS was applied to the back, two trials with application to acupuncture points, and two trials with application to the cranium.[38] Overall, there was no significant difference between TENS and control groups in pain ratings, although the two trials of TENS applied to acupuncture points indicated reduction in severe pain. Some studies reported lower use of added pain medications in the TENS groups than in the control groups. No adverse events were reported. Despite the lack of objective evidence of pain reduction with the most common applications of TENS, most women using it were satisfied and stated they would use it again in a future labor.

TENS may be more effective for relief of back pain than labor pain in general, but only a few observational studies have investigated this possibility.[3]

The satisfaction expressed by people with TENS appears to relate to benefits other than pain relief. TENS allows the laboring person to be in control of the intervention, allows ambulation, does not affect decision making or cognition has no effects on their mental state, and provides an inexpensive option for those who wish to avoid medications. There are no known side effects from TENS when used as directed for normal healthy individuals.[3]

TENS provides modest benefits in reduction of pain relief medications and is a satisfying option for many who use it. Its efficacy when applied in early labor and in relieving back pain deserves further study. Individual preferences regarding its use should be respected.[39,40,41]

Sterile water injections for back labor

When the baby is in an OP position, the laboring person often experiences significant lower back pain, sometimes referred to as "back labor." Back labor, no matter what the cause, can be severely painful. Intradermal or intracutaneous sterile water injections injected into four specific points on the laboring person's back can be used as a non-pharmacologic approach for relief of back pain in labor. The mechanism of action is not fully understood but appears to be linked to the Gate Control Theory of pain relief.[3,42] More specifically, it appears that the sterile water acts as a mild irritant stimulating localized discomfort. The use of sterile water injections does not preclude the use of epidural anesthesia. Therefore, for those who would like to avoid epidural anesthesia, sterile water injections may be used in a stepwise attempt to address overwhelming back pain. Formerly, the sterile water injections were administered intracutaneously (0.05 to 0.1 mL) and were considered to cause significant acute pain that lasted about 30 seconds, followed by 60 to 90 minutes of back pain relief.[3,42] A single intradermal sterile water injection is an alternative approach using the same technique. The laboring person identifies the place of the most pain, to determine the injection site. Lee and colleagues conducted a randomized clinical trial comparing the single to the four intradermal injection techniques with 305 laboring people with lower back pain (Lee et al., 2013). While injection pain was significantly less with the single-site technique, those who experienced the injections at four sites experienced significantly greater pain relief at 30 minutes.

Subcutaneous injections (0.5 mL) have been studied in comparison to intra-cutaneous injections. A randomized controlled trial compared 0.5 mL of sterile water injected subcutaneously in each of the four sites to 0.1 mL injected intracutaneously in each site and 1 mL of placebo (saline solution) in each site (Fig 12.22). The subcutaneous injections were found to be as effective as intracutaneous injections in relieving back pain and significantly less painful during administration.[42] Another confirmed this finding.[43] Therefore, experts now recommend giving subcutaneous sterile water injections rather than intradermal injections for back pain relief in labor.[42] Hutton and colleagues[40] conducted a meta-analysis of sterile water injections that included eight randomized controlled trials. They found that those who received the sterile water injections had a significant reduction in cesarean birth. This finding suggests broader benefits of sterile water injections and warrants further study. A randomized control trial by Genc and colleagues[44] found laboring people who received sterile water injections had both less back pain and higher maternal satisfaction scores than the control group.

Procedure for subcutaneous sterile water injections

Saline cannot be used for this procedure as it will have no effect.[42] Sterile water is drawn up into one or more tuberculin syringes (in an amount sufficient to allow for four injections of 0.5 mL each).[45] The skin is cleansed with isopropyl alcohol, and the water is injected subcutaneously into four points located in the sacral region of the back (Fig. 8.10). Even though subcutaneous injections are less painful than the intracutaneous injections, the discomfort of the procedure can be further reduced if two health professionals administer the injections

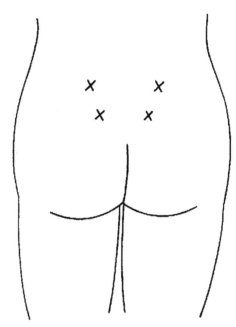

Fig. 12.22.   Sterile water injection points.

simultaneously and administer them during, rather than between, contractions. Pain relief is often noticed within minutes.

BREATHING FOR RELAXATION AND A SENSE OF MASTERY

Breathing rhythmically during contractions, sometimes combined with moaning, is a widespread labor coping ritual.[34] Many people have already learned some breathing techniques from books or childbirth preparation classes.[37] The caregiver should ask them what they learned and encourage them to use what is already familiar. Many people discover their own unique rhythms of breathing and numerous other coping rituals, especially in active labor. People who have their own rituals do not need correction or instruction. They need support and freedom from disturbance (within the realistic context of clinical care). However, people who do not know what to do may feel overwhelmed and out of control, anxious, or tense. They can be taught simple, effective breathing rhythms and assisted in using them during contractions.

Simple breathing rhythms to teach on the spot in labor

How   We recommend that the caregiver be able to teach both slow and light breathing. These can be taught quickly between contractions.

   Slow breathing should be initiated at the point in labor when the laboring person cannot walk or talk through the peaks of the contractions. Teach them to "sigh" their way through the contractions with full, easy, audible breaths that may or may not be accompanied by moaning. Combine breathing with imagery. Here are some examples:

"Every out-breath is a relaxing breath."
"Send each in-breath to a tense area and on the out-breath, send that tension away…"

"Imagine that each breath is another step up the mountain that is your contraction. When you get to the peak, you can breathe your way down."

"Let's count your breaths as you go through the contractions. Then (assuming the contractions follow a fairly consistent pattern) we'll be able to tell when you are about halfway through. It will make your contractions seem shorter."

Light breathing is reserved for a time in active labor when the laboring person becomes discouraged or finds that the slow breathing is no longer helping very much, even with your encouragement and help. Teach them to breathe more shallowly and more quickly but still at a speed at which they are comfortable through the contractions (e.g., one quick light in-breath followed by an audible out-breath every 1 to 3 seconds. They pause briefly after each out-breath to keep from breathing too fast). It may be easier for the laboring person if you pace them with rhythmic hand or head movements, and talk to them soothingly and in the rhythm of their breathing: "Good … that's the way … just like that … that's right … yes. …" Hyperventilation is unlikely if you pace them and encourage them to keep their inhalations silent and shorter than their exhalations, which should be audible or accompanied by moaning. (If hyperventilation occurs, the laboring person may need to breathe in and out of their cupped hands, a paper bag, or a surgical mask until the symptoms—light-headedness, gulping for air—disappear. Help them slow their breathing and move less air, while maintaining a steady rhythm.) You can continue the use of guided imagery if they respond well to it. Most people, after being helped with rhythmic breathing through several contractions, can then continue without guidance.

Of course, you will want the laboring person to adapt these rhythmic patterns in whatever way suits them best.

Note: If the laboring person is in advanced labor when they arrive, it may be impossible to teach them very much if they lack rhythm in breathing in breathing or moaning, help them find a rhythm. Get them to look at your hand, move your hand up and down in rhythm, and say (in the same rhythm), "Breathe with my hand … that's right … stay with it … good …" and so forth. How breathing techniques help: Breathing in a consistent rhythmic pattern is self-calming; it encourages tension release and a sense of wellbeing. This rhythmic self-calming behavior helps to quiet the cortical activity of the brain, putting the laboring person in a more instinctual state of mind.

When to use breathing techniques

- Whenever the laboring person seems distressed by the contractions.
- If they have not mastered any other techniques for coping with labor pain.

When not to use breathing techniques

- If the laboring person is successfully using other coping or breathing techniques.
- If they resist trying them, or cannot respond to your teaching.

BEARING-DOWN TECHNIQUES FOR THE SECOND STAGE

To help people push more effectively when they have received epidural anesthesia.

Spontaneous bearing down (pushing)

Spontaneous bearing down is unplanned and unrehearsed by the laboring person before birth, and undirected during the birth. The laboring person's strong involuntary urge to push usually compels them to bear down effectively in synchrony with strong contractions.

How: When the contraction begins, the laboring person begins breathing in any way that is satisfying to them, and bear down when they have the reflexive urge, for as long and as forcefully as their urge demands. Each bearing-down effort usually lasts no more than 5 to 7 seconds.[46,47,48,49] The laboring person may hold their breath, moan, release air, or bellow during contractions, and breathe quickly and lightly for several seconds between bearing-down efforts. This breathing helps ensure adequate fetal oxygenation.

Note: Although some experts prescribe "open glottis pushing" (releasing air during bearing-down efforts), we are reluctant to prescribe any specific pushing techniques during contractions; rather, we support spontaneous behavior, and only if that is non-productive do we suggest corrective actions, described later.[50]

Self-directed pushing

Sometimes, due to fear, pain, or "holding back," spontaneous bearing-down efforts are ineffective, and self-directed pushing is more productive.

How: Self-directed pushing is used when the laboring person has a spontaneous urge to push but their bearing-down efforts are unfocused, ineffective, and "diffuse," without apparent progress for 30 minutes. Often you will observe that their eyes are clenched shut, and they seem afraid or unwilling to bear down into the pelvis.

First, the caregiver encourages the laboring person to try a new position. Gravity-enhancing positions seem to help the laboring person focus their attention. If that does not help, the caregiver may instruct the laboring person to open their eyes and direct their gaze and their efforts downward toward their vaginal the vaginal canal outlet. Without any further direction, the laboring person frequently responds impressively, becoming much more effective in their bearing-down efforts.

Lastly, the caregiver may have to tell the laboring person to "Push to the pain and right through it. It hurts less on the other side."

CONCLUSION

The comfort measures described in this chapter exemplify the non-pharmacologic approach to labor pain relief. They reduce pain while maintaining a sense of mastery and participation by the laboring person. They make it possible for the use the positions and movements to maintain labor progress and, one hopes, to reduce the likelihood of a cesarean for dystocia.

REFERENCES

1. Simkin P, Klein M. (2015) Nonpharmacological approaches to management of labor pain, parts 1 and 2. *UpToDate* 17(3), 1–11. Retrieved from: http://www.uptodate.com/contents/nonpharmacologic-approaches-to-management-of-labor-pain (accessed August 28, 2016).
2. Fahami F, Behmanesh F, Valiani M, Ashouri E. (2011) Effect of heat therapy on pain severity in primigravida women. *Iranian Journal of Nursing and Midwifery Research* 16(1), 113–116.
3. Lehmann JF. (1990) *Therapeutic Heat and Cold*, 4th edn. Baltimore: Williams & Wilkins.
4. Klein M, Lorenzo C. (2013) Superficial heat and cold. Medscape. Retrieved from: http://emedicine.medscape.com/article/1833084 (accessed May 21, 2016).
5. Lieberman E, O'donoghue C. (2002) Unintended effects of epidural analgesia during labor: A systematic review. *American Journal of Obstetrics and Gynecology* 186(5 Suppl Nature), S31–S68. doi: 10.1067/mob.2002.122522
6. Osborne C, Ecker JL, Gauvreau K, Davidson KM, Lieberman E. (2011) Maternal temperature elevation and occiput posterior position at birth among low-risk women receiving epidural analgesia. *Journal of Midwifery & Women's Health* 56(5), 446–451. doi: 10.1111/j.1542-2011.2010.00064.x
7. Enwemeka CS, Allen C, Avila P, Bina J, Konrade J, Munns S. (2002) Soft tissue thermodynamics before, during, and after cold pack therapy. *Medicine and Science in Sports and Exercise* 34(1), 45–50. doi: 10.1097/00005768-200201000-00008
8. Ganji Z, Shirvani MA, Rezaei-Abhari F, Danesh M. (2013) The effect of intermittent local heat and cold on labor pain and child birth outcome. *Iranian Journal of Nursing and Midwifery Research* 18(4), 298–303.
9. Odent M. (1997) Can water immersion stop labor? *Journal of Nurse-midwifery* 42(5), 414–416. doi: 10.1016/s0091-2182(97)00051-7
10. Cluett ER, Burns E. (2009) Immersion in water in labour and birth. *The Cochrane Database of Systematic Reviews*, (2), CD000111. doi: 10.1002/14651858.CD000111.pub3
11. Benfield RD, Hortobágyi T, Tanner CJ, Swanson M, Heitkemper MM, Newton ER. (2010) The effects of hydrotherapy on anxiety, pain, neuroendocrine responses, and contraction dynamics during labor. *Biological Research for Nursing* 12(1), 28–36. doi: 10.1177/1099800410361535

12. The Royal Australian and New Zealand College of Obstetricians and Gynaecologists. (2008) *College Statement 24: Warm Water Immersion during Labour and Birth*. East Melbourne: RANZCOG.

13. Katz VL, Ryder RM, Cefalo RC, Carmichael SC, Goolsby R. (1990) A comparison of bed rest and immersion for treating the edema of pregnancy. *Obstetrics and Gynecology* 75(2), 147–151.

14. Harper B. (2005) *Gentle Birth Choices*. Rochester, VT: Healing Arts Press.

15. Cluett ER, Pickering RM, Getliffe K, St George Saunders NJ. (2004) Randomised controlled trial of labouring in water compared with standard of augmentation for management of dystocia in first stage of labour. *BMJ (Clinical Research Ed.)* 328(7435), 314. doi: 10.1136/bmj.37963.606412.EE

16. Committee on Obstetric Practice, & American Academy of Pediatrics. (2014) ACOG Committee Opinion no. 594: Immersion in water during labor and delivery. *Obstetrics and Gynecology* 123(4), 912–915. doi: 10.1097/01.AOG.0000445585.52522.14

17. American College of Nurse-Midwives. (2014) *Position Statement. Hydrotherapy during Labor and Birth*. Silver Spring, MD: American College of Nurse-Midwives.

18. Harding C, Munro J, Jokinen M. (2012). Evidence based guidelines for midwifery-led care in labour: Immersion in water for labour and birth. Royal College of Midwives. Available at: https://www.azdhs.gov/documents/licensing/special/midwives/training/guidelines-for-water-immersion-water-birth.pdf (accessed May 21, 2016)

19. Field T. (2010) Pregnancy and labor massage. *Expert Review of Obstetrics & Gynecology* 5(2), 177–181. doi: 10.1586/eog.10.12

20. Chang MY, Chen CH, Huang KF. (2006) A comparison of massage effects on labor pain using the McGill Pain Questionnaire. *The Journal of Nursing Research: JNR* 14(3), 190–197. doi: 10.1097/01.jnr.0000387577.51350.5f

21. Schlaeger JM, Gabzdyl EM, Bussell JL, Takakura N, Yajima H, Takayama M, Wilkie DJ. (2017) Acupuncture and acupressure in labor. *Journal of Midwifery & Women's Health* 62(1), 12–28. doi: 10.1111/jmwh.12545

22. Smith CA, Collins CT, Levett KM., Armour M, Dahlen HG, Tan AL, Mesgarpour B. (2020) Acupuncture or acupressure for pain management during labour. *The Cochrane Database of Systematic Reviews* 2(2), CD009232. doi: 10.1002/14651858.CD009232.pub2

23. Chung UL, Hung LC, Kuo SC, Huang CL. (2003) Effects of LI4 and BL 67 acupressure on labor pain and uterine contractions in the first stage of labor. *The Journal of Nursing Research: JNR* 11(4), 251–260. doi: 10.1097/01.jnr.0000347644.35251.c1

24. Lee MK, Chang SB, Kang DH. (2004) Effects of SP6 acupressure on labor pain and length of delivery time in women during labor. *Journal of Alternative and Complementary Medicine (New York, N.Y.)* 10(6), 959–965. doi: 10.1089/acm.2004.10.959

25. Hamidzadeh A, Shahpourian F, Orak RJ, Montazeri AS, Khosravi A. (2012) Effects of LI4 acupressure on labor pain in the first stage of labor. *Journal of Midwifery & Women's Health* 57(2), 133–138. doi: 10.1111/j.1542-2011.2011.00138.x

26. Klaus MH, Kennell JH. (1997) The doula: An essential ingredient of childbirth rediscovered. *Acta Paediatrica (Oslo, Norway: 1992)* 86(10), 1034–1036. doi: 10.1111/j.1651-2227.1997.tb14800.x

27. Bertsch TD, Nagashima-Whalcn L, Dykcman S, Kennell JH, McGrath S. (1990) Labor support by first-time fathers: Direct observations with a comparison to experienced doulas. *Journal of Psychosomatic Obstetrics & Gynecology* 11(4), 251–260.

28. Hodnett ED, Gates S, Hofmeyr GJ, Sakala C. (2013) Continuous support for women during childbirth. *The Cochrane Database of Systematic Reviews* 7, CD003766. doi: 10.1002/14651858.CD003766.pub5

29. Hodnett ED, Gates S, Hofmeyr GJ, Sakala C. (2013) Continuous support for women during childbirth. *The Cochrane Database of Systematic Reviews* 7, CD003766. doi: 10.1002/14651858.CD003766.pub5

30. Hodnett E. (1996) Nursing support of the laboring woman. *Journal of Obstetric, Gynecologic, and Neonatal Nursing: JOGNN* 25(3), 257–264. doi: 10.1111/j.1552-6909.1996.tb02434.x

31. Hodnett ED, Lowe NK, Hannah ME, Willan AR, Stevens B, Weston JA, Ohlsson A, Gafni A, Muir HA, Myhr TL, Stremler R, & Nursing Supportive Care in Labor Trial Group. (2002) Effectiveness of nurses as providers of birth labor support in North American hospitals: A randomized controlled trial. *JAMA* 288(11), 1373–1381. doi: 10.1001/jama.288.11.1373

32. Jones L. (2012) Pain management for women in labour: An overview of systematic reviews. *Journal of Evidence-Based Medicine* 5(2), 101–102.

33. Butler J, Abrams B, Parker J, Roberts JM, Laros RK, Jr. (1993) Supportive nurse-midwife care is associated with a reduced incidence of cesarean section. *American Journal of Obstetrics and Gynecology* 168(5), 1407–1413. 10.1016/s0002-9378(11)90773-x

34. Simkin P. (2002) Supportive care during labor: A guide for busy nurses. *Journal of Obstetric, Gynecologic, and Neonatal Nursing: JOGNN* 31(6), 721–732.

35. Sinclair C. (1989) The clinical significance of pain and cognitive activity in latent labor. *Obstetrics and Gynecology* 73(6), 1054. doi: 10.1097/00006250-198906000-00037

36. Cook L. (2010) Cook's counterpressure as a comfort method in labor. Unpublished manuscript and personal communication. Birthing Basics (www.birthingbasics.net).

37. Simkin P, Whalley J, Keppler A, Durham J, Bolding A. (2016) *Pregnancy, Childbirth, and the Newborn: The Complete Guide*, 6 edn. Deephaven, MN: Meadowbrook.

38. Dowswell T, Bedwell C, Lavender T, Neilson JP. (2009) Transcutaneous electrical nerve stimulation (TENS) for pain relief in labour. *The Cochrane Database of Systematic Reviews* (2), CD007214. doi: 10.1002/14651858.CD007214.pub2

39. Derry S, Straube S, Moore RA, Hancock H, Collins SL. (2012) Intracutaneous or subcutaneous sterile water injection compared with blinded controls for pain management in labour. *The Cochrane Database of Systematic Reviews* 1, CD009107. doi: 10.1002/14651858.CD009107.pub2

40. Hutton EK, Kasperink M, Rutten M, Reitsma A, Wainman B. (2009) Sterile water injection for labour pain: A systematic review and meta-analysis of randomised controlled trials. *BJOG: An International Journal of Obstetrics and Gynaecology* 116(9), 1158–1166. doi: 10.1111/j.1471-0528.2009.02221.x

41. Mårtensson L, Wallin G. (2008) Sterile water injections as treatment for low-back pain during labour: A review. *The Australian & New Zealand Journal of Obstetrics & Gynaecology* 48(4), 369–374. doi: 10.1111/j.1479-828X.2008.00856.x

42. Mårtensson L, Nyberg K, Wallin G. (2000) Subcutaneous *versus* intracutaneous injections of sterile water for labour analgesia: a comparison of perceived pain during administration. *BJOG: An International Journal of Obstetrics & Gynaecology* 107, 1248–1251. doi: 10.1111/j.1471-0528.2000.tb1161

43. Bahasadri S, Ahmadi-Abhari S, Dehghani-Nik M, Habibi GR. (2006) Subcutaneous sterile water injection for labour pain: A randomised controlled trial. *Australian and New Zealand Journal of Obstetrics and Gynaecology* Apr; 46(2), 102–106. doi: 10.1111/j.1479-828X.2006.00536.x. PMID: 16638030.

44. Genç Koyucu R, Demirci N, Ender Yumru A, et al. (2018) Effects of intradermal sterile water injections in women with low back pain in labor: A randomized, controlled, clinical trial. *Balkan Medical Journal* 35(2), 148–154. doi: 10.4274/balkanmedj.2016.0879

45. Mårtensson L, Wallin G. (1999) Labour pain treated with cutaneous injections of sterile water: A randomised controlled trial. *British Journal of Obstetrics and Gynaecology* Jul; 106(7), 633–637. doi: 10.1111/j.1471-0528.1999.tb08359.x. PMID: 10428516

46. Benyon CL. (1957) The normal second stage of labour; a plea for reform in its conduct. *The Journal of Obstetrics and Gynaecology of the British Empire* 64(6), 815–820. doi: 10.1111/j.1471-0528.1957.tb08483.x

47. Roberts J, Hanson L. (2007) Best practices in second stage labor care: Maternal bearing down and positioning. *Journal of Midwifery & Women's Health* 52(3), 238–245. doi: 10.1016/j.jmwh.2006.12.011

48. Hanson L. (2009) Second-stage labor care: Challenges in spontaneous bearing down. *The Journal of Perinatal & Neonatal Nursing* 23(1), 31–41. doi: 10.1097/JPN.0b013e318196526b

49. Lemos A, Amorim MM, Dornelas de Andrade A, de Souza AI, Cabral Filho JE, Correia JB. (2015) Pushing/bearing down methods for the second stage of labour. *The Cochrane Database of Systematic Reviews* (10), CD009124. doi: 10.1002/14651858.CD009124.pub2

50. Osborne K, Hanson L. (2014) Labor down or bear down: A strategy to translate second-stage labor evidence to perinatal practice. *The Journal of Perinatal & Neonatal Nursing* 28(2), 117–126.

Index

Please note, page numbers in *italics* refer to figures and page numbers in **bold** reference tables.

Simkin's Labor Progress Handbook: Early Interventions to Prevent and Treat Dystocia, Fifth Edition. Edited by Lisa Hanson, Emily Malloy, and Penny Simkin.
© 2024 John Wiley & Sons Ltd. Published 2024 by John Wiley & Sons Ltd.